U0599825

# 口腔颌面肿瘤外科手术彩色图谱

# A Colour Atlas of Oral and Maxillofacial Oncologic Surgery


翦新春　著

Xinchun Jian

审校　汪济广



世界图书出版公司

西安 北京 广州 上海

**图书在版编目（CIP）数据**

口腔颌面肿瘤外科手术彩色图谱/翦新春编.
－西安：世界图书出版西安公司，2003.11
ISBN 7－5062－6211－8

Ⅰ.口... Ⅱ.翦...
Ⅲ.口腔颌面部疾病:肿瘤－外科手术－图谱
Ⅳ.R739.8－64

中国版本图书馆 CIP 数据核字（2003）第 092355 号

**口腔颌面肿瘤外科手术彩色图谱**

主　　编　翦新春
审　　校　汪济广
责任编辑　侯清高
封面设计　范晓荣

出版发行　世界图书出版西安公司
地　　址　西安市南大街 17 号　　邮　编　710001
电　　话　029－7279676　7233647　7214941(发行部)
电　　话　029－7235105(总编室)
传　　真　029－7279675　7279676
E－mail　wmcrxian@public.xa.sn.cn
经　　销　各地新华书店
制　　版　陕西工人报社彩色输出中心
印　　刷　人民日报社西安印务中心
开　　本　889×1194　　1/16
印　　张　14.25
字　　数　240 千字

版　　次　2003 年 11 月第 1 版　2003 年 11 月第 1 次印刷
书　　号　ISBN 7－5062－6211－8/R·637
定　　价　138.00 元

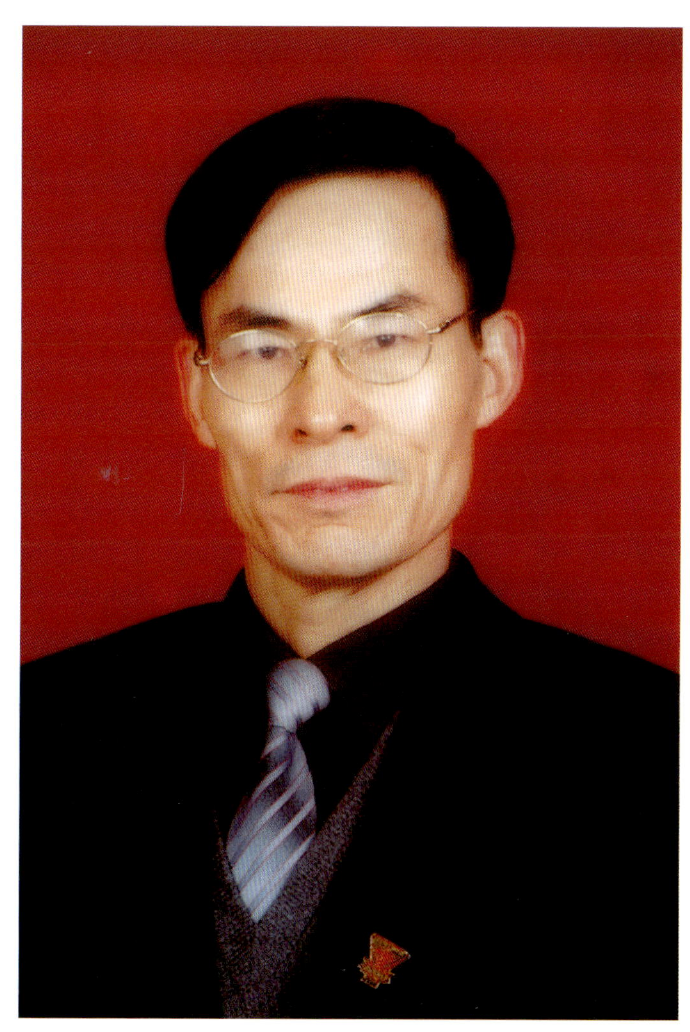

翦新春教授

Xinchun Jian，DDS，MD

# 口腔颌面肿瘤外科手术彩色图谱

A Colour Atlas of Oral and Maxillofacial Oncologic Surgery

著　者

翦新春

中南大学湘雅医院外科学博士生导师

中南大学湘雅医院口腔颌面外科教授

中南大学口腔医学院口腔颌面外科教研室主任

中南大学口腔医学院院长

# A Colour Atlas of Oral and Maxillofacial Oncologic Surgery

Editor
Xinchun Jian, DDS, MD

*Professor, Department of Oral and Maxillofacial Surgery.*
*Director, Department of Oral and Maxillofacial Surgery.*
*Xiang Ya Hospital, Central South University, Changsha, Hunan.*
*Dean, School of Stomatology, Central South University, Changsha, Hunan.*

# 前　言

在近代外科学中，最为刺激和最具挑战性的新技术之一是颅底部和头颈部肿瘤经外科手术切除后的即刻重建技术。发生在颅底、口腔、颌面部或颈部的良恶性肿瘤，在处理时往往需要神经外科和头颈外科医师们通力合作，对发生在这一边缘区域的病变进行联合外科处理，使这些病变的治疗得到了革命性的改变。本书主要内容集中在对颅底及口腔颌面颈部良、恶性肿瘤的外科处理上，特别是恶性肿瘤；有时认为不能处理或处理不当会造成患者死亡，由于有了神经外科和头颈外科医师，有时还有整形外科医师合作进行手术，使得这些具有挑战性的肿瘤得到了完整、干净的切除。

本书由10章组成，包括了口腔、颌面、颈部发生的大部分良恶性肿瘤，对其手术切除及重建的方法进行了详细的描述。在重建中，因为有些皮瓣适应于多个区域的重建，因此某一皮瓣的手术方法可能在多章节中描述。

本书每章每节对手术的进路是我们对每个患者选择的个性化手术方法，手术技术是以每步每步的描述呈现给读者的，这种描述有助于指导外科医师进行良好的外科手术。

在该书出版之际，首先感谢对我个人从事口腔颌面颈部肿瘤外科治疗起到关键性指导作用的前辈们。邱蔚六、张孟殷教授是鼓励和为我从事口腔颌面颈部肿瘤外科树立榜样的向导者。袁贤瑞教授、马建荣教授是对我从事颅底肿瘤外科得以实施造成影响的神经外科方面的伙伴。我感谢原湖南医科大学湘雅医院口腔颌面外科，现中南大学湘雅医院口腔颌面外科的同事们，如果没有他们的努力工作和熟练的技术合作，我的成功是不可能的。

我要特别感谢原湖南医科大学湘雅医院前院长、神经外科主任刘运生教授，原湖南医科大学湘雅医院副院长、耳鼻咽喉科主任肖健云教授，原中南大学湘雅医院院长、现湘雅医学院院长田勇泉教授对我各方面的指导、帮助和支持。

我要感谢吴林艳女士在我的书稿整理和打印上所做的杰出而不知疲倦的努力。

我要感谢高兴与我合作的患者们，他们的真诚给我的职业进取提供了极大的力量。

最后，我要特别感谢我的生活和家庭中最重要的人们，他们永恒的支持、关爱和热情点燃着我每天生活和工作的活力。

我相信这本书对口腔颌面肿瘤外科医师的手术操作能够起到一定的帮助，然而，本书只在手术如何进行上起指导作用，并不能取代对知识的继续追求。

翦新春

2003. 5. 8

# Preface

One of the most exciting and challenging innovations in modern surgery is the advent of skull base surgery and immediate reconstructive techniques after excision of the tumors of the head and neck. The well-coordinated, integrated surgical attack on tensions afflicting this transitional area between neurologic and head and neck surgery has revolutionized the management of these lesions. This book is primarily focused on the surgical treatment of neoplasms on the oral and maxillofacial regions. These tumors, especially malignancies, were often considered inoperable and the patients doomed to die. The cooperative surgical attack by the neurosurgeon and the head and neck surgeon, followed by the expertise of the reconstructive surgeon, has resulted in complete resection of these challenging tumors and a safe watertight closure.

There are 10 chapters in this book that most tumors occured in the head and neck regions are included and the reconstructive methods after the excisions are descriped. On the reconstruction methods, because similar flaps may be indicated for multiple problems, certain flaps may be described in more than one chapter. The approach descriped in each chapter has followed our approach to individual patient. The operative technique section provides the reader with step-by-step description of the procedure. It is our intention that this descriptive method will guide the surgeon during operative procedure.

When this book will be published, I would like to acknowledge the pionners in oral and maxillofacial oncologic surgery who have had a personal influence on my career in this adventurous endeavor. Prof. Weiliu Qiu、Mengyin Zhang were among the forerunners in oral and maxillofacial oncologic surgery whose example and encouragement stimulated me to embark on my career in oral and maxillofacial oncologic surgery. Prof. Xianrui Yuan、Jianrong Ma are neurosurgery colleagues who have significantly influenced the shaping of my thought processes as skull base surgery has evolved.

I would like to thank the members of Department of Oral and Maxillofacial Surgery, Former Hunan Medical University. The success of my career would have been impossible without their skill and hard work.

I would further like to thank Prof. Yunsheng Liu, former President, Director, Department of Neurosurgery, Xiang Ya Hospital, former Hunan Medical University; Prof. Jianyun Xiao, former vice-President, Xiang Ya Hospital, former Hunan Medical University; Prof. Yongquan Tian, former President, Xiang Ya Hospital, for their support and assistances.

I would like to thank Mrs. Linyan Wu for her outstanding, tireless efforts and hard work in the typing of the manuscript. I would like to thank the patients with whom I have had a pleasure to interact. Their trust and honesty has kept me humble and encouraged me to remain in the health care profession. Finally, I would especially like to thank the most important people in my life, my family. Their undying support, love, and enthusiasm refresh my spirit to meet each day with a renewed level of excitement.

I believe that this book can be of some assistance in the development of the oral and maxillofacial oncologic surgeon's operative career. However, it should serve only as a guide to getting started and is in no way a replacement for a continuing quest for further knowledge.

Xinchun Jian

May. 8. 2003

# 目　录

# Contents





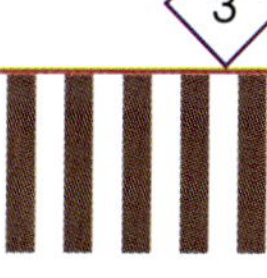

# I. 颅内及颅底肿瘤

1. 颞窝及脑膜恶性淋巴瘤的外科手术治疗
2. 中颅窝脑膜瘤继发侵犯翼下颌间隙的手术治疗
3. 中颅底炎性假瘤的外科手术治疗
4. 翼腭窝及中颅窝底肿瘤面部组织异位进路切除术
5. 翼腭窝神经纤维瘤摘除术
6. 前及中颅窝底复发性软骨肉瘤切除颞肌瓣转移即刻重建修复术

# I. Intracranial and skull base tumors

1. Surgical excision of malignant lymphoma in the temporal fossa and dura
2. Surgical treatment of intracranial meningioma secondarily involving infratemporal fossa and pterygomandibular space
3. Surgical treatment of the inflammatory pseudotumor under inferior surface of the middle skull base
4. Facial translocation: a new approach to the middle cranial base and pterygopalatine fossa
5. Excision of neurofibroma in the pterygopalatine fossa
6. Excision of recurrent chondrosarcoma in the anterior and middle cranial base and immediate reconstruction with temporal muscle

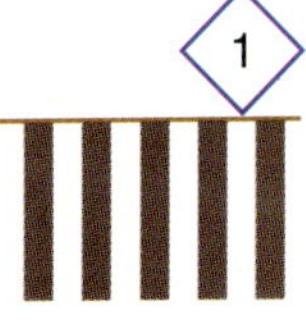

# 1. 颞窝及脑膜恶性淋巴瘤的外科手术治疗

# 1. Surgical excision of malignant lymphoma in the temporal fossa and dura

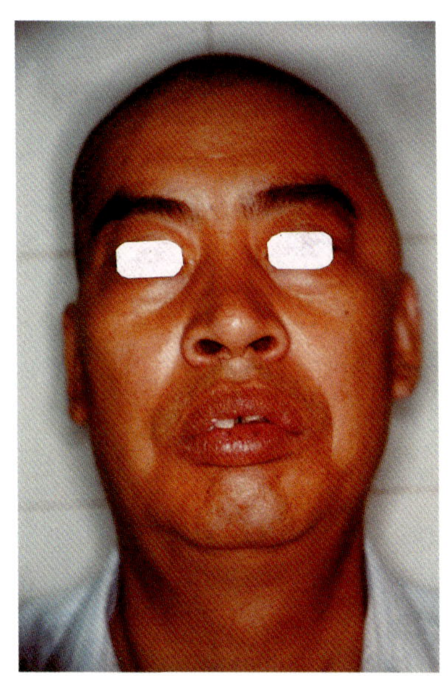

图 1

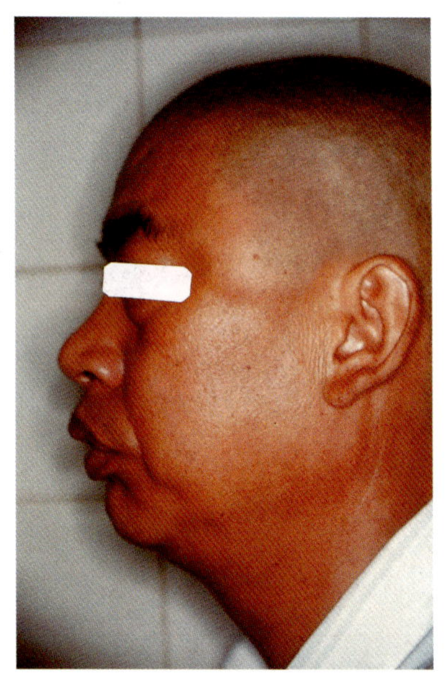

图 2

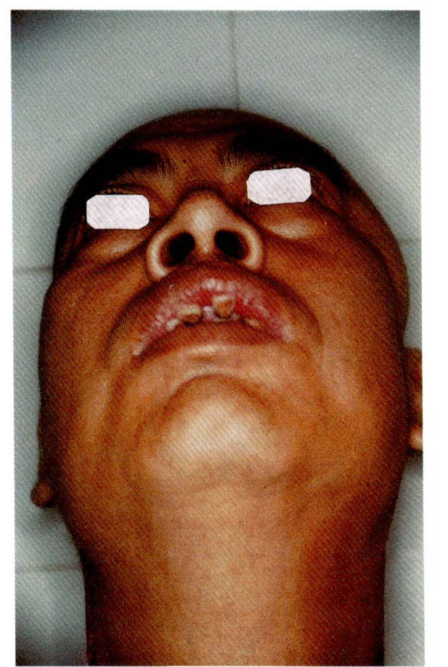

图 3

**图 1，2** 患左颞部及颅中窝恶性淋巴瘤 48 岁患者的正面及侧面观。

图 1 正面观显示双侧颞部不对称，左侧明显膨隆；图 2 侧面观显示左侧颞部丰满，表面皮肤正常。

Fig. 1, 2 Frontal and lateral views of a 48-year-old male patient with malignant lymphoma in the temporal region and middle cranial fossa.

Frontal view shows both temporal asymmetry and the left temporal expansion obviously. Fig. 2 shows left temporal expansion. The surperficial skin is normal.

**图 3** 仰面观左侧颞部膨隆。

Fig. 3 Submental view shows left temporal expansion.

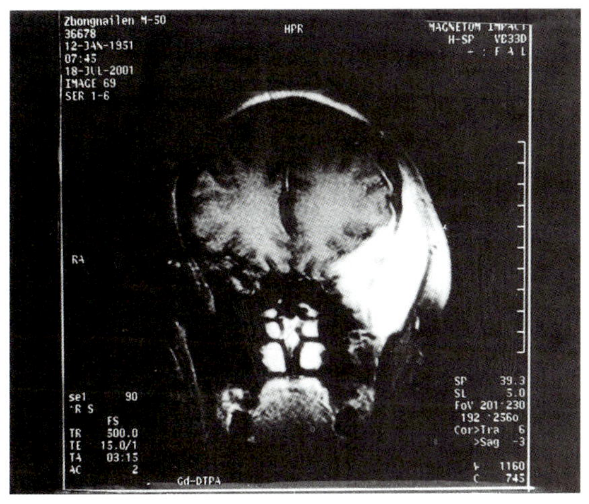

图 4

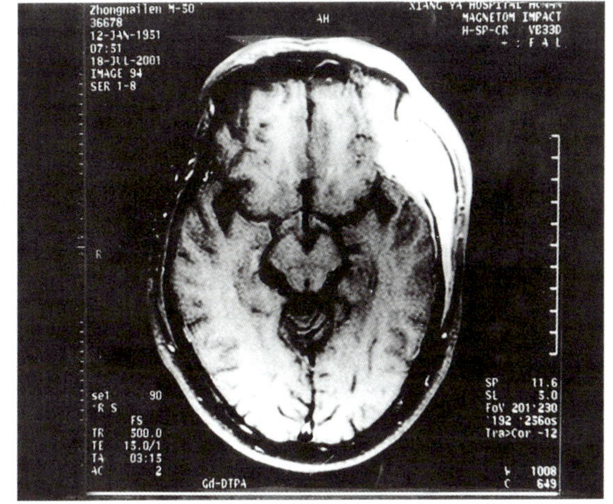

图 5

**图 4, 5** 冠状及横断磁共振扫描显示肿瘤通过颞骨侵入颅内硬脑膜。

Fig. 4, 5 Coronal and axial magnetic resonance image shows penetration of tumor through temporal bone into overlying dura.

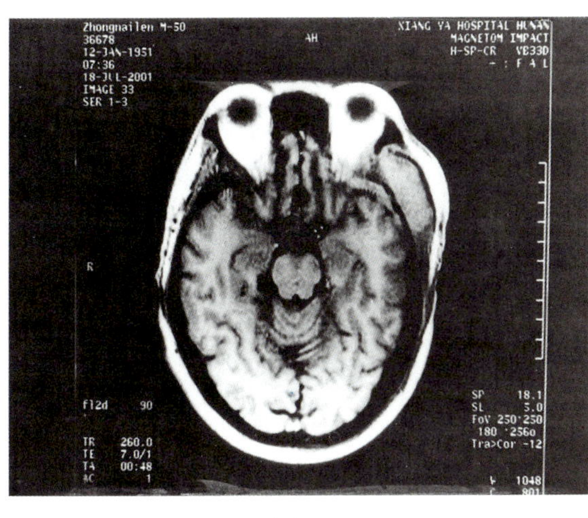

图 6

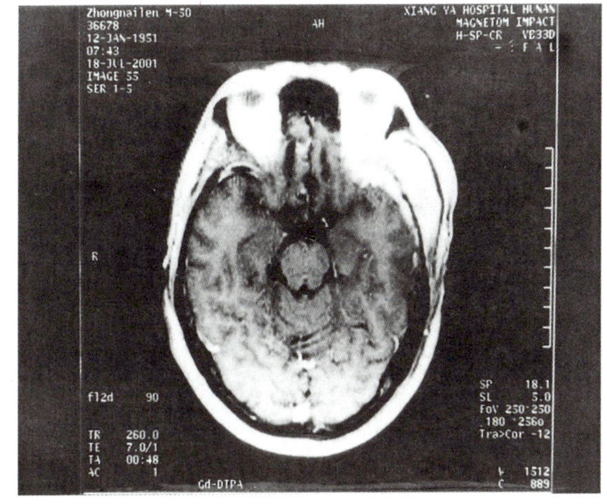

图 7

**图 6, 7** 横断磁共振显示肿瘤侵犯眼球外侧部及眼球后部结构。

Fig. 6, 7 Axial magnetic resonance image shows extension of the tumor into lateral orbital wall and postocular tissue.

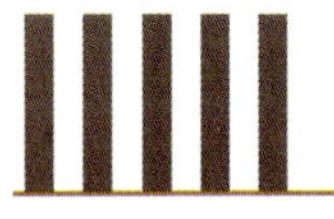



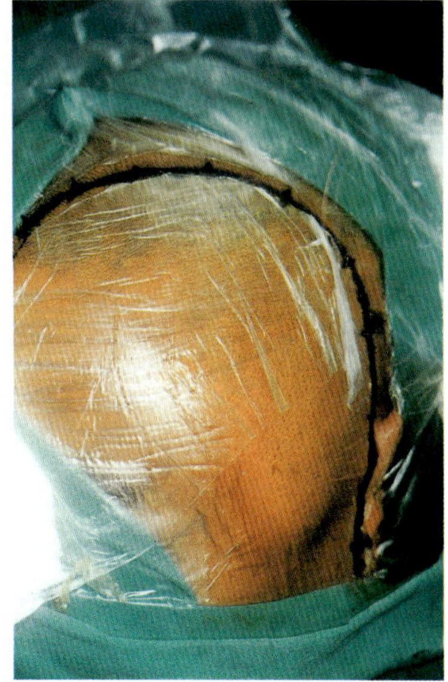

图 8

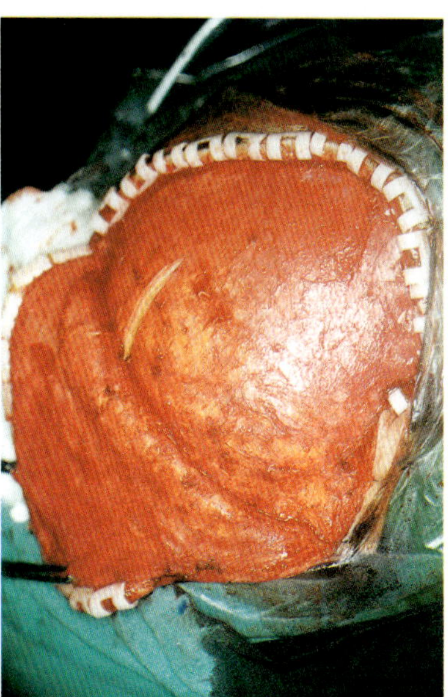

图 9

**图 8** 用美蓝画出半冠状切口的切口线。

**图 9** 按标准的方法掀起头皮瓣，向前解剖达眶外侧缘。切断颞浅动脉的前支并电凝，保留颞浅动脉的后支以供颞肌之血运。切口在颧弓之下的部分应在腮腺筋膜浅面以避免损伤腮腺浅叶及面神经的分支。

**Fig. 8** The standard hemi-coronal incision line is marked out by the methylene blue.

**Fig. 9** The scalp flap is raised in the standard way, anteriorly the dissection is taken to the lateral orbital rim. The anterior branch of the superficial temporal artery is coagulated and sharply transected. The posterior branch of the superficial temporal artery is left undisturbed along the temporalis fascia to provide vascularization to the temporalis muscle. The incision is extended inferiorly beneath the pinna of the ear. The subzygomatic portion of the incision is made superficially to avoid injury to the parotid gland and the branches of the facial nerve.

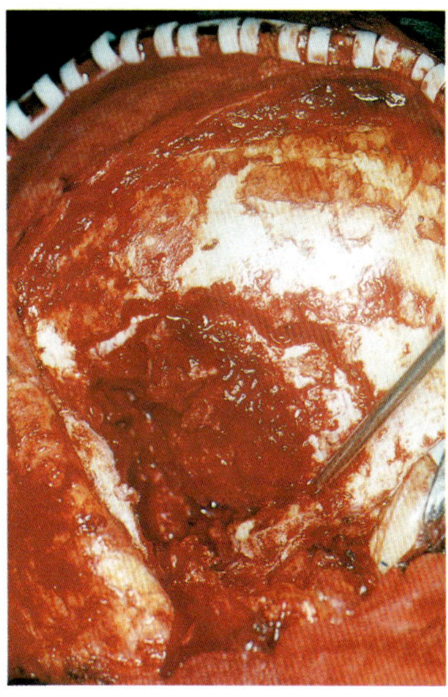

图 10

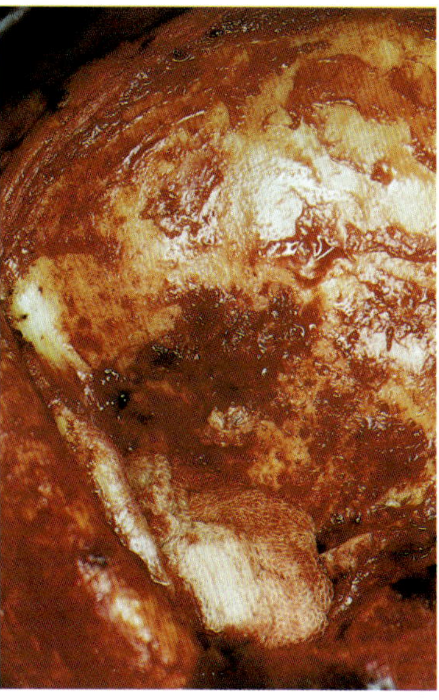

图 11

**图 10** 切开颞肌浅及深筋膜层，在行此切口时，应从眶外侧缘后 1cm 与颧弓平行切开，其目的是避免损伤面神经额支。从颧弓上在骨膜下分离颞肌筋膜，并将此筋膜向前反折。在颧突和颧弓根部行颧弓截断术，在截断颧弓之前，在截骨的两端分别钻孔以便颧弓复位时的固定。沿颞上线切开颞肌及颞肌筋膜，用一宽而扁的骨膜剥离器沿颅骨膜深面分离颞肌骨膜瓣。此时，颞部及颞下窝的肿瘤完全被暴露于手术野中。

**图 11** 在肿瘤周围至少 1cm 去除颅外肿瘤部分；见颞骨部分骨质破坏。

**Fig. 10** A subficial incision is made through the superficial and deep temporalis fascia layers, 1cm posterior to the lateral orbital rim, parallel to the course of the zygoma, to avoid injury to the frontalis branch of the facial nerve. The temporalis fascia is then dissected from the zygoma in a subperiosteal fashion and this fascia is reflected anteriorly. A zygomatic osteotomy is made at the malar eminence and at the root of the zygoma. Drill holes are placed in the two ends of each osteotomic line in anticipation of placing miniplates for later reconstruction.

The temporalis muscle/fascia along the superior temporal line is incised and is reflected the temporalis inferiorly.

**Fig. 11** The tumor is completely exposed in the operative field. After partial tumor of out of the cranium is removed, the destruction of the temporal bone is obvious.

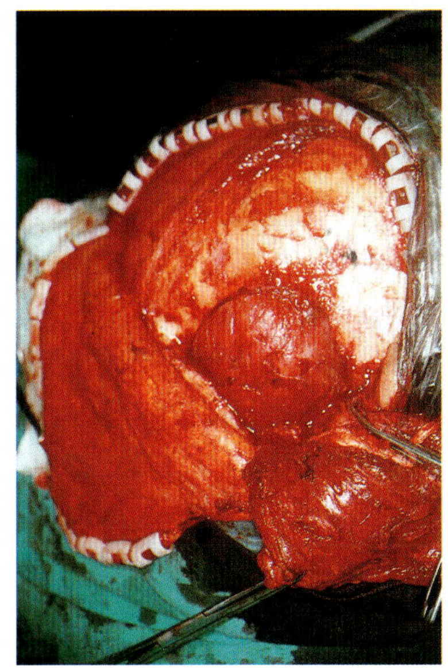

图 12

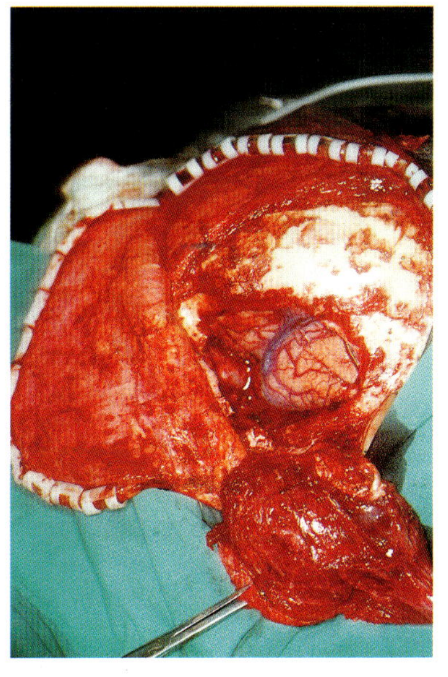

图 13

**图 12** 截开颞部骨板。暴露中颅窝和中颅窝内的下部结构的关键是要行 L－型的颅骨截开术，该术式截开的颅骨包括蝶骨大翼、颞骨鳞部、圆孔和椭圆孔端的水平部分。通常，一个中等大小的截骨就能提供足够的暴露。脑膜的肿瘤侵犯随肿瘤在血管和神经进入颅内的孔道处累及较少，如果肿瘤行放射治疗后复发而往往有广泛累及，有时甚至半侧脑膜被肿瘤组织所替代。

**图 13** 在正常脑膜 5－10mm 之内切除脑膜组织，并对切除边缘的脑膜组织行冰冻切片活组织检查。通常，肉眼认为正常的脑膜组织也有肿瘤的扩散，而且需要在病理学报告指导下一步的切除范围。图 13 为受累硬脑膜切除之后的情景，中脑浅静脉明显可见。

在中颅区行手术时，有两点应特别注意，那就是生命中枢结构和某些重建的困难而使切除受到限制。

在中颅窝妨碍进一步脑膜切除的两个主要结构是下吻合静脉和上矢状窦，下吻合大脑静脉在不同的距离将矢状窦的静脉血引流进入侧窦。假如上吻合静脉不能耐受或管腔过小的话，下吻合静脉将是整个同侧大脑半球惟一的引流静脉。如果将它损伤的话，将会导致同侧大脑半球的栓塞甚至造成病人的死亡。这可在手术前脑静脉造影确定静脉类型而避免该并发症。

在前颅窝从前颅窝底向上到冠状缝的上矢状窦可以被安全地结扎。中颅窝的血管不能被结扎，否则将会导致偏瘫和死亡。幸运的是颅底肿瘤扩散达此处的病变极罕见。

切除脑膜的另一个限制是脑膜修复和脑脊液漏的预防。当沿其下的脑干行脑膜切除时，在获得良好的脑膜关闭上困难会逐渐增加，在此部位的脑脊液漏与鼻咽部相通，鼻咽部是整个上呼吸道病源菌高度集中的部位之一。组织胶可以应用，但在强度上仍以缝线为优，大多数纤维胶约在 1 周内粘附强度丧失。

**Fig. 12** Temporal bone is osteotomied. The key to the exposure to the middle fossa and its immediate subcranial structures is an L-shaped craniotomy that has a vertical component comprised of the greater wing of the sphenoid and squamosal aspect of the temporal bone, and a short horizontal component that ends at the foramen ovale and foramen spinosum. Often a modest-sized craniotomy provides adequate exposure.

Dural invasion varies from minimal involvement at the neural and vascular foramen at the sites of entry into the intracranial space to widespread involvement characteristic of recurrent tumors after full-course radiation therapy. Sometimes the half dura is replaced almost entirely by tumor tissue.

**Fig. 13** A cuff of 5 to 10mm of grossly healthy dura is excised and the periphery examined by frozen-section analysis. Often grossly normal dura has tumor extensions and requires further resection as dictated by the pathologist's report. Fig. 13 shows the condition after the involved dura has been resected and the superficial middle cerebral vein may be seen in the operative field.

Certain limitations to resection are imposed by vital central structures and the restrictions of certain reconstructive options. In the middle fossa, the two major structures that impede further dural excision are the vein of Labbé and the superior sagittal sinus. The vein of Labbé, or inferior anastomotic cerebral vein, drains into the lateral sinus at a variable distance from the sigmoid sinus. If the superior anastomotic vein of Trolard is not patent or is of small caliber, the vein of Labbé will be the only vein draining the entire ipsilateral cerebral hemisphere. To sacrifice it would then result in massive infarction and often death. Cerebral venography may establish the venous drainage pattern in those patients in whom the vein of Labbé is in jeopardy.

The superior sagittal sinus can usually be safely obliterated in the anterior fossa from the anterior fossa floor up to the coronal suture. The middle fossa component cannot be ligated because in most instances it will lead to quadriplegia and often death. Fortunately, few skull base tumors extend that far.

The second dural restriction concerns the potential for dural reconstruction and the provision of a watertight seal. As dural resection along the clivus and under the brainstem increases in extent, there is a progressive increase in difficulty in obtaining a sound dural closure. A cerebrospinal fluid leak at this site is an open avenue to the nasopharynx, which possesses one of the highest concentrations of pathogenic bacteria in the entire upper aerodigestive tract. Tissue glue helps, but a suture line is superior in strength. For most fibrin glues, the adhesive strength is lost in about 1 week.

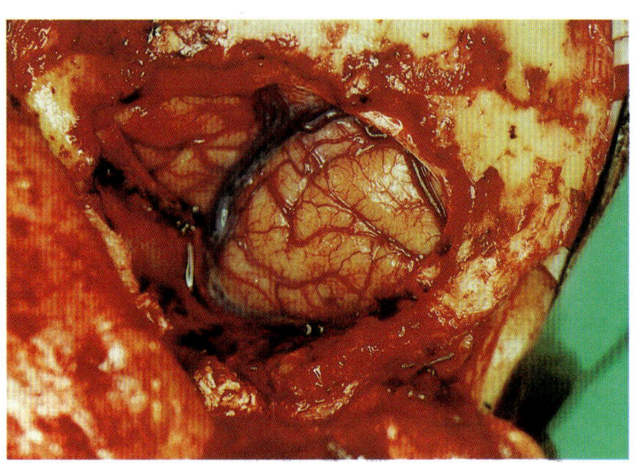

图 14

**图 14** 部分硬脑膜切除之后的情景，大脑浅中静脉清晰可见。

**图 15** 为了防止脑脊液漏，颞筋膜被用来修复被切除的脑膜。缝合应仔细，尤其是在斜坡上的下面。缝合之后擦干创面，涂布组织胶以增加缝合强度。第二层由肌肉组成，假如颞肌被保留的话，可以被用来修复颅底和覆盖在截开的颅骨部位。在通过此种处理后，由切除蝶骨之下的软组织遗留的浅在死腔得以消失。

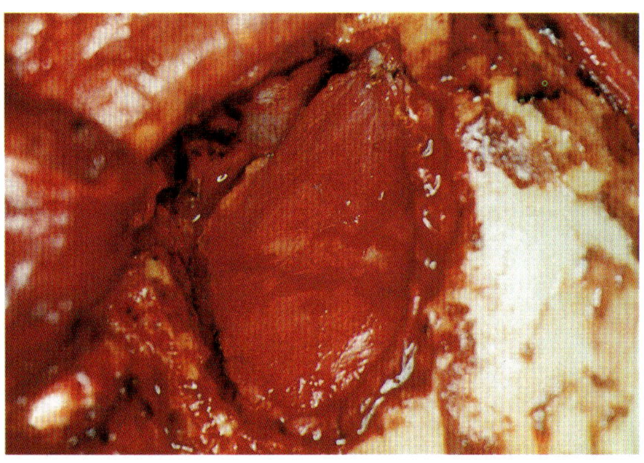

图 15

**Fig. 14** The condition after the partial dura has been excised. Superficial middle cerebral vein may be seen.

**Fig. 15** To prevent cerebrospinal fluid leek, fascia lata, temporalis fascia, or allograft may be used to patch resected dura. Careful suture, especially on the inferior aspects above the clivus, is essential. The closure may be enhanced with tissue glue.

The next layer comprises muscle. The temporalis muscle, if preserved, is placed under and across the craniotomy site. The pericranial cuff is sutured to the basipharyngeal fascia of the nasopharynx. In this way, the potential dead space left by resected soft tissue under the sphenoid bone can be obliterated. The integrity of the muscle is carefully ensured before this step.

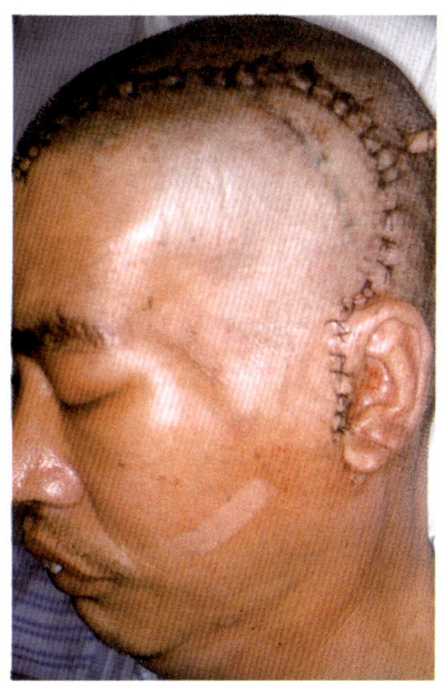

图 16

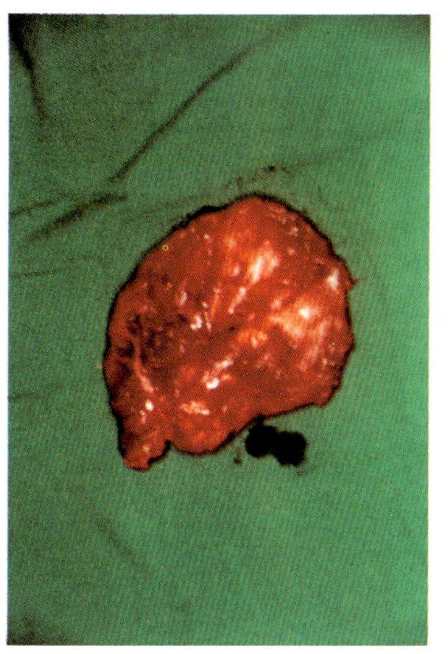

图 17

**图 16** 将颧骨和截开的颅骨瓣还回，用微型钛板固定，L 型颅骨切开瓣通常部分被丧失是因为骨被肿瘤破坏和保证肿瘤在安全缘被切所致，应当由肌瓣充填。

缝合皮肤，创口放置负压引流，除非有脑脊液漏形成，一般引流在术后 72 小时被拔除。

如果脑脊液漏在术后 3 天还不停止，病人应被送入手术室行脑脊液漏修补。

**图 17** 被切除的肿瘤标本。

**Fig16** The zygoma and the craniotomy bone flaps are returned and fixed with mini-plates. The inferior aspect of the L-shaped craniotomy flap is often partially missing because of bone erosion by tumor and subsequent osseous resection to ensure tumor-free margins. The muscle flap fills in the dead space and adds support.

Skin closure is then done and the wound drained with a closed system of suction drainage.

The lumbar drain is usually discontinued at about 72 hours unless a cerebrospinal fluid leak occurs. If a leak does not step in 3 days, the patient should be sent back to the operating room for repair.

**Fig17** The specimen excised tumor.

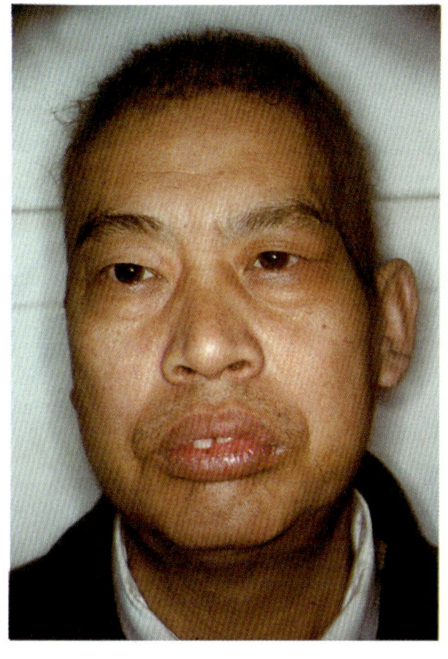

图 18

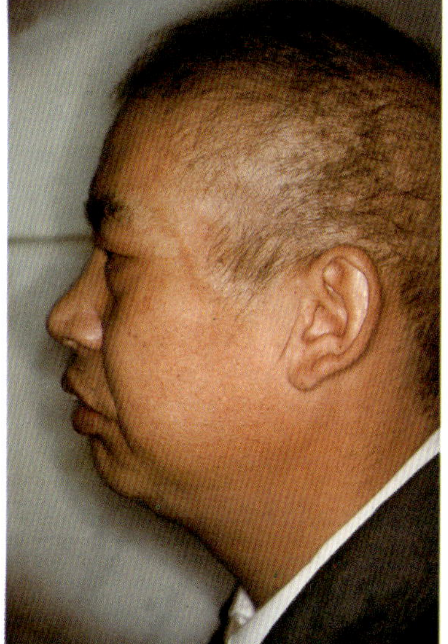

图 19

**图 18，19** 患者行颞窝及颅中窝肿瘤切除后 6 个月的情景。

**Fig18, 19** Patient, 6 months after temporal fossa-middle cranial fossa tumor resection.

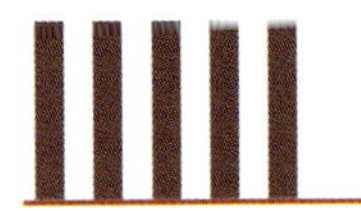



# 2. 中颅窝脑膜瘤继发侵犯翼下颌间隙的手术治疗

# 2. Surgical treatment of intracranial meningioma secondarily involving infratemporal fossa and pterygomandibular space

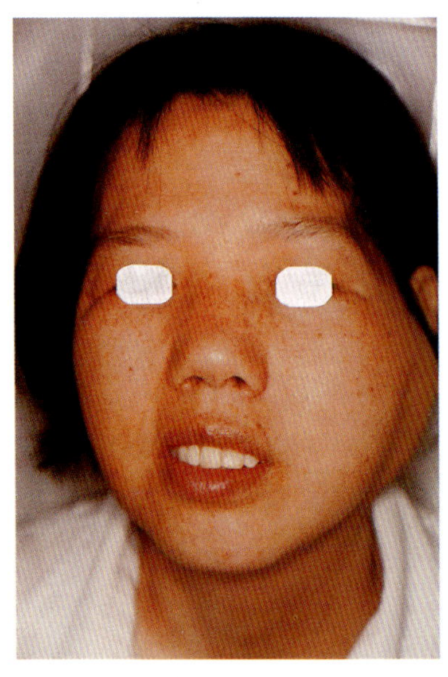

图 20

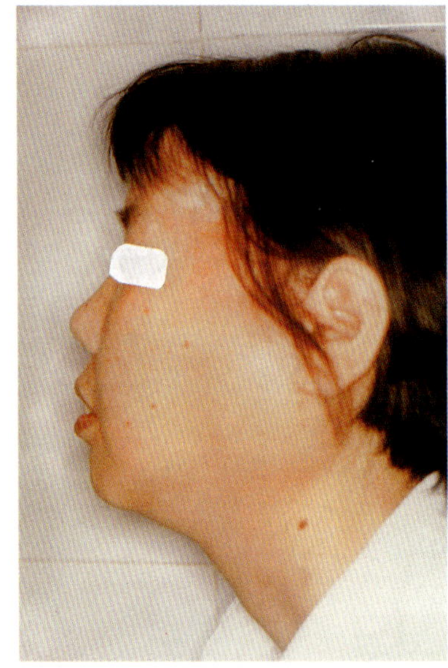

图 21

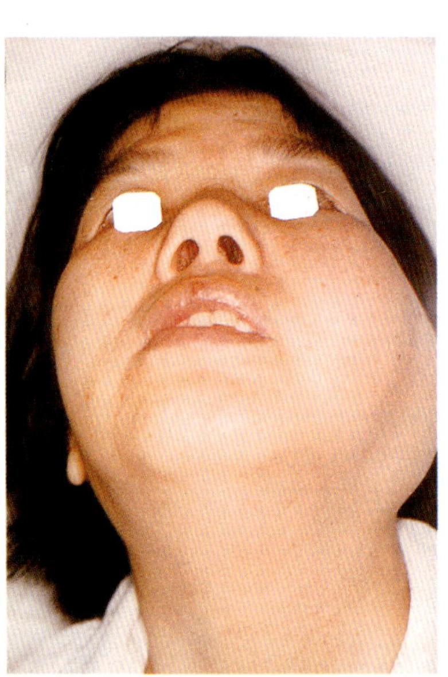

图 22

**图 20** 左中颅窝脑膜瘤继发侵犯颞下颌间隙的 53 岁一女性患者，正面观显示两侧面颊部明显不对称，左侧明显膨隆。

**图 21** 侧面观见左侧颞下及左面部明显膨隆，表面皮肤正常；左侧眼裂变小。

**Fig. 20** A 53-year-old women patient with left middle cranial fossa meningioma secondarily involving infratemporal fossa and pterygomandibular space.

**Fig. 21** Frontal view shows that both sides of the face are asymmetry and left side is expansive. Lateral view shows that left face is expansive and facial skin is normal.

**图 22** 仰面观见两侧面部不对称，左侧面部极度膨隆。

**Fig. 22** Submental view shows that both sides of the face are asymmetry and the left side is expansive extremely.

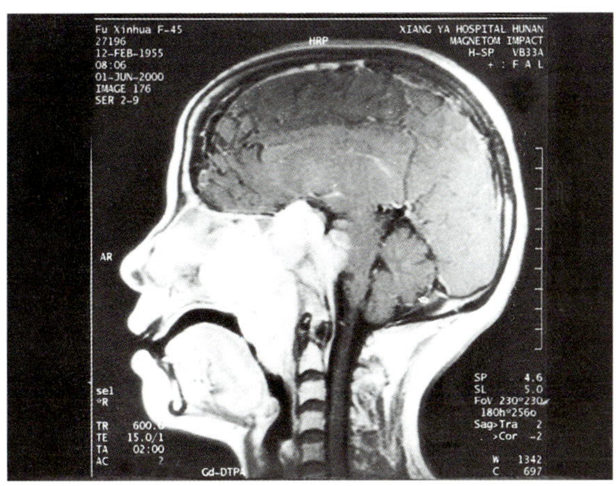

图 23

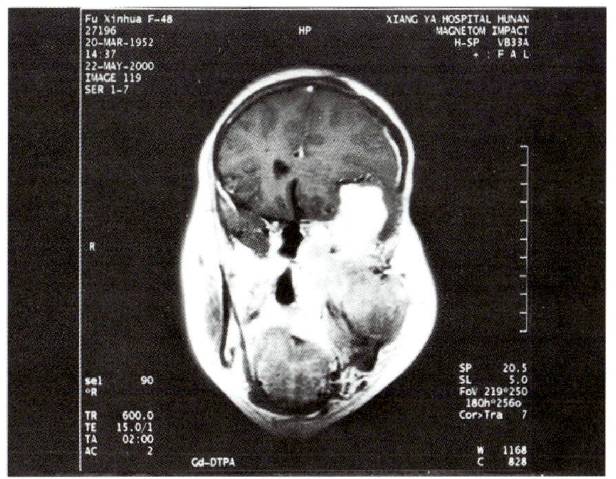

图 24

**图 23** 磁共振矢状切面显示肿瘤通过中颅窝底的圆孔进入颞下窝和翼下颌及咽旁间隙内。
**图 24** 磁共振冠状切面显示肿瘤通过中颅窝底的圆孔、卵圆孔进入颞下及翼下颌间隙中。

**Fig. 23** Sagittal magnetic resonance image shows the extension of the tumor through the foramen ovale, rotumdum into the infratemporal fossa, parapharyngeal space and pterygomandibular space.

**Fig. 24** Coronal magnetic resonance image shows the tumor extending through the floor of the middle fossa via the foramen ovale, rotumdum into the infratemporal fossa and pterygomandibular space.

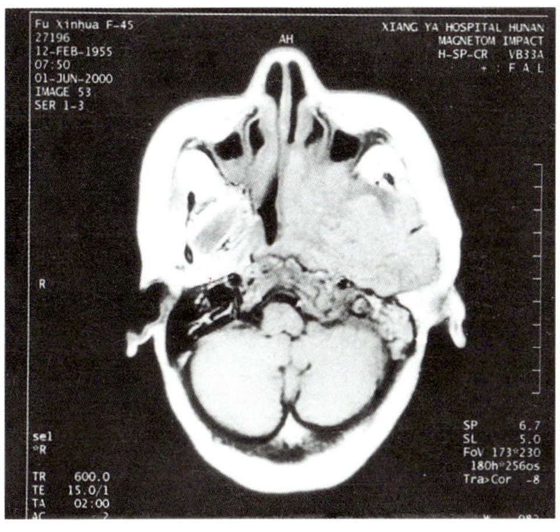

图 25

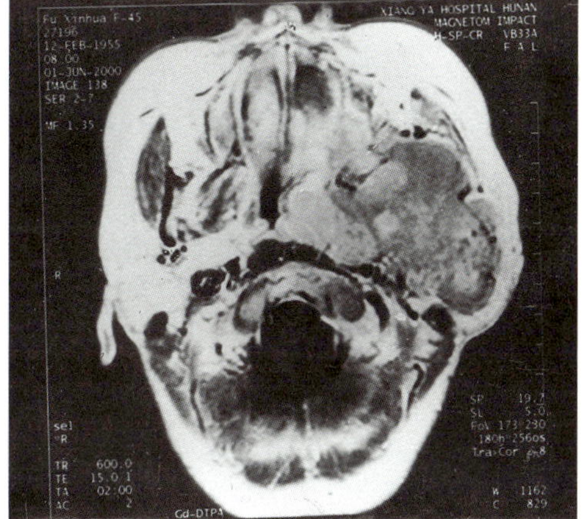

图 26

**图 25** 横断磁共振片显示肿瘤侵入颞下翼腭间隙。
**图 26** 横断磁共振片显示肿瘤扩展进入咽旁及翼下颌间隙。

**Fig. 25** Axial magnetic resonance image shows the extension of the tumor into the infratemporal fossa and pterygopalatine space.

**Fig. 26** Axial magnetic resonance image shows the tumor extending into the parapharyngeal and pterygomandibular space.

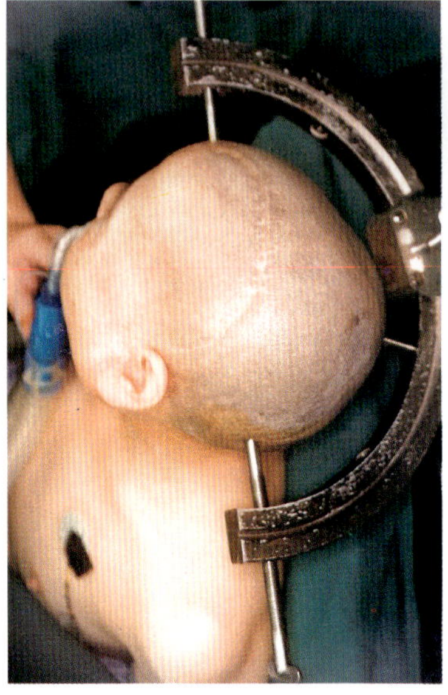
图 27

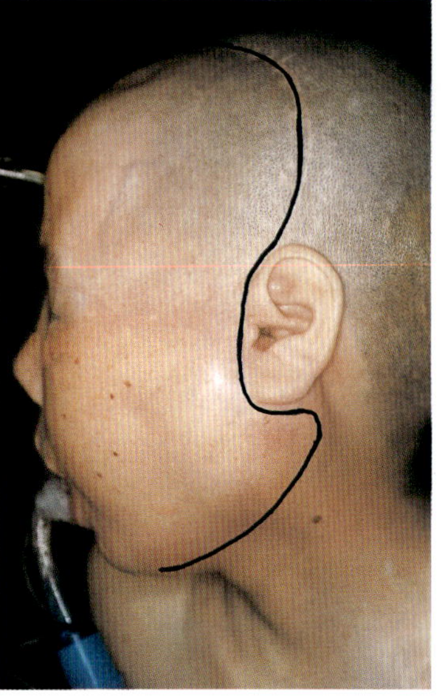
图 28

**图 27,28** 病人仰卧,头偏健侧。头颅用头架固定以防手术中移动。用美蓝画出颅面颈部切口线。

**Fig. 27, 28** The patient is placed with the head at the foot end of the table and with the table rotated 180 degrees away from the anesthesiologist, rotating the operating field away from the anesthetic equipment increases the degree of operative maneuverability. The patient's head is fixed with three-point pin. Incisive line is marked out with methylene blue.

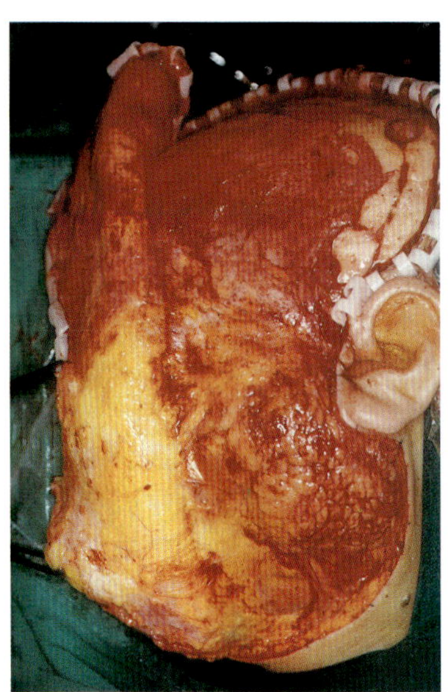
图 29

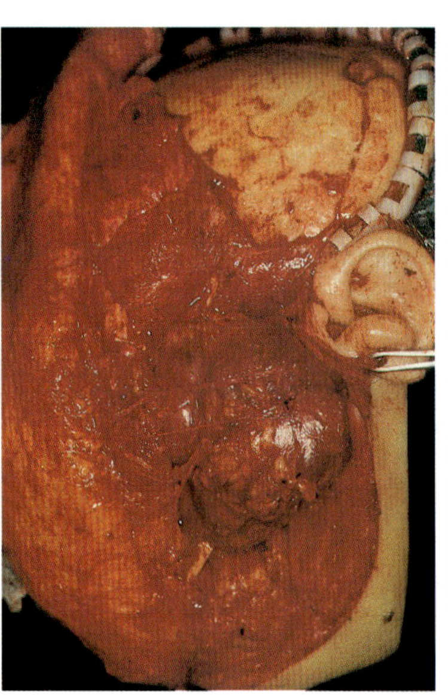
图 30

**图 29** 采用向下延至耳前的半冠状切口。如行同期颈清扫术的话,可将切口向下延续达颈部呈 S 型。头皮瓣按标准的方法掀起。在面颈部侧向前掀开皮瓣,前面解剖至眶外侧缘及嚼肌前缘。

**图 30** 做保留面神经的全腮腺切除术。将下颌升支去除,以获得良好的暴露。如果计划将升支重新放回,则应保留其嚼肌附着,以维持它的血供。同样,将颧弓前、后端截断并移去。如此,其深层的肿瘤可暴露于手术野中。

**Fig. 29** The hemicoronal incision continues down in front of the ear as for a face lift. If a simultaneous neck dissection is to be performed, it is taken down to the neck in an S fashion. The scalp flap is raised in the standard way. Anteriorly the dissection is taken to the lateral orbital rim and the anterior border of the masseter.

**Fig. 30** A total parotidectomy is performed, preserving the facial nerve. This dissection is aided by magnification and a nerve stimulator. The ascending ramus is removed to make the exposure convenient. If the ramus is to be replaced, its masseteric attachment should be left intact to maintain its blood supply. Similarly, the zygomatic arch is divided anteriorly and posteriorly and then removed. At this point it may be possible to see the tumor.

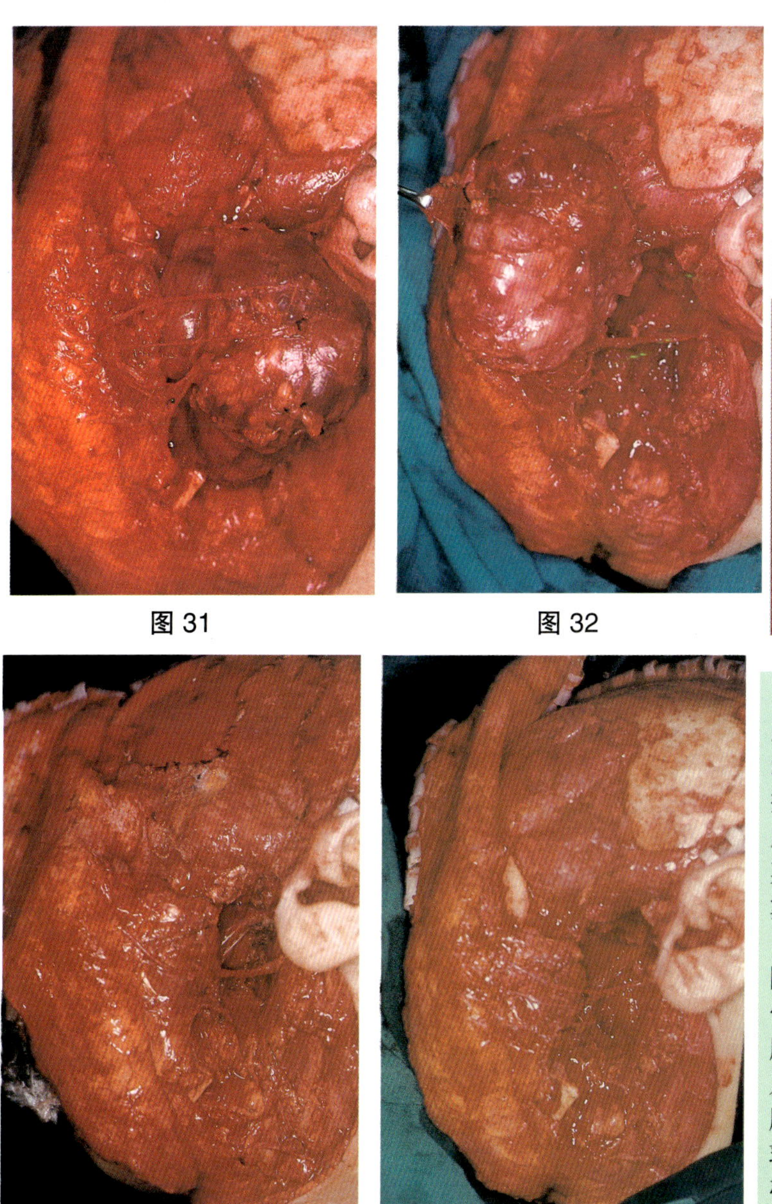

图 31 图 32 图 33 图 34

**图 31** 本图显示颅底及肿瘤。从耳前开始，在面神经的深面沿颅底部解剖至肿瘤所在的部位。

**图 32** 在大多数情况下，可以在肿瘤从颅底穿出的周围完全分离而切除，但面神经的主要分支仍然被保留。

**Fig. 31** This photograph shows how this dissection leads conveniently to the base of the skull and the tumor. Beginning in frontal of the ear, deep to the facial nerve a dissection is made along the skull base until the tumor is located.

**Fig. 32** It is possible in most tumors to dissect completely around the area of tumor exit from the skull, but the main branches of the facial nerve is still preserved.

**图 33** 按 Pieper 和 Al-Mefty 的术式切除颅内肿瘤。颅内、外肿瘤被切除之后，必须仔细检查三叉神经的各分支和骨骼肌是否有肿瘤的侵犯，如果有，就必须将其切除。肿瘤的颅外部分被切除之后，发现被肿瘤累及的骨，其中包括眶底，都应该被去除。同时也必须对翼腭窝、翼板进行检查。

**图34** 颅外肿瘤和被累及的骨一旦被去除，就必须考虑重建问题。眼眶可用金属网、骨或二者重建。用带血管蒂的颞肌瓣修复，把脑膜与曾暴露过的气窦/和鼻咽部分开。颞下及翼颌肿瘤摘除后遗留的死腔，容易形成血肿和导致感染，因此要用有良好血运的胸锁乳突肌瓣填塞。如截断的下颌支保留着肌肉蒂，应放回原处做固定。还回颧骨、用金属丝或钛板固定。

**Fig. 33** The intracranial tumor is resected or enucleated according to Pieper and Al-Mefty's operative approach*. After the intracranial and extracranial tumor has been resected, the branches of the trigeminal nerve and skeletal muscle must be assessed for tumor invasion and resected aggressively. Once the extracranial component of the tumor has been removed, any involved bone should be drilled away including the floor of the orbit. We carefully inspect the pterygopalatine fossa as well as the pterygoid plates for the presence of tumor.

**Fig. 34** Once the extracrainal tumor and involved bone have been removed, meticulous reconstruction is necessary. The orbit can be reconstructed with mesh, bone, or both. The temporalis muscle provides a viscularized flap to provide a barrier between any exposed air sinus/nasopharynx and dura. The dead space resulting from the resection of the extracranial tumor is a potential source of hematoma and infection and is filled with well-vascularized sternomastoid muscle flap. If the ascending ramus of the mandible has been preserved on a muscular pedicle, it is replaced and wired or plated at the osteotomy site. Zygoma restored and fixed in place with miniplates.

*: Pieper DR, Al-Mefty O.: Management of intracranial meningiomas secondarily involving the infratemporal fossa: Radiographic characteristics. Pattern of tumor invasion, and surgical implications, Neurosurgery. 45; 231 - 238, 1999.

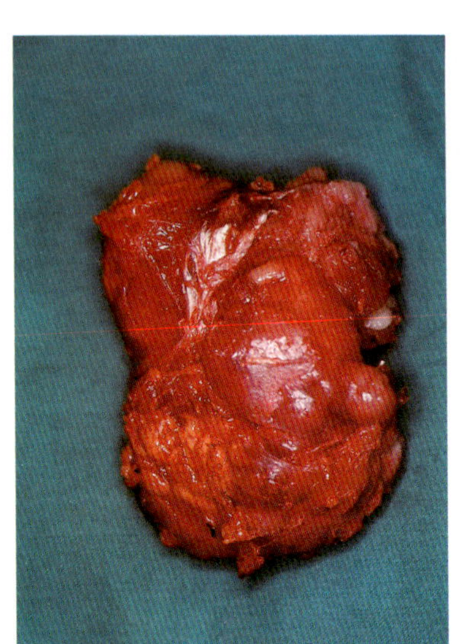

图 35

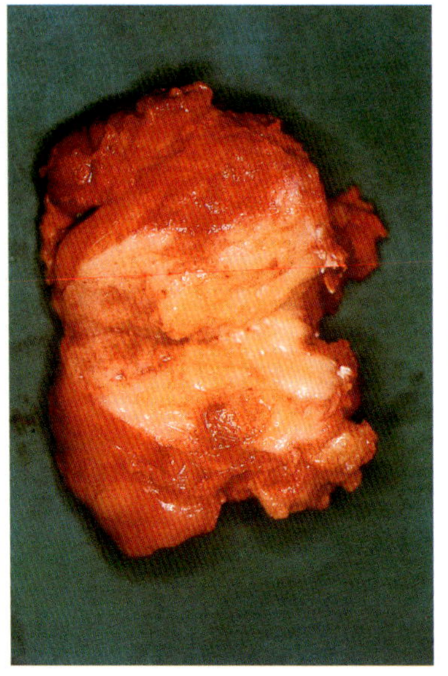

图 36

图 35，36 术后颅外脑膜瘤手术标本显示表面呈结节状，肿瘤切面呈黄色。

Fig. 35, 36 The specimen of post-operative extracranial meningioma shows nodular form on the tumor surface, and incisive surface is yellow.

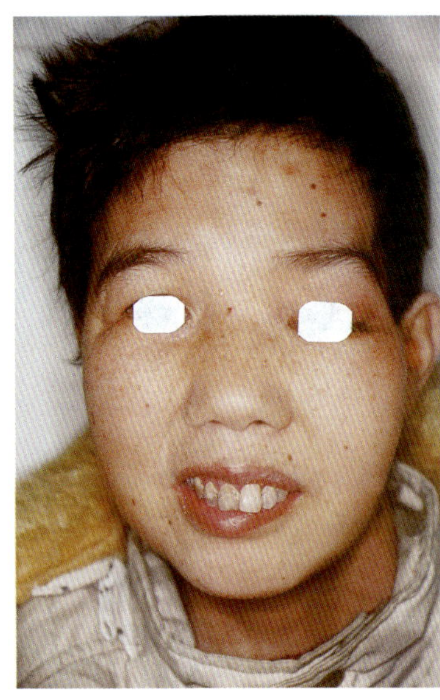

图 37

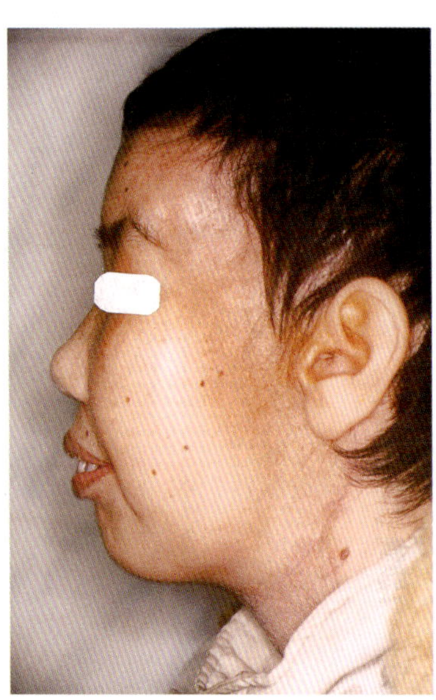

图 38

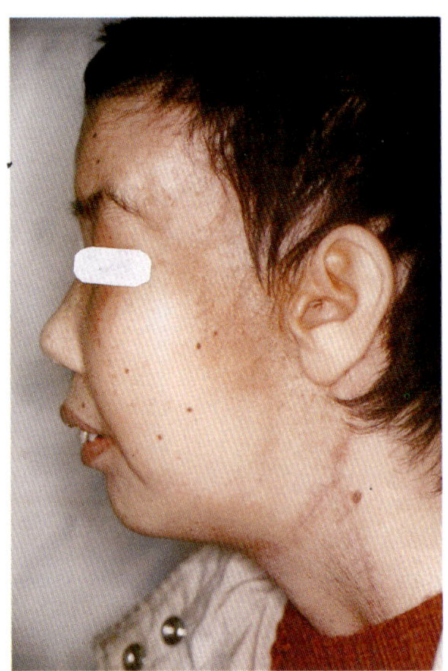

图 39

图 37, 38 患者手术后 1 年的正面和侧面观。

Fig. 37, 38 Frontal and lateral views of a 53-year-old women patient with intracranial meningioma secondarily involving the infratemporal fossa and pterygomandibular space 1 year after surgery.

图 39 患者术后 1 年的颈部侧面观。

Fig. 39 Lateral view of neck of a 53-year-old women patient 1 year after surgery.

# 3. 中颅底炎性假瘤的外科手术治疗

# 3. Surgical treatment of inflammatory pseudotumor under inferior surface of the middle skull base

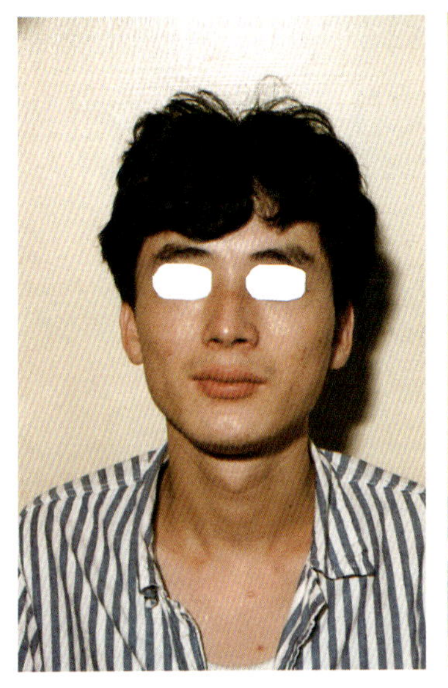

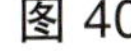

图 40

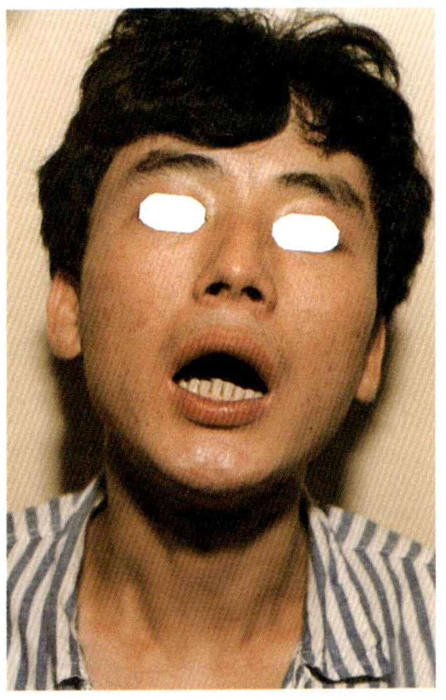

图 41

**图 40, 41** 一患左侧翼腭窝区炎性假瘤的28岁患者正面观及张口受限情况。

**Fig. 40, 41** Frontal view and condition of the openning mouth degree of a 28-year-old male patient with inflammatory pseudotumor in inferior surface of the middle skull base.

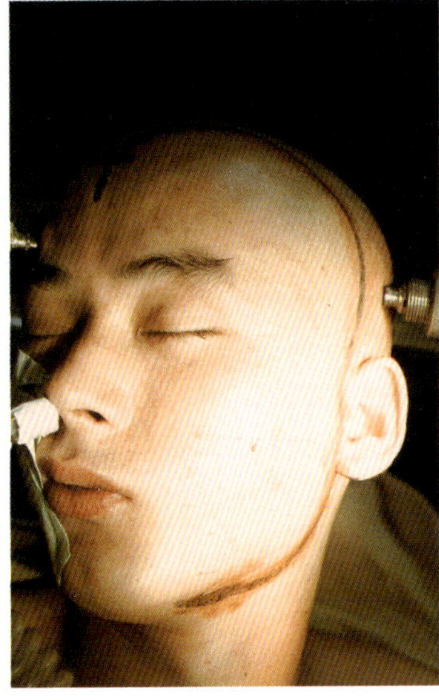

图 42

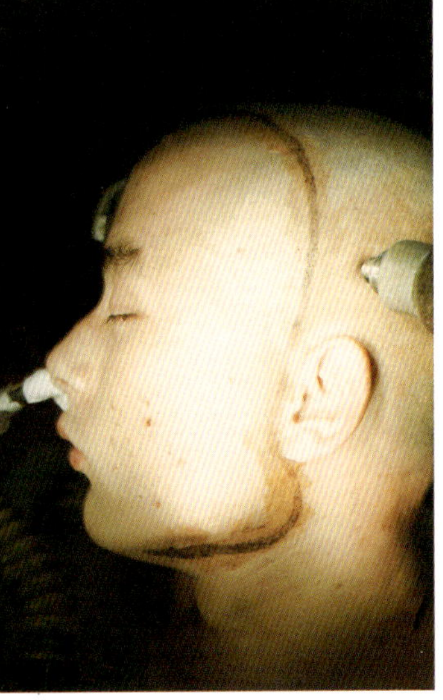

图 43

**图 42, 43** 颅面部切口的正面及侧面观。头部用头架固定。采用向下延至耳前的半冠状切口。如行同期颈清扫术的话，可将切口向下延续达颈部呈S形。

**Fig. 42, 43** The frontal and lateral views of the craniofacial incision line drawing. The head is fixed by three-point pin. The standard hemicoronal incision continues down in front of the ear as for a face lift. If a simultaneous neck dissection is to be performed, it is taken down to the neck in an S fashion. Alternatively, a McFee incision may be used.



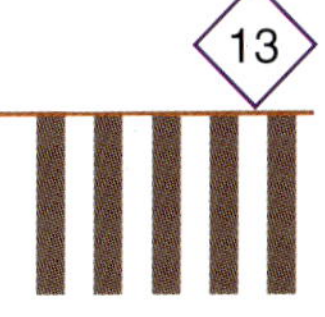

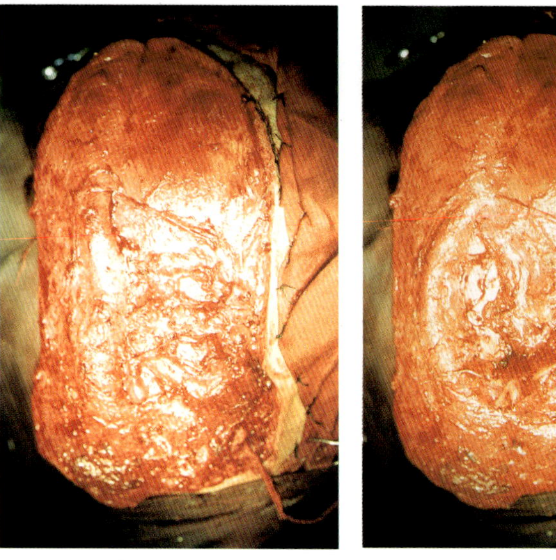

图 44　　图 45

**图 44,45** 按常规方法将皮瓣掀起,向前解剖达眶外侧缘。做保留面神经的全腮腺摘除术。将下颌升支去除以获得良好的显露。如果计划将升支重新放回,则应保留其嚼肌附着,以维持它的血供。同样,将颧弓前、后端截断并移去。

**Fig. 44, 45** The scalp flap is raised in the standard way. In the face and neck it is lifted. Anteriorly the dissection is taken to the lateral orbital rim. A total parotidectomy is performed, preserving the facial nerve. This dissection is aided by magnification and a nerve stimulator. The ascending ramus is removed to make the exposure convenient. If the ramus is to be replaced, its masseteric attachment should be left intact to maintain its blood supply. Similarly, the zygomatic arch is divided anteriorly and posteriorly and then removed.

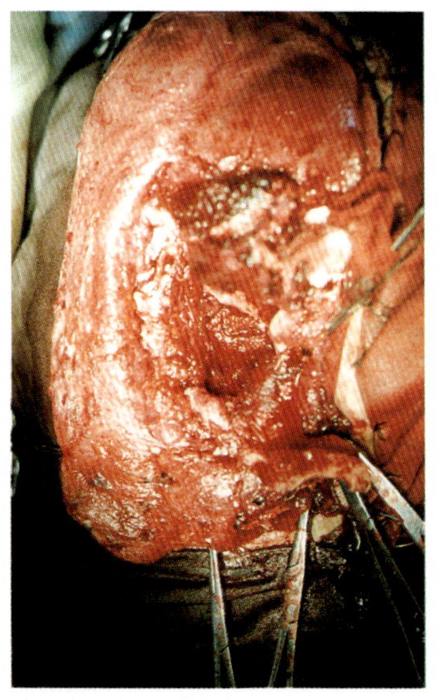

图 46

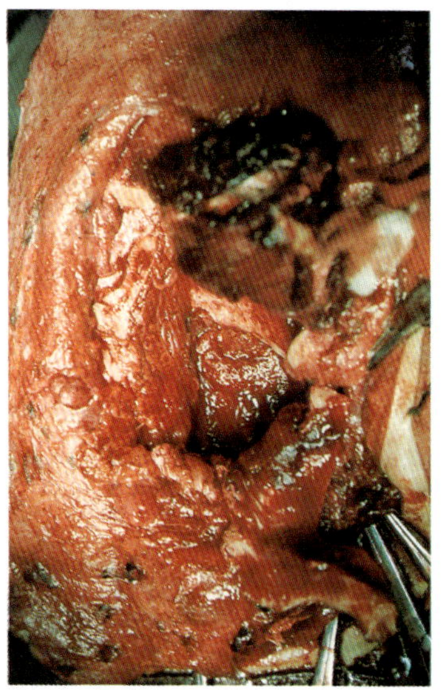

图 47

**图 46, 47** 如此，肿瘤便可暴露在视野中。在某些病例,由于肿瘤向下延伸至颈部或为了识别进入颅底的组织，作根治性颈淋巴清扫术。本图显示颅底及肿瘤。

**Fig. 46, 47** At this point it may be possible to see the tumor. In some cases, because the tumor extends well down into the neck or in order to facilitate identification of the structures entering the skull base, a radical neck dissection is performed. These photographes show how this dissection leads conveniently to the base of the skull and the tumor.

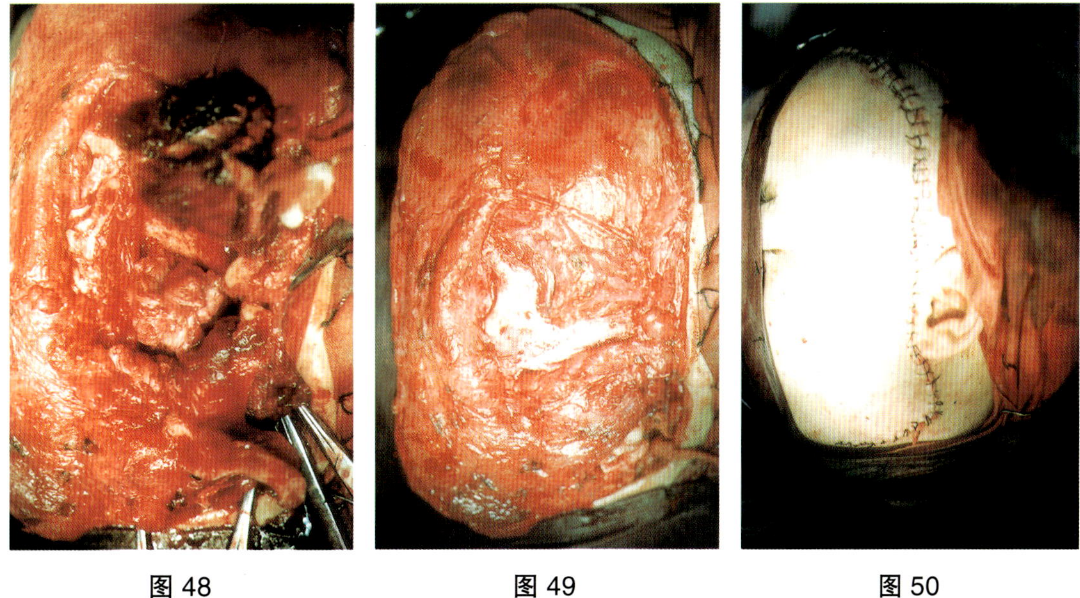

图 48　　图 49　　图 50

**图 48** 从耳前开始，在面神经的深面沿颅底部解剖至肿瘤所在的部位。切断颈内静脉，保留颈总动脉。在大多数情况下，可以在肿瘤从颅底穿出的周围完全切除。在良性肿瘤，如像神经纤维瘤，可将其剜除。

**图 49** 肿瘤摘除后所遗留的死腔，容易形成血肿和导致感染，因此要用有良好血运的胸锁乳突肌瓣填塞。如截断的下颌支保留着肌肉蒂，应放回原处并作固定。如果完全截下，则不应放回原处，因为会形成死骨。还回颧骨，用金属丝或钛板固定。

**Fig. 48** Beginning in front of the ear, deep to the facial nerve a dissection is made along the skull base until the tumor is located. The jugular vein is divided, and the carotid artery preserved. It is possible in most tumors to dissect completely around the area of tumor exit from the skull, benign tumors such as neurofibromas can frequently be enucleated.

**Fig. 49** The dead space resulting from the resection is a potential source of hematoma and infection and is filled with well-vascularized sternomastoid muscle flap. If the ascending ramus of the mandible has been preserved on a muscular pedicle, it is replaced and wired or plated at the osteotomy site. If it has been totally removed, it should not be replaced. Zygoma restored and fixed in place with miniplates.

**图 50** 放引流管后放回皮瓣，分层缝合。

**Fig. 50** The skin flap is closed with suction drainage unless there has been an extensive dural repair. The skin flap is sutured with silk line in the layers.

# 4. 翼腭窝及中颅窝底肿瘤面部组织异位进路切除术

# 4. Facial translocation: a new approach to the middle cranial base and pterygopalatine fossa

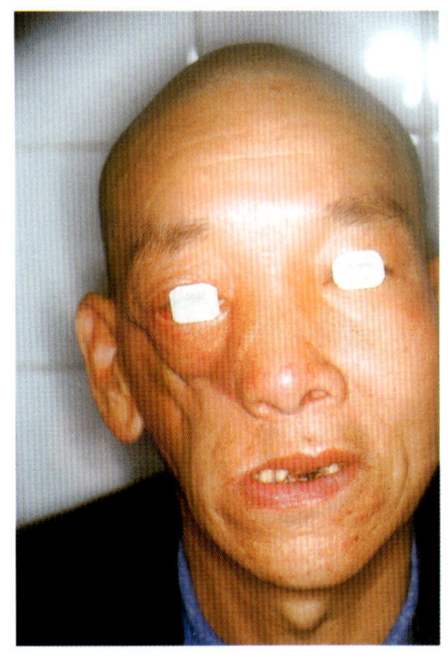

图 51

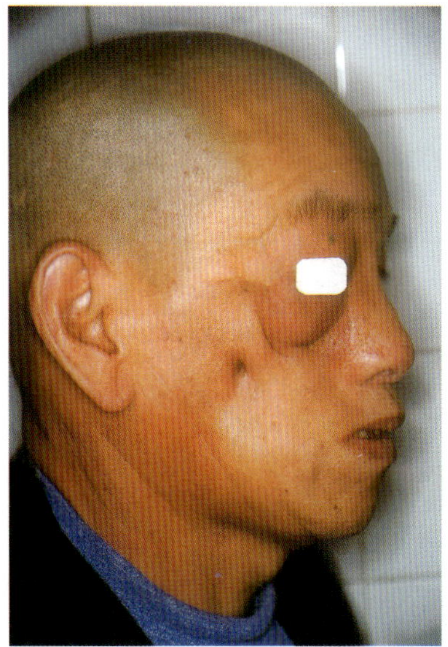

图 52

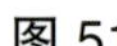

图 51，52 患右侧上颌及颅中窝底恶性纤维组织细胞瘤 65 岁患者的正面及侧面观。

Fig. 51, 52 Frontal and lateral views of a 65-year-old male patient with malignant fibrohistocytic tumor in the pterygomaxillary fossa and middle cranial fossa.

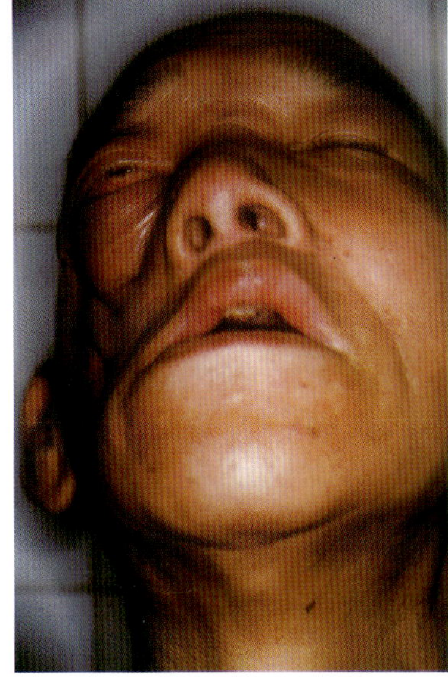

图 53

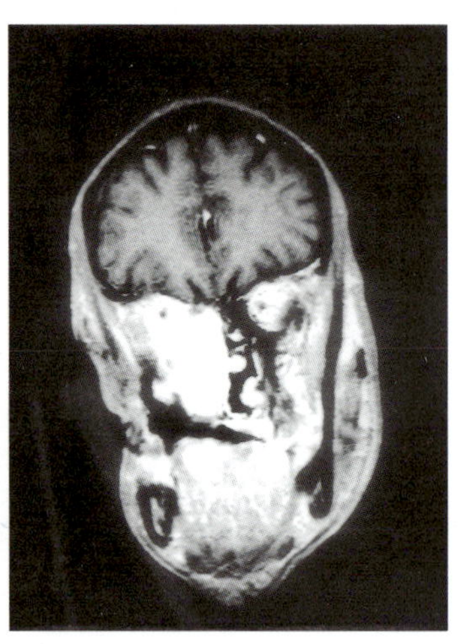

图 54

图 53 仰面观显示右侧面部明显畸形。

图 54 冠状磁共振扫描显示右侧中颅底、右眶内侧壁、右上颌窦及右侧鼻腔被肿瘤累及。

Fig. 53 Submental view shows right facial deformities.

Fig. 54 Coronal MRI scan demonstrates involvement of right middle cranial base, right orbital internal wall, right maxillary sinus and right nasal cavity.

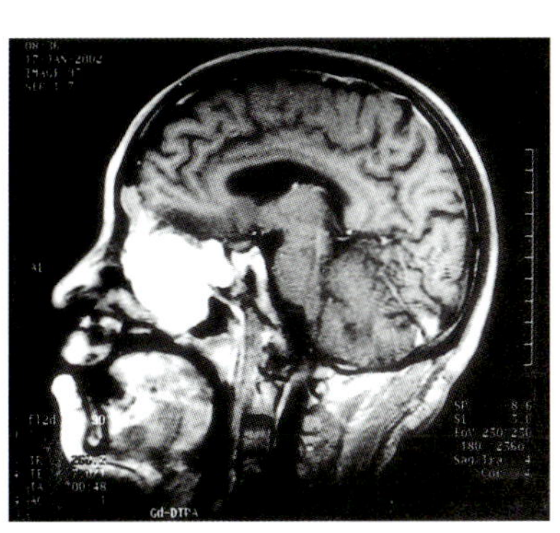

图 55

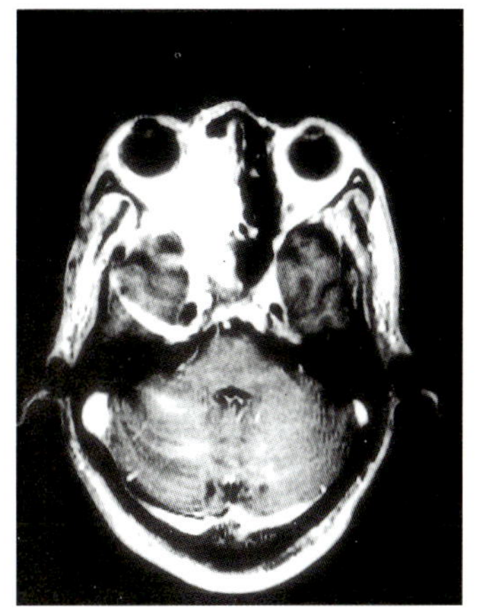

图 56

**图 55** 矢状磁共振扫描示肿瘤累及上颌窦、鼻腔、筛窦及蝶窦。
**图 56** 水平扫描见肿瘤累及眶内侧壁、右侧鼻腔及眶尖。

**Fig. 55** Sagittal MRI scan shows a tumor involving the maxillary sinus, nasal cavity, ethmoid and sphenoid sinuses.

**Fig. 56** Preoperative axial MRI scan shows a tumor involving middle cranial base, medial wall of the right orbit and right nasal cavity.

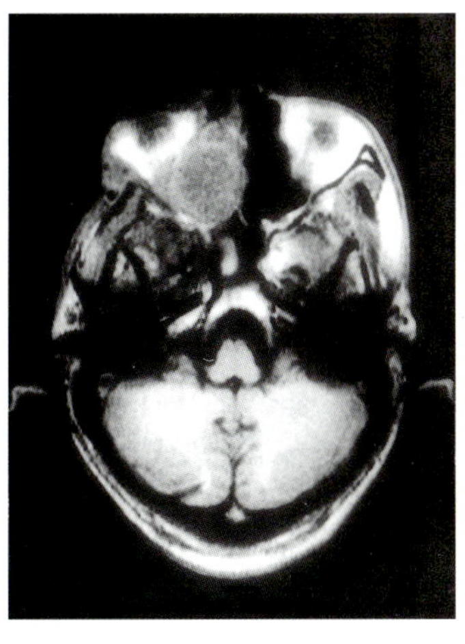

图 57

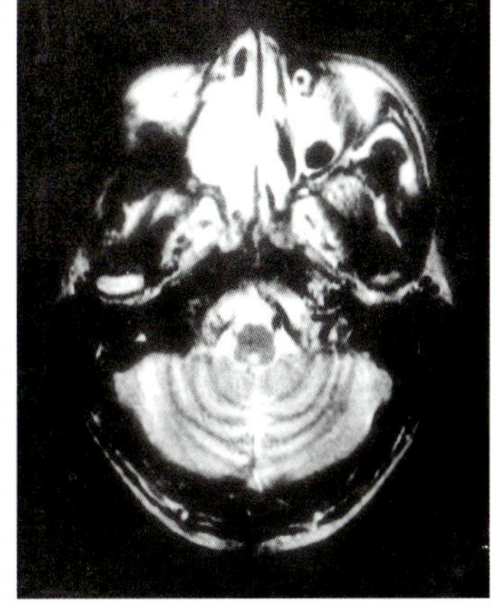

图 58

**图 57, 58** 不同水平 MRI 扫描显示肿瘤累及不同部位。
图 57 示轴性平扫肿瘤累及右眶内侧壁及右侧鼻腔；图 58 示轴性平扫肿瘤累及右侧上颌窦和鼻腔。

**Fig. 57, 58** Different axial MRI scans show tumor involving different part.

Figure 57 shows a tumor involving medial wall of the right orbit and right nasal cavity; Figure 58 shows a tumor involving medial wall of the right orbit, the right nasal cavity, sphenoid sinus.

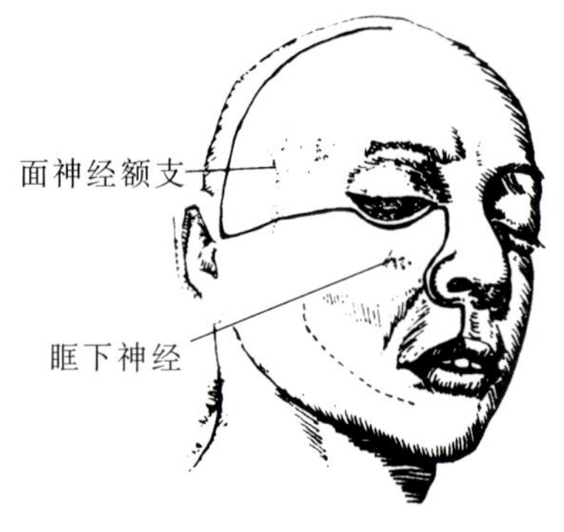


图 59

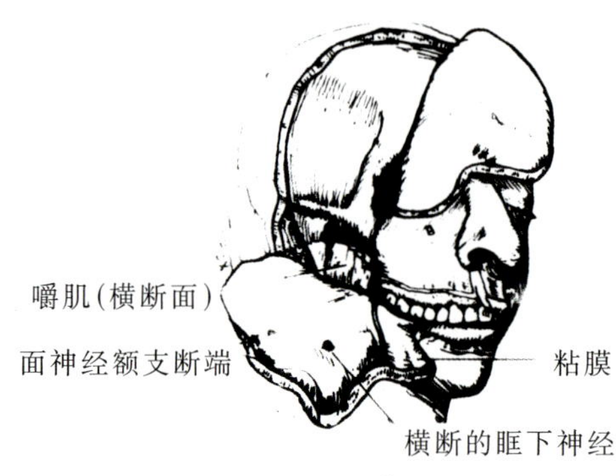


图 60

**图 59** 使用面部组织异位进路的切口设计。
**图 60** 显示被掀起的颊部和额颞瓣。

Fig. 59 Outline of incisions used in facial translocation approach.
Fig. 60 Cheek and frontotemporal flaps are elevated.

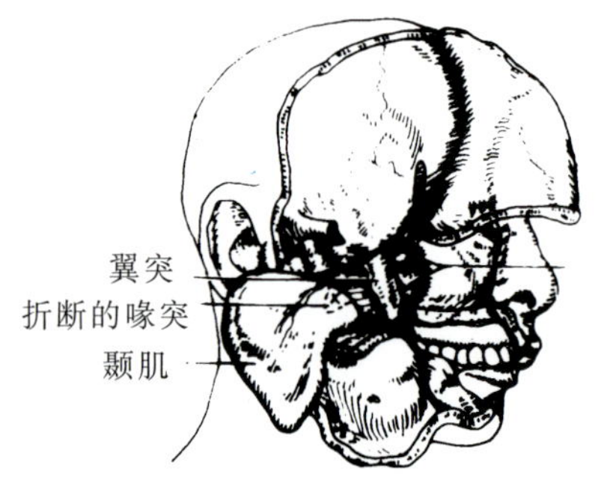


图 61

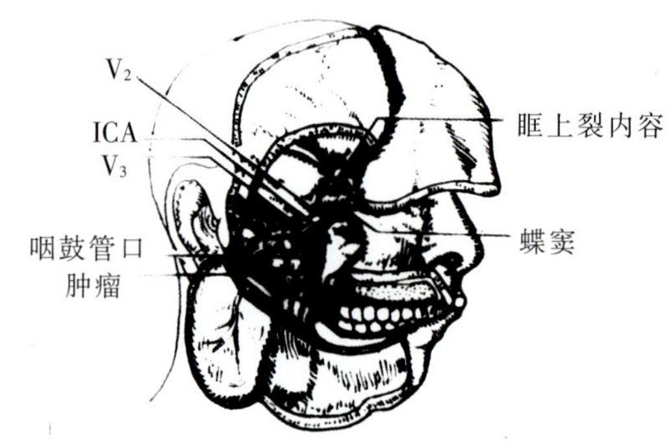


图 62

**图 61** 颞肌移位后,显示颞下窝和翼腭区域。
**图 62** 额颞颅骨切开术完成整个鼻咽和相关结构的上部暴露。

Fig. 61 After transposition of temporalis muscle, infratemporal fossa content and pterygoid region are seen.

Fig. 62 Frontotemporal craniotomy completes superior exposure of the entire nasopharynx and related structures.

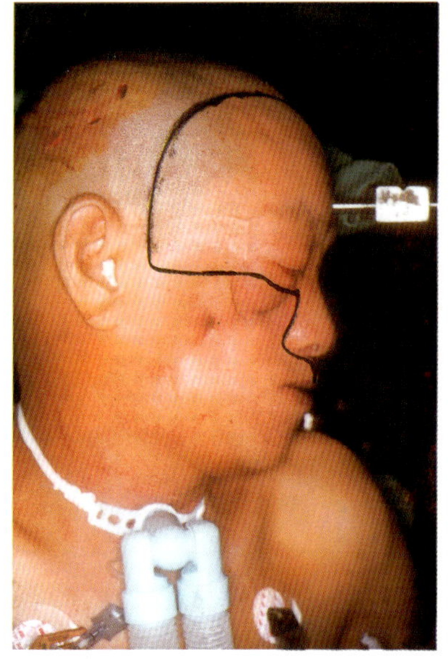

图 63

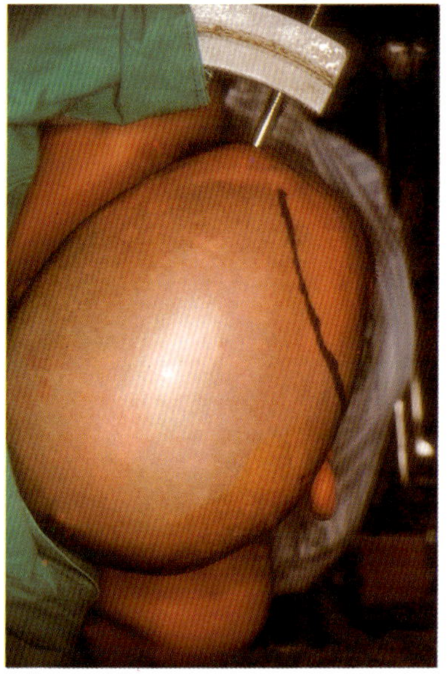

图 64

**图 63, 64** 切口设计

用美蓝在上唇患侧开始向上达鼻底，绕鼻翼向上达内眦，在下睑下缘由内向外达耳屏前向上作半冠状切口画线。

**Fig. 63, 64** Outline of incision.

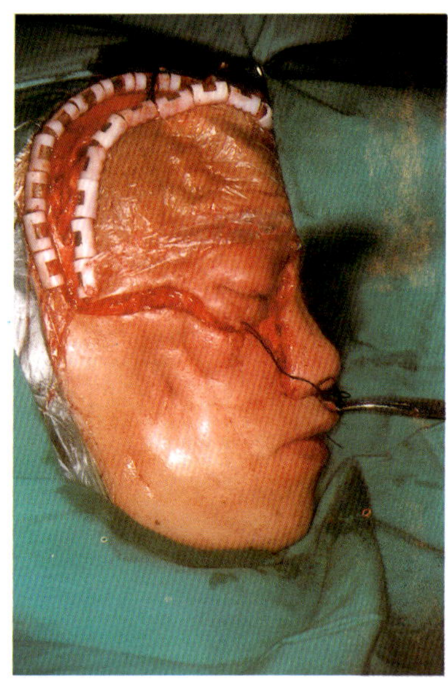

图 65

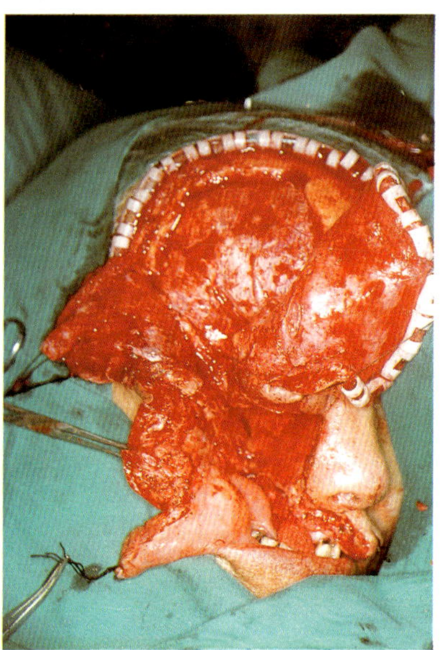

图 66

**图 65** 从上唇红唇缘开始切开上唇，绕鼻翼及鼻外侧向上达内眦，由内眦水平向外达耳屏前，然后沿耳前向上作半冠状切开。

**图 66** 在完成横跨颞部的横切口及半冠状切口之后，向中线翻转颞额头皮瓣。在上颌骨骨膜下由上向下掀起并翻转颊瓣达硬腭以下。该瓣是一个以面和下唇血管为蒂蒂在下的颊瓣，这个瓣包含上唇的外 1/3、整个颊部软组织、面神经和腮腺在内。

从中线暴露颅面部骨骼，包括额骨、鼻根、上颌骨鼻突、眶上、外侧和颧弓。此时，锯开额颅颞骨，鉴别棘孔、卵圆孔和圆孔及眶上裂。截断眶及上颌骨各连接以游离上颌骨的前面、颧突、颧弓、眶下和外侧缘及眶底。在骨膜下横形截骨后将颞肌向下翻转，此时可见到鼻中隔的后部、对侧鼻咽部的起端，上颌窦后壁、翼外板及其肌肉和颞下窝。

**Fig. 65** The first incision divides the upper lip in the midline, passes under the nasal pyramid, and extends laterally, reaching the level of the temporomandibular joint, at which point it exits to meet the vertical coronal/preauricular incision. An incision is then made along the maxillary buccogingival fold on the involved side, running from the midline to the retromolar area. Another incision is made along the mandibular buccogingival fold on the involved side, running from canine to retromolar area.

**Fig. 66** The frontotemporal scalp flap is reflected toward the midline after completion of the hemicoronal incision. The cheek flap is reflected inferiorly to the level of the angle of mandible after the elevation of the maxillary and mandibular periosteum and the masseteric fascia in a downward fashion. An inferiorly based cheek flap is developed on the facial and inferior labial vascular pedicles. It includes the lateral third of the upper lip and the entire cheek soft tissue.

Craniofacial skeleton is exposed from the midline (forehead, nasion, nasal process of the maxilla, superior, lateral and inferior orbital rim, maxilla, and the zygomatic arch) to the external aspect of the temporomandibular joint, the masseter and the mandibular ramus. A frontotemporal craniotomy is performed at this time, identifying foramina spinosum, ovale, and rotundum, as well as the superior orbital fissure. Osteotomies of the orbitomaxillary skeleton are performed to free the anterior face of the maxilla, malar eminence, zygomatic arch, and inferior and lateral orbital rims, as well as the orbital floor. This permits an inferior translocation of the temporalis muscle after a transverse subperiosteal osteotomy at the middle segment of the ramus. A view available at this point includes the posterior end of the nasal septum, beginning of the contralateral nasopharynx, posterior wall of the maxillary sinus, pterygoid plate and muscles, and the infratemporal fossa.

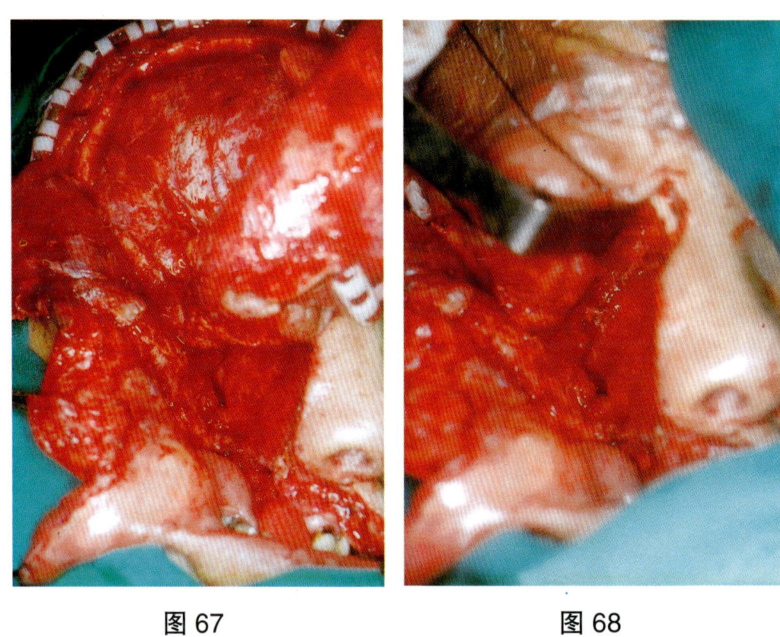

图 67　　图 68

**图 67, 68** 内侧暴露技术提供了到达整个鼻咽、双侧蝶窦、翼上颌间隙、斜坡、筛窦、眶内侧壁及下缘的外科进路；使用旁侧暴露技术，外科医师能切除颞下窝、关节窝、翼腭窝、斜坡、全眶、同侧蝶窦、颞骨、下颌升支和髁状突区的肿瘤。这两种技术的结合使从颞骨到对侧咽鼓管的颅底肿瘤得到良好的暴露，也使颅内解剖变得容易。

**Fig. 67, 68** The technique for "medial exposure" provides surgical access to entire nasopharynx, both sphenoid sinuses, the pterygomaxillary space, clivus, ethmoid sinus, and medial and inferior orbit. Using the "lateral exposure" technique, the surgeon can access the infratemporal fossa, glenoid fossa, pteygopalatine fossa, clivus, entire orbit, ipsilateral sphenoid, temporal bone, mandibular ramus and condyle. A combination of two techniques exposes the cranial base from the temporal bone to the contralateral eustachian tube. Note that with either approach, the corresponding intracranial anatomy can be easily accessed.

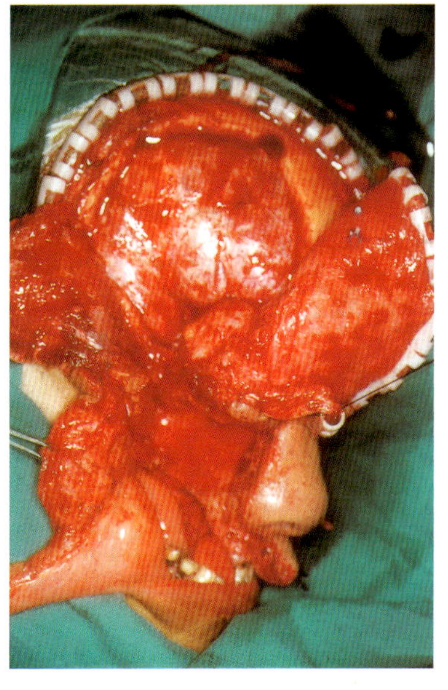

图 69

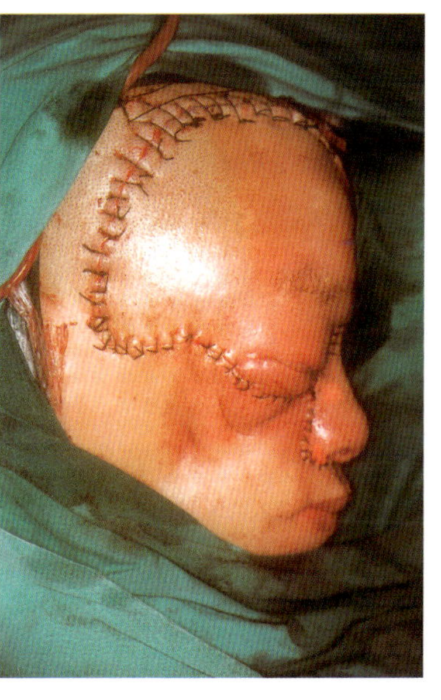

图 70

**图 69** 肿瘤的边界及其组织学指导着肿瘤的摘除，因为有极良好的视野而使肿瘤及病变结构切除变得容易。肿瘤被摘除之后，对肿瘤的边缘结构进行检查。如有脑膜缺损，可使用移植体即刻修复。

**图 70** 还回在手术时截下的颅眶颞骨，用微型钛板固定。沿术前的标记分层间断缝合。

**Fig. 69** The tumor perimeter and its histology guide the three-dimensional tumor resection, which is well-controlled because of the excellent visualization. The reconstructive phase begins after tumor resection and margin verification. If there is defect of the dura, the dura may be repaired with a graft primarily.

**Fig. 70** After reconstruction of the cranial base, the osteoplastic unit is repositioned. The miniplates are fastened with appropriate screws. The maxillary periosteum and subcutaneous tissues are closed in layers with interrupted 4 – 0 chromic sutures. All skin incisions are closed with 5 – 0 or 6 – 0 monofilament sutures.

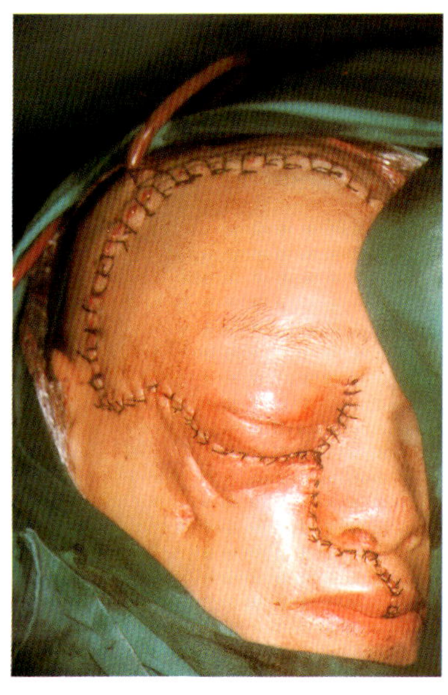

图 71

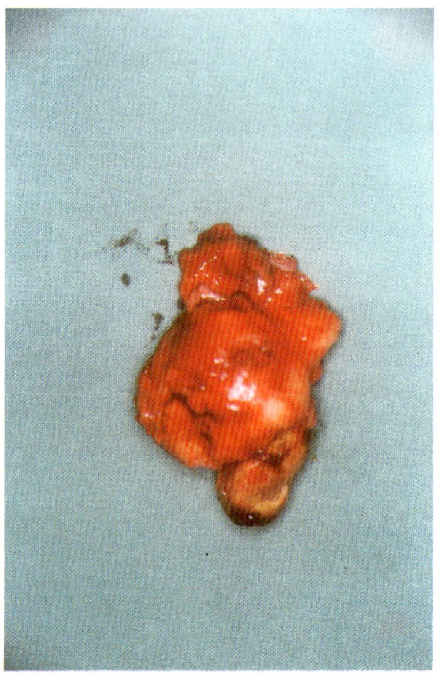

图 72

**图 71** 缝合后的正面观。

**图 72** 手术后的肿瘤标本。

**Fig. 71** Frontal view postoperatively.

**Fig. 72** The tumor specimen postoperatively.

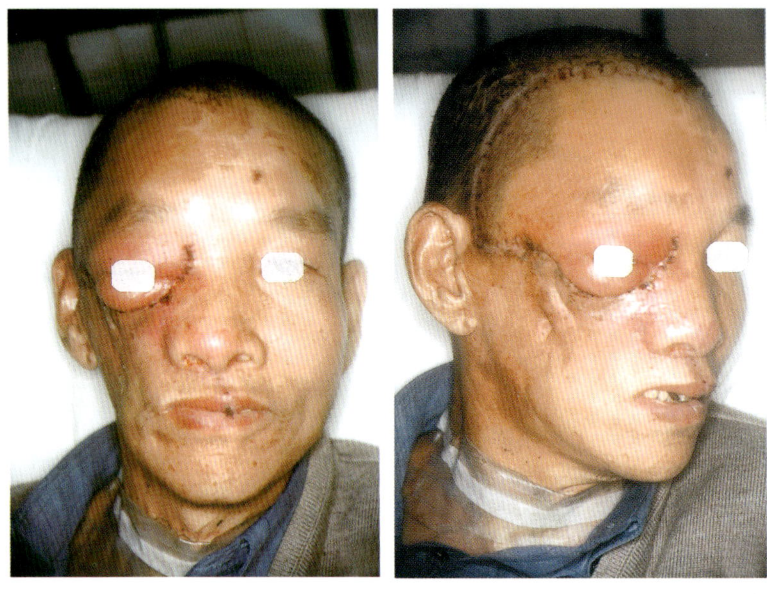

图 73　　图 74

图 73,74　手术后 10 天,患者的正、侧面观。

Fig. 73, 74　The patient's frontal and lateral views 10 days postoperatively.

# 5. 翼腭窝神经纤维瘤摘除术

# 5. Excision of neurofibroma in the pterygopalatine fossa

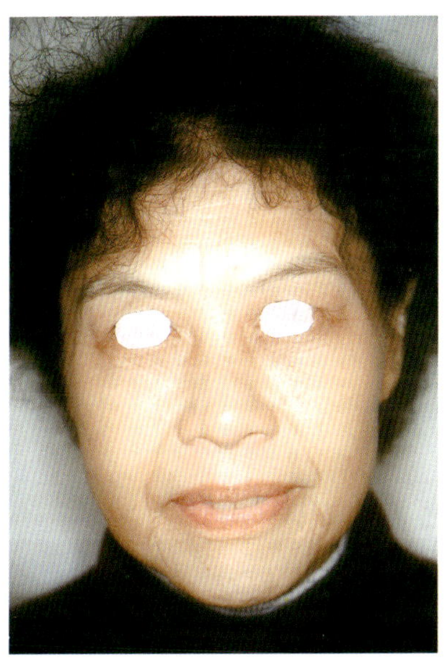

图 75

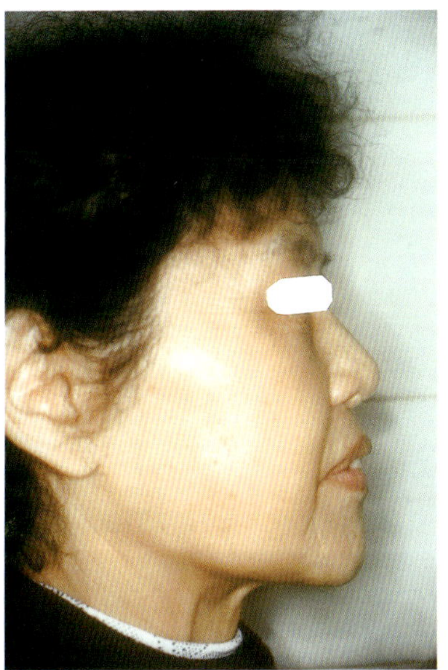

图 76

图 75, 76 患右侧翼腭窝神经纤维瘤 58 岁患者的正面及侧面观。

Fig. 75, 76 Frontal and lateral views of a 58-year-old female patient with neurofibroma in the pterygopalatine fossa.

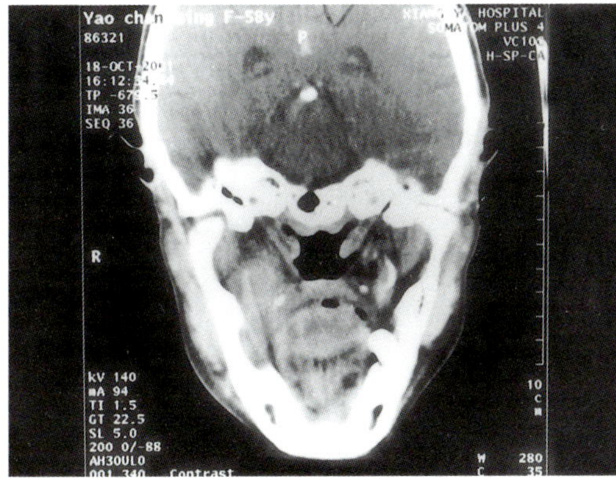


图 77

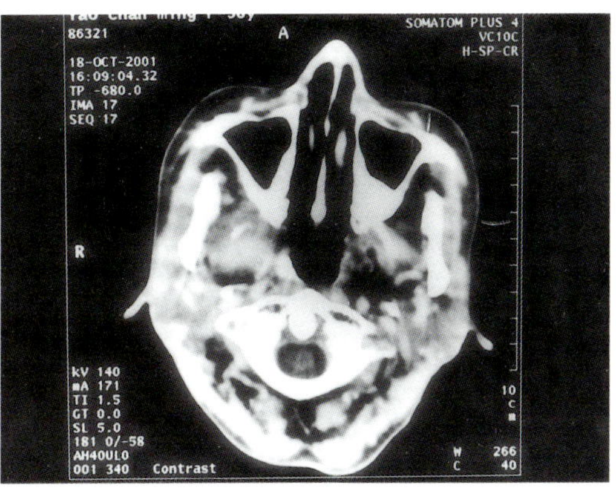


图 78

图 77 冠状 CT 扫描显示右翼腭窝区占位性病变。
图 78 轴性平扫显示右侧翼腭窝由肿瘤所占据。

Fig. 77 Coronal CT scan shows a lesion occupied pterygopalatine fossa.
Fig. 78 Axial CT scan shows that the right pterygopalatine fossa is occupied by the tumor.

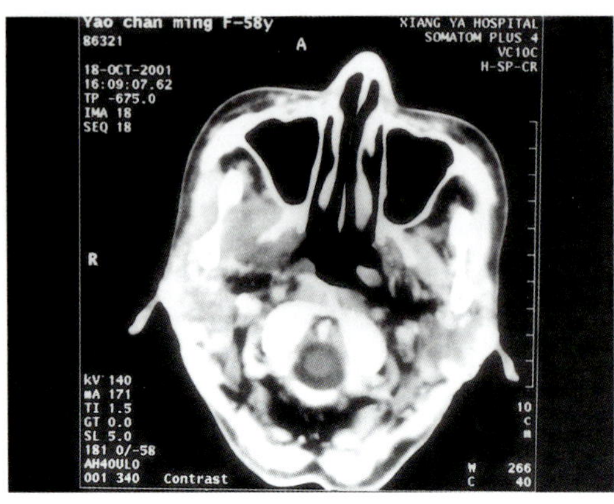



图 79

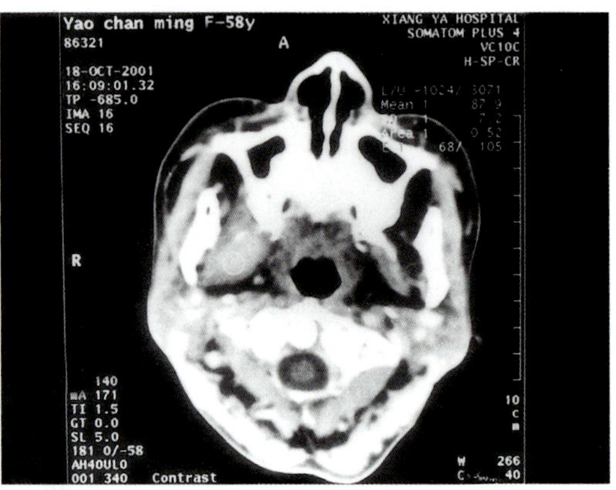



图 80

图 79, 80　不同轴性 CT 平扫显示右翼腭窝占位性病变。

Fig. 79, 80　Different axial CT scans show the lesion occupied the right pterygopalatine fossa.

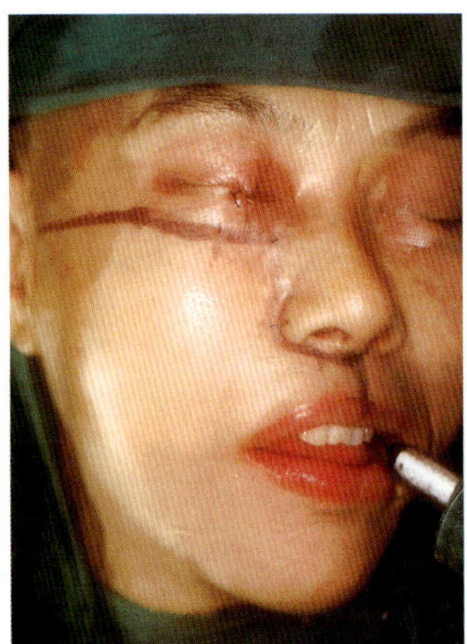

图 81

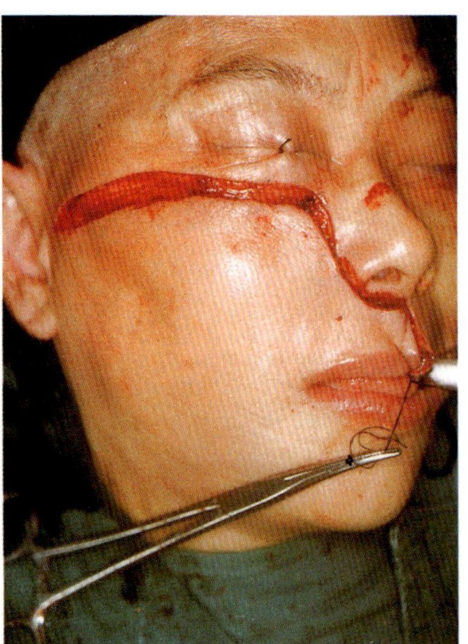

图 82

图 81　用美蓝在上唇患侧开始向上达鼻底，绕鼻翼向上达内眦，在下睑下缘由内向外达耳屏前画线。

图 82　从上唇红唇缘开始切开上唇，绕鼻翼及鼻外侧向上达内眦，由内眦水平向外达耳屏前切开。

Fig. 81　The patient is placed in a recumbent position with the head rotated 45° to the uninvolved side. Intravenous anesthesia, with endotracheal intubation via oral cavity, is used. A incision design is made through upper lip in the philtrum from the nasolabial groove to the vermilion border, the external skin incision is extended transversely from the upper end of the lip incision in the nasolabial groove to beyond the nasal ala and then superiorly along the nasofacial groove to the lower eyelid. Horizontal extension of this incision placed near the lid margin to reaching the level of the temporomandibular joint with methylene blue.

Fig. 82　The first incision divides the upper lip in the midline, passes under the nasal pyramid, and extends laterally, reaching the level of the temporomandibular joint. An incision is then made along the maxillary buccogingival fold on the involved side, running from the midline to the retromolar area. Another incision is made along the mandibular buccogingival fold on the involved side, running from canine to retromolar area.

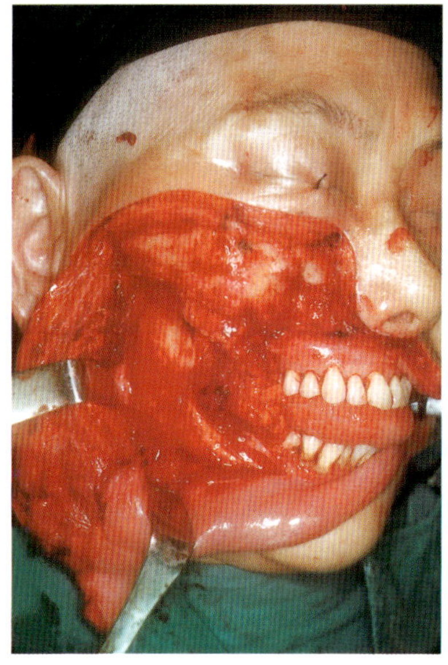
图 83

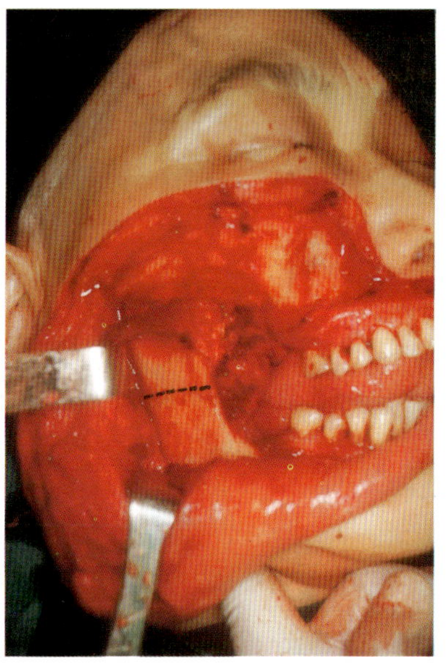
图 84

图 83 用骨膜剥离器由上向下分离颊部软组织瓣，分离达眶下孔时，结扎切断眶下神经血管束。继续向下分离达患侧前庭沟，向后分离达磨牙后区，沿翼下颌韧带外侧向下分离达下颌磨牙后垫并继续向前达第一前磨牙处。

图 84 将下颌升支的外侧面分开，暴露患侧上颌骨及下颌升支外侧面。在下颌升支中段水平截断下颌升支上部。

Fig. 83 A large flap is raised at the level of the mimetic muscles with an electrosurgical knife. The flap is reflected to yield adequate exposure of the anterior aspect of the maxilla, the inferior half of the orbital rim, the inferior portion of the temporalis muscle, the zygomatic bone and zygomatic arch, the external aspect of the temporomandibular joint, and the masseter and the mandibular ramus.

Fig. 84 The masseter muscle is sectioned with an electrosurgical knife a little below the zygomatic arch, and temporalis muscle is sectioned a little above the zygomatic arch. The mandibular ramus is sectioned transversely with a Gigli saw above the angle of the mandible, and disarticulation of the temporomandibular joint is done using the electrosurgical knife.

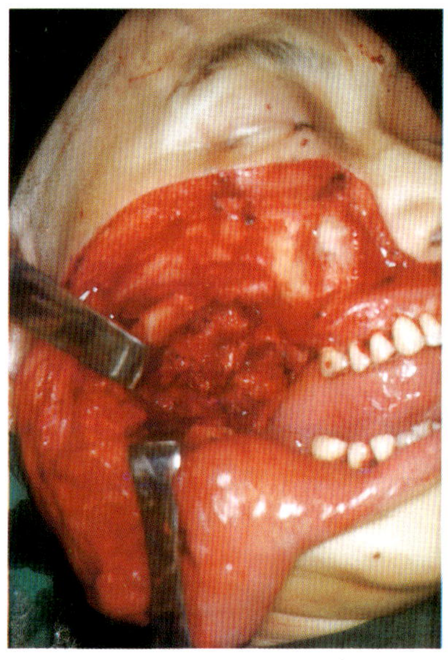
图 85

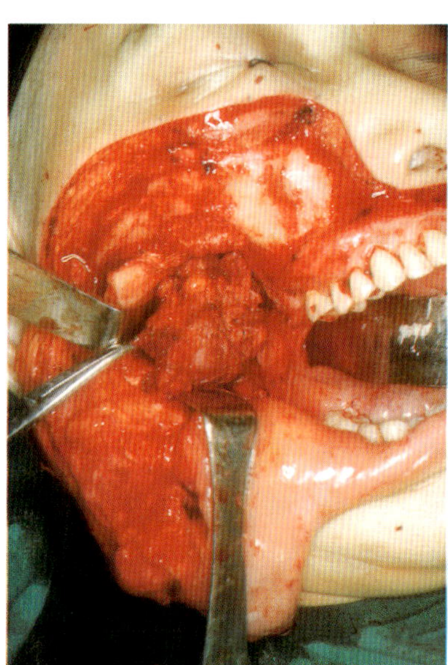
图 86

图 85 该手术对肿瘤的外侧面、翼突的外表面、翼腭窝和翼内肌的外表面提供足够的暴露，同时也使肿瘤后极的周围有足够的边缘。

图 86 当截骨被完成之后，肿瘤摘除极为容易。

Fig. 85 This maneuver provides adequate exposure of the external aspect of the tumor, the lateral surface of the lateral pterygoid process, the pterygopalatine fossa, and the lateral surface of the internal pterygoid muscle, allowing an adequate margin around the posterior limit of the tumor.

Fig. 86 After all the bone cuts are completed, the surgical specimen of the tumor is easily removed.

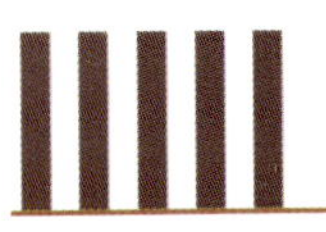



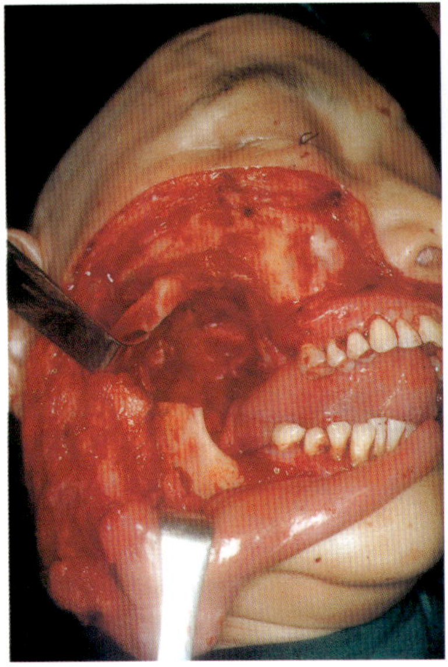

图 87

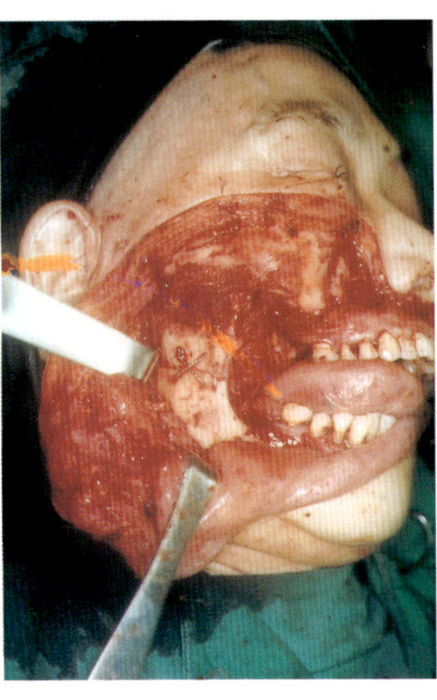

图 88

**图 87** 当肿瘤被完全摘除之后，腔内填入可吸收明胶海绵。

**图 88** 还回被截断的下颌升支部分，用微型钛板或不锈钢丝固定。

**Fig. 87** After the tumor in the pterygopalatine fossa has been excised, the surgical cavity is packed with absorbable gelatin sponge.

**Fig. 88** The mandibular ramus is returned and is fixed with miniplates or stainless steel wire.

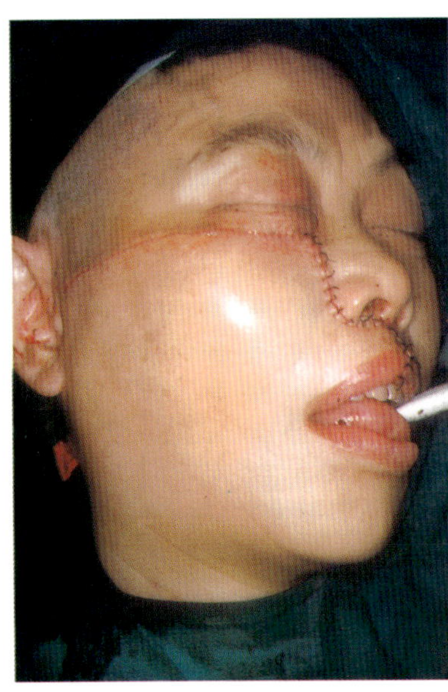

图 89

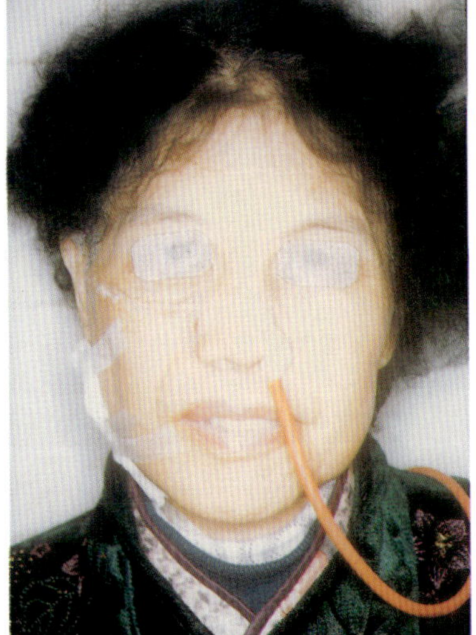

图 90

**图 89** 还回颊瓣后分层间断缝合，局部轻加压包扎。

**图 90** 术后插鼻胃管进流质饮食10天。7天拆除全部缝线。

**Fig. 89** The buccal flap is returned and is sutured with numerous fine interrupted silk sutures.

**Fig. 90** Tube feedings are required for 10 days. Suture lines are removed 7 days postoperatively.

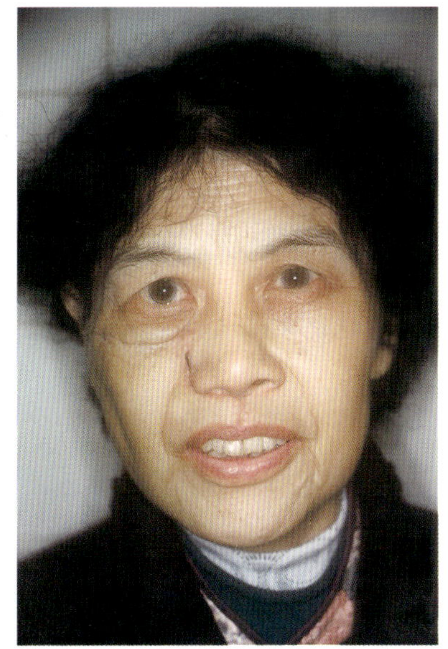
图 91

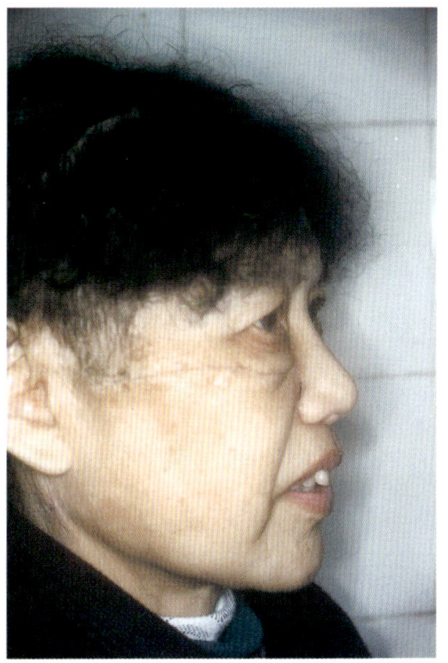
图 92

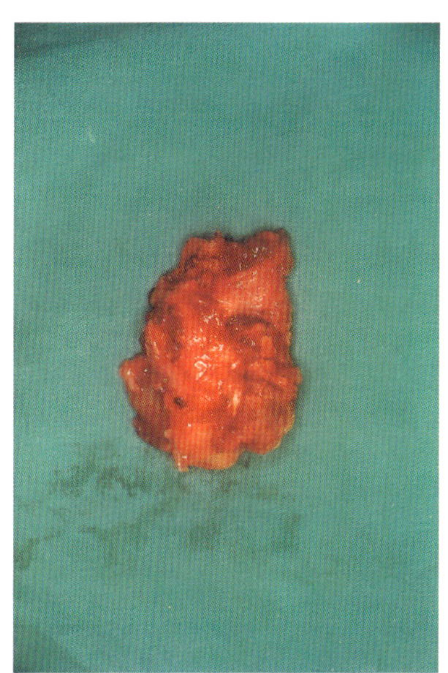
图 93

图 91, 92 患者术后第 11 天正、侧面观。

Fig. 91, 92 The patient's frontal and lateral views 11 days postoperatively.

图 93 手术后的外科标本。

Fig. 93 The surgical specimen postoperatively.

# 6. 前及中颅窝底复发性软骨肉瘤切除颞肌瓣转移即刻重建修复术

# 6. Excision of recurrent chondrosarcoma in the anterior and middle cranial base and immediate reconstruction with temporal muscle

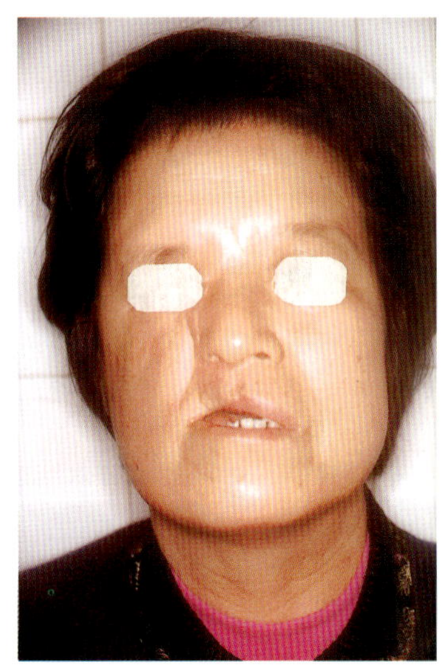

图 94

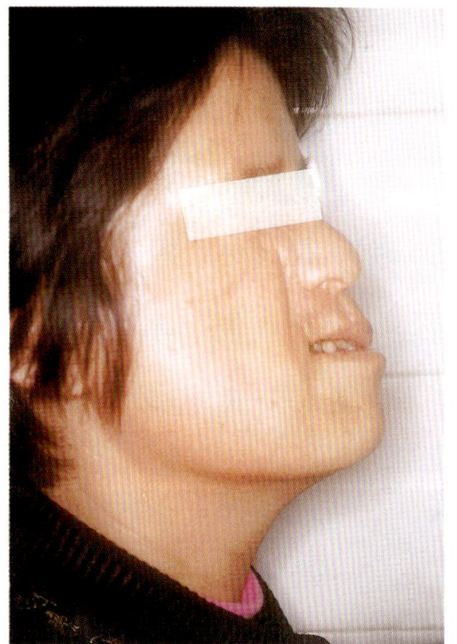

图 95

图 94，95 患右上颌及中颅窝底复发性软骨肉瘤的一 48 岁女性患者的正面及侧面观。

Fig. 94, 95 Frontal and lateral views of a 48-year-old female patient with recurrent chondrosarcoma in the right maxilla and the right anterior and middle cranial base.

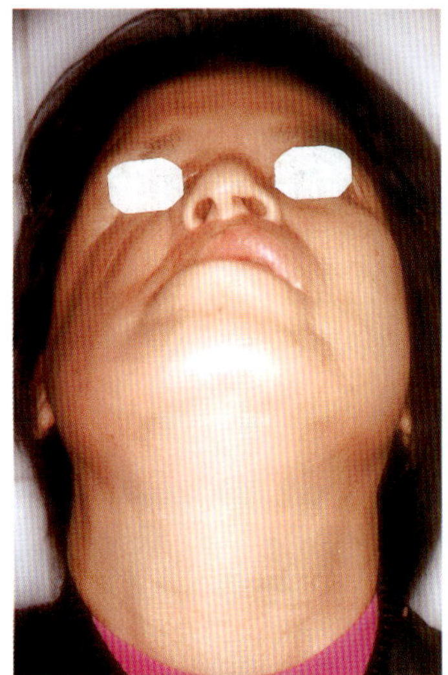

图 96

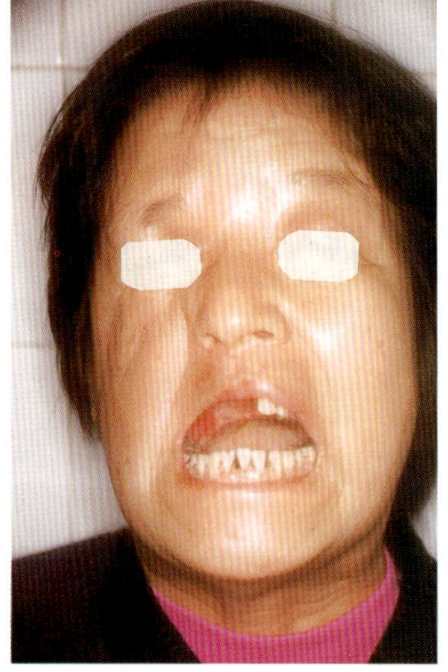

图 97

图 96 患者仰面观见右面部明显畸形，右眼裂及眼球缺如。

图 97 患者术前张口明显受限。

Fig. 96 The patient' submental view shows obvious deformity in the right face and loss of the right ocular orb and ocular fissure.

Fig. 97 Preoperative frontal view shows that opening mouth is small.

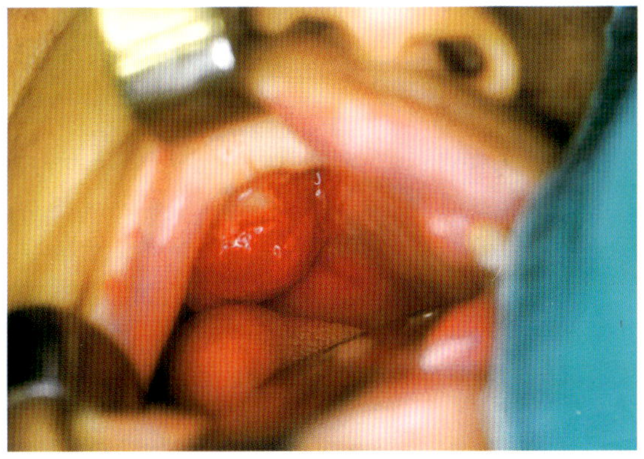

图 98

图 98 复发性肿瘤突入口腔内。

Fig. 98 Recurrent tumor protruding into the mouth.

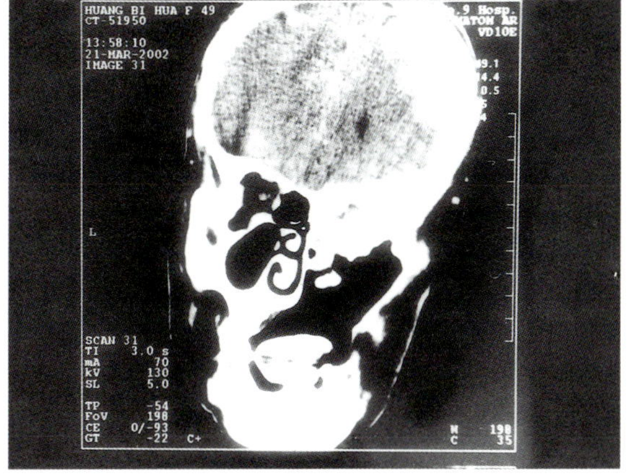


图 99

图 99 冠状 MRI 扫描显示右侧颅底复发性软骨肉瘤。

Fig. 99 Coronal MRI scan shows a recurrent cartilaginous sarcoma of the central cranial base on the right side.

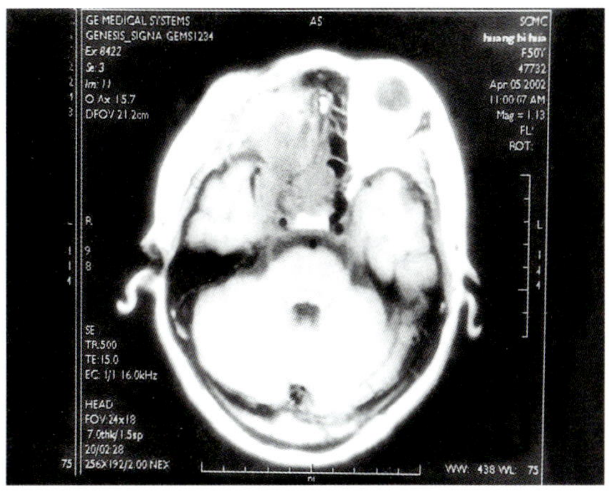


图 100

图 100 轴性 MRI 平扫显示右侧颅中窝底及右眶区和上颌窦区域被复发性软骨肉瘤所占位。

Fig. 100 Axial MRI scan shows that the right central skull base, the right orbital area and the right maxillary sinus are occupied by the recurrent cartilaginous sarcoma.

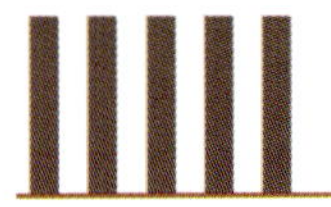



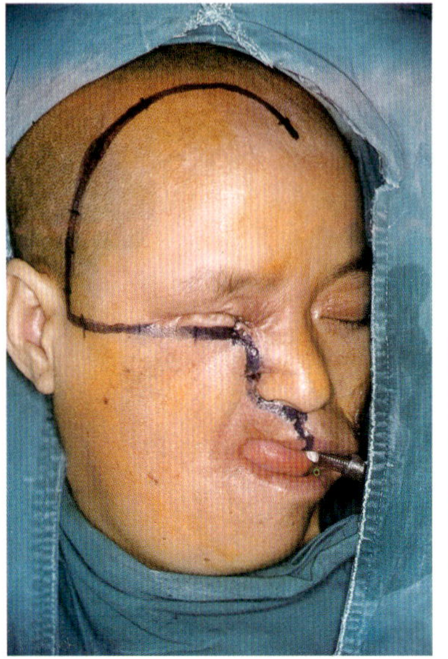

图 101

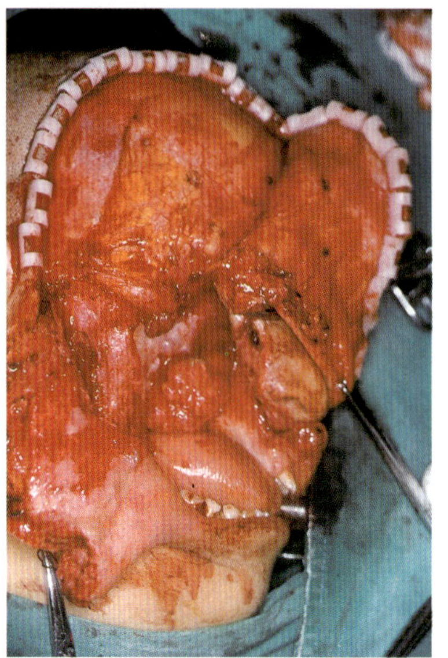

图 102

**图 101** 切口设计。

**图 102** 从上唇红唇缘开始切开上唇，绕鼻翼及鼻外侧向上达内眦，由内眦水平向外达耳屏前，然后沿耳前向上作半冠状切开。在完成横跨颞部的横切口及半冠状切口之后，向中线翻转颞额头皮瓣和颊瓣。颊瓣包含上唇的 1/3，整个颊部软组织、面神经和腮腺在内。

从中线暴露颅面部骨骼，包括额骨、鼻根、眶上、外侧壁和颧弓及其肿瘤的外侧面。

**Fig. 101** Outline of incision.

**Fig. 102** The first incision divides the upper lip in the midline, passes under the nasal pyramid, and extents laterally, reaching the level of the temporomandibular joint, at which point it exits to meet the vertical coronal preauricular incision. An incision is then made along the maxillary buccogingival fold on the involved side, running from the midline to the retromolar area. Another incision is made along the mandibular buccogingival fold on the involved side, running from canine to retromolar area.

The frontotemporal scalp flap is reflected toward the midline after completion of the hemicoronal incision. The cheek flap is reflected inferiorly to the level of the angle of mandible. An inferiorly based cheek flap is developed on the facial and inferior labial vascular pedicles. It includes the lateral third of the upper lip, the entire cheek soft tissue.

Craniofacial skeleton is exposed from the midline, which includes forehead, nasal process of the maxilla, superior, lateral orbital rim, zygomatic arch and the external aspect of the temporomandibular joint, and the masseter and the mandibular ramus, and the external surface of the tumor.

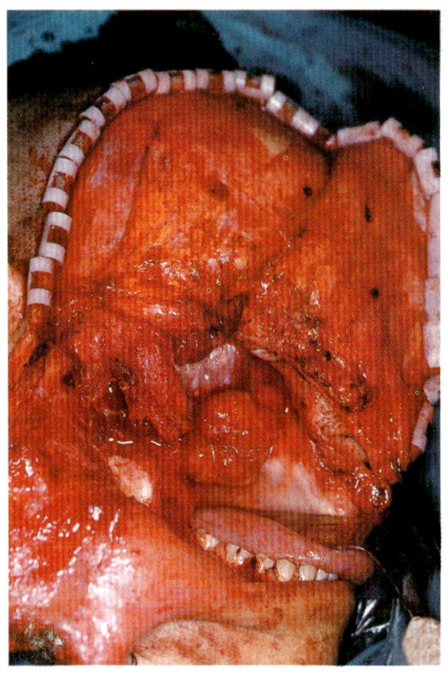

图 103

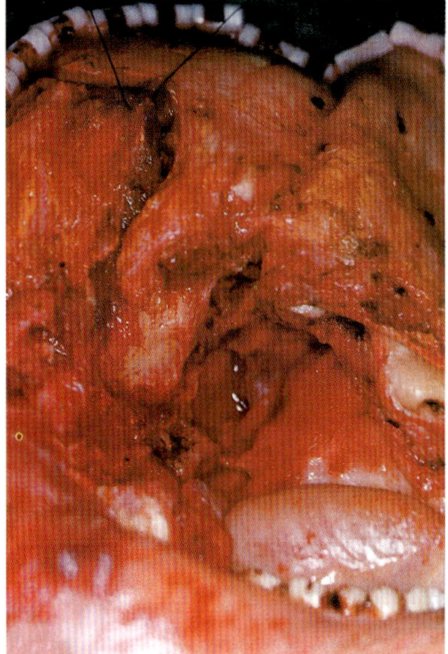

图 104

**图 103** 复发的肿瘤及其周围结构被清楚地暴露在手术野中。采用电刀由后向前，由下向上达颅中窝底完全切除肿瘤及受侵的骨质。

**图 104** 肿瘤被去除后的情景。暴露的颅底结构使用颞肌瓣进行修复。

**Fig. 103** Recurrent chondrosarcoma and around the structures are clearly exposed in the operative field. The entire tumor and involved bone are excised from backward to toward, and from downward to the middle cranial base by electrosurgery.

**Fig. 104** The condition of the right middle cranial base after the tumor has been removed.

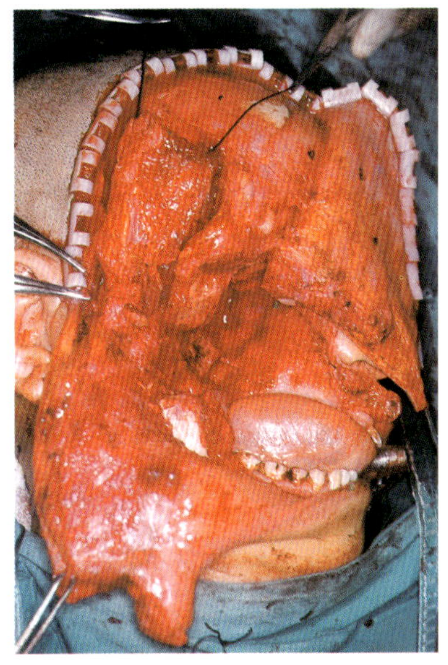

图 105

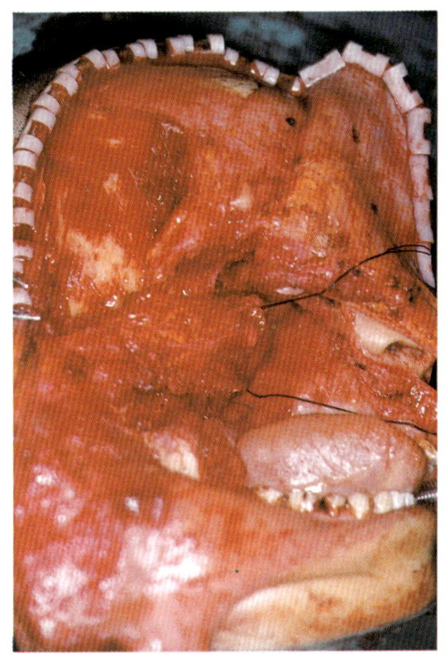

图 106

**图 105** 一旦中颅窝底的肿瘤和受累的骨已经被切除后，必须进行认真的修复重建。颞肌为任何暴露的气窦/鼻咽和脑膜之间提供了一个带血管的屏障瓣。如果颅底缺损小于或等于 5cm，带血管的颞肌为修复提供了良好的组织，为其提供的血供动脉主要是不间断的颌内动脉。如果缺损扩大或超过中线，颞肌瓣可带同侧颅骨膜或帽状腱膜以提供足够的软组织覆盖长度。如果颞肌不能被应用或缺损超过 5cm，游离组织转移是最好的重建方法。

**图 106** 从颞骨或蝶骨翼上掀起整个颞肌或颞肌的前半和颅骨骨膜及颞深筋膜。完成了从下颌骨及颧骨上分离肌肉之后，在其前后缘各穿过一针，使肌肉向下旋转以维持血管蒂的适当关系。在把肌肉与其下的骨膜分开时必须细心以避免损伤来自于颌内动脉及其穿枝的血液供应，这种掀起至少应扩展至颞下嵴甚至更下为好。从颧骨上将嚼肌分离使颞肌更好地松弛进入下颌和颅底缺损区而仍然保持颞肌的血液供应。肌肉与脑膜和邻近结构缝合，而颞肌筋膜与颅底缺损边缘相缝合。

**Fig. 105** Once the infratemporal tumor and involved bone have been removed, meticulous reconstruction is necessary. The temporalis muscle provides a vascularized flap to provide a barrier between any exposed air sinus/ nasopharynx and dura. For skull base defects less than or equal to 5cm, the vascularized temporalis muscle provides excellent tissue for reconstruction, providing its blood supply from the internal maxillary artery is not interrupted. If the defect extends to or beyond the midline, the temporalis flap can be harvested with the ipsilateral pericranium or galea to provide additional flap length for adequate soft-tissue coverage. If the temporalis muscle is unavailable or if the defects exceed 5cm, free-tissue transfer is the best reconstructive option.

**Fig. 106** The entire temporalis muscle, or its anterior half, with the attached pericranium, deep temporalis fascia, and skull periosteum are elevated from the temporal bone and sphenoid wing. The muscle detachment from the mandible and zygoma is completed. A silk suture through its anterior and posterior fascial margins will assist in transporting the muscle beneath the intact zygomatic arch and maintain its proper relationship to its vascular pedicle. Care is taken to elevate the temporalis muscle from the underlying periosteum to avoid injury to its blood supply from the internal maxillary artery and its perforating branches. This elevation may extend at least to the infratemporal crest and even beyond. Separation of the masseter muscle from the zygoma permits the mobilized temporalis muscle to be delivered beneath the zygoma into the mandibular and skull-base defects while maintaining its vascular connection. The temporalis fascia is sutured to the margin of the skull-base defect as the muscle is allowed to rest against the dura and adjacent structures.

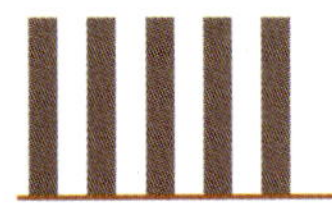



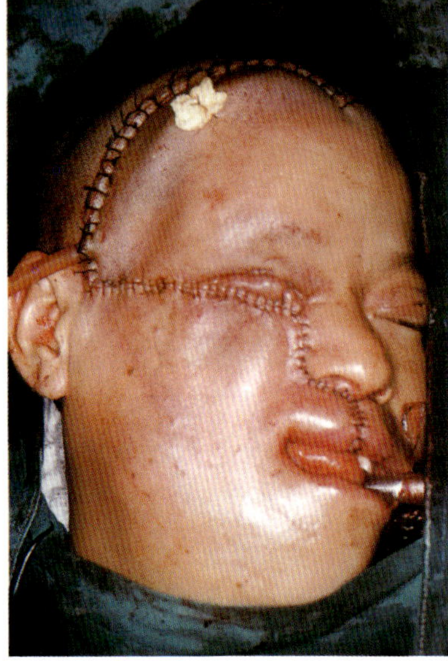

图 107

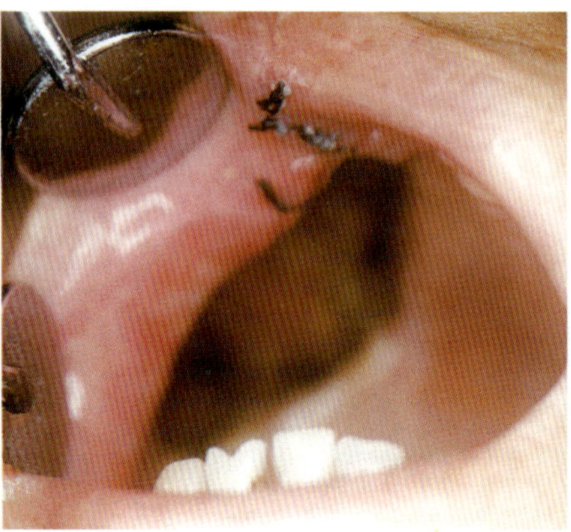

图 108

图 107 用 1－0 线缝合口内及头面部创口。

图 108 缝合后的口内情景。

Fig. 107 The oral cavity incision is closed with interrupted 1－0 silk line sutures. The facial wound is closed with 5－0 chromic and 6－0 nylon. The scalp wound is closed interrupted suture.

Fig. 108 The condition of the oral cavity after suture.

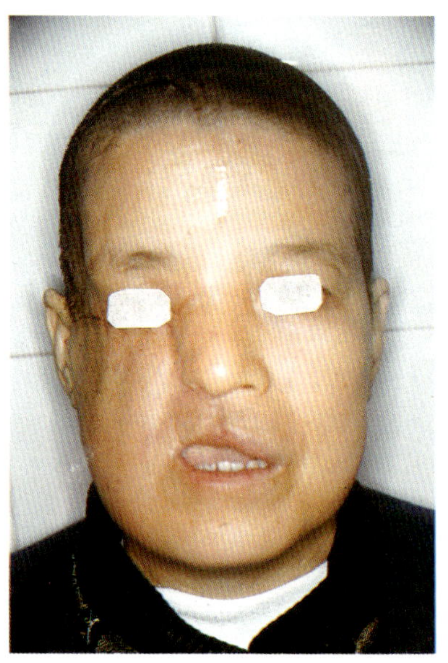

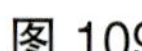

图 109

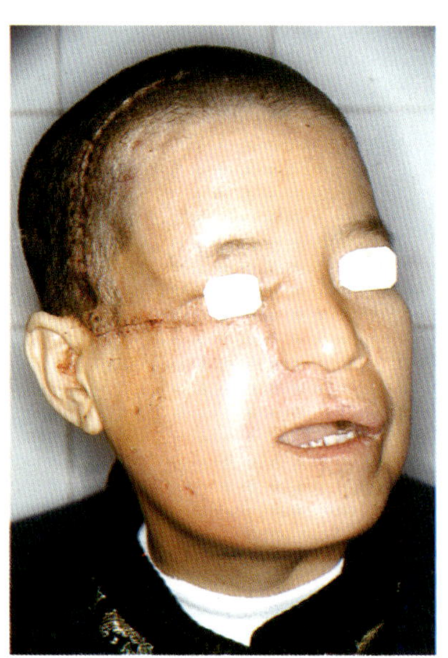

图 110

图 109, 110 拆线后患者的正、侧面观。

Fig. 109, 110 The patient's frontal, lateral views after sutured lines have been removed.

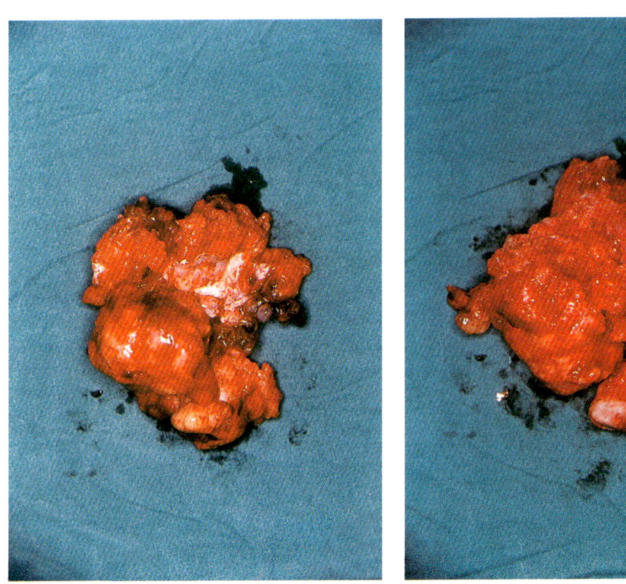

图 111　　图 112

图 111, 112　术后标本的内、外侧面观。

Fig. 111, 112　The internal and external views of postoperative specimen.

# Ⅱ. 上颌骨肿瘤

7. 上颌根尖囊肿刮除羟基磷灰石植入术
8. 上颌骨骨纤维异常增殖症的手术切除术
9. 上颌骨骨化纤维瘤的外科手术治疗
10. 上颌骨恶性纤维组织细胞瘤的外科治疗

# Ⅱ. Maxilla tumors

7. Excision of radicular cyst and implantation of hydroxyapatite in the maxilla
8. Excision of fibrous dysplasia in the maxilla
9. Surgical excision of ossifying fibroma in the maxilla
10. Surgical excision of the malignant fibrohystoblastoma in the maxilla

# 7. 上颌根尖囊肿刮除羟基磷灰石植入术

# 7. Excision of radicular cyst and implantation of hydroxyapatite in the maxilla

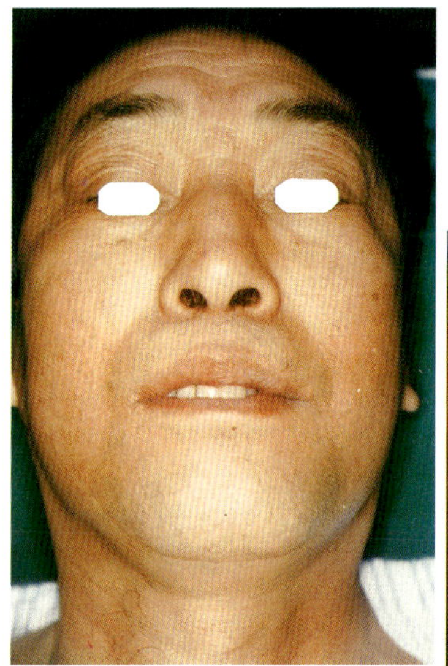

图 113

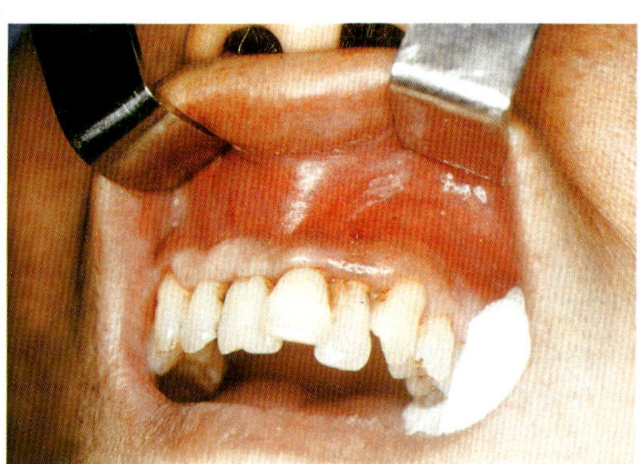

图 114

**图 113** 左上颌前牙根尖囊肿患者的正面观显示上唇丰满。

**图 114** 左上颌侧切牙根尖囊肿，唇侧牙龈上有一瘘管存在。

Fig. 113 Frontal view of a 54-year-old male patient with radicular cyst shows expension of the labiculogingival sulcus of the left maxillary anterior alveolar bridge.

Fig. 114 Radicular cyst of the left maxillary lateral incisor. There is a fistula on the gingiva of the left maxillary anterior labilar side.

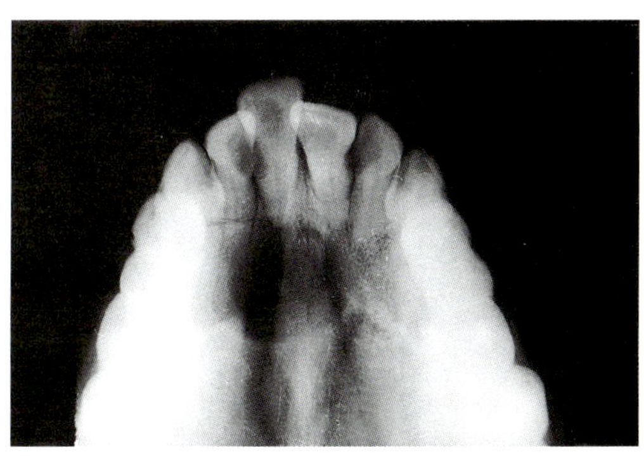

图 115

**图 115** 根端囊肿的 X 光片显示一个圆形、囊肿周围有骨质阻射线的放射透光区。

Fig. 115 Radiograph of radicular cyst shows that the lesion appears as a circumscribed radiolucency with a well defined outline at the apices of several teeth roots.

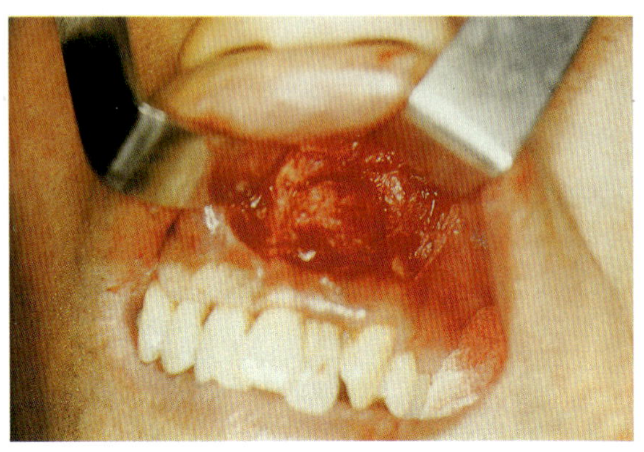

图 116

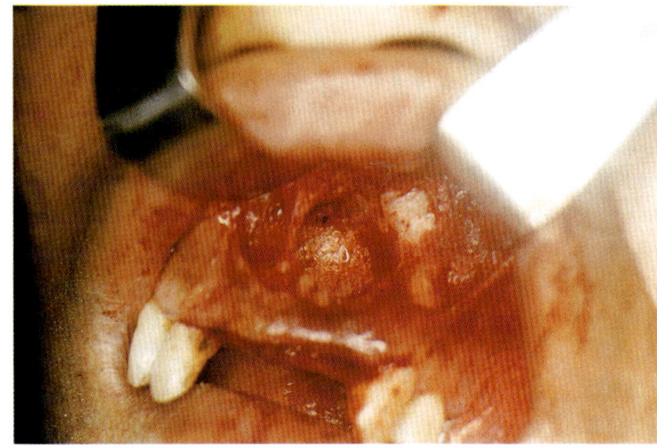

图 117

**图 116** 在囊肿之上做一半月形切口，切开粘骨膜，用小的骨膜剥离器将粘骨膜掀起。

**图 117** 用一小的咬骨钳将囊壁之上的骨质咬去，然后用一小骨膜剥离子在囊壁与骨质之间将囊壁完整剥离下来。

**Fig. 116** A curved incision is made over the site of the cyst and flap of mucosa and periosteum is elevated.

**Fig. 117** Small chisels and rongeurs are used to remove a window of bone over the cyst. An attempt is made to avoid perforating the cyst wall, curettes and small curved elevators are then used to enucleate the intact cyst. The bony cavity is irrigated.

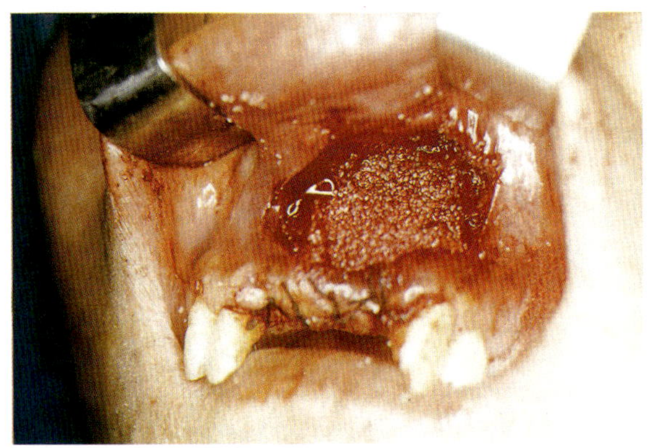

图 118

**图 118** 囊腔内放入羟基磷灰石人工骨，将唇侧粘骨膜瓣复位后用细丝线缝合。如囊腔极小，也可直接缝合而不会感染，但必须拔除患牙。

**Fig. 118** Hydroxyapatite is placed in the cavity and mucoperiosteal flap partly sutured in place with fine silk. Small cavities which are not infected may be closed without packing, but the tooth (or teeth) of the lesions must be extracted.

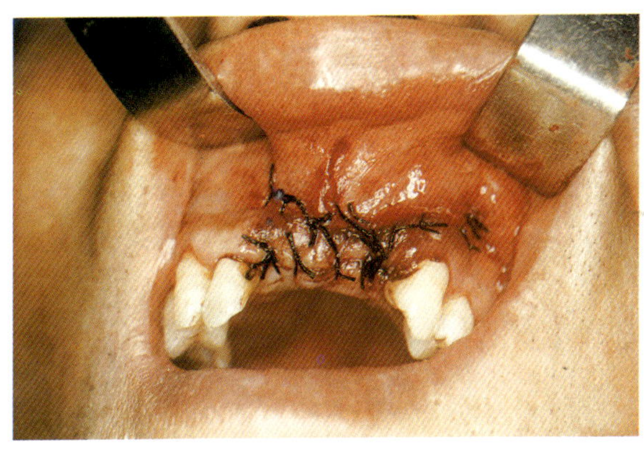

图 119

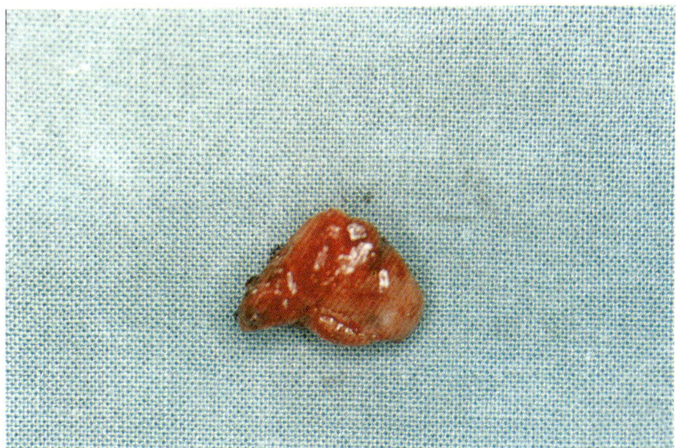

图 120

图 119 粘骨膜瓣被缝合后的情景。
图 120 手术刮除的完整囊肿标本。

Fig. 119 Condition after mucoperiosteal flap has been sutured with fine silk.
Fig. 120 The enucleated intact cyst specimen.

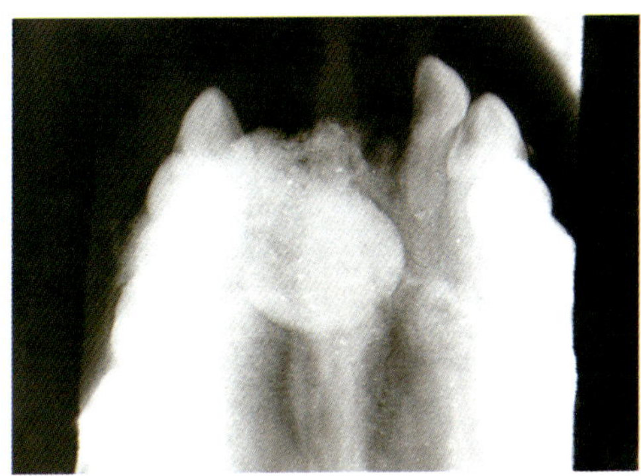

图 121

图 121 手术后 1 年患者病变区愈合的 X 光片表现。

Fig. 121 Finding of radiograph 1 year after operation.

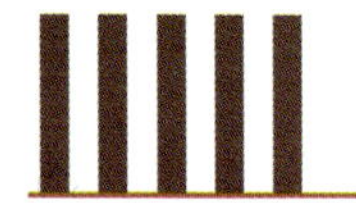



# 8. 上颌骨骨纤维异常增殖症的手术切除术

# 8. Excision of fibrous dysplasia in the maxilla

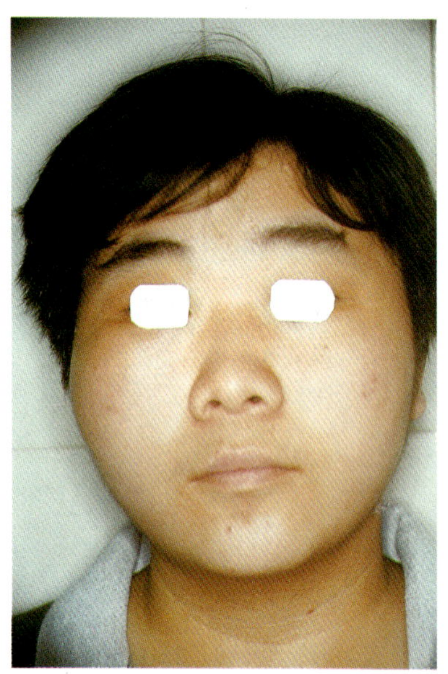

图 122

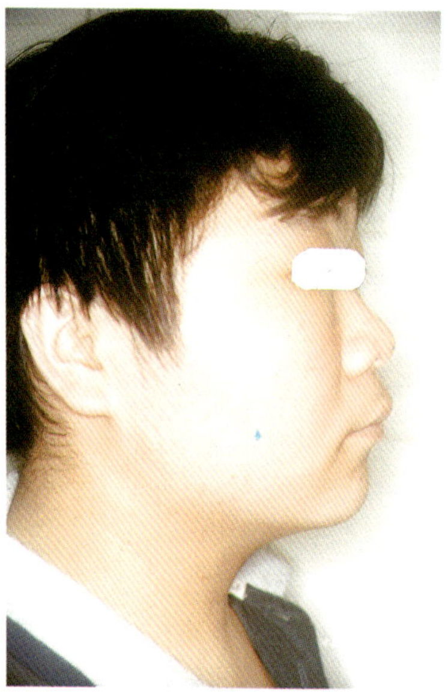

图 123

**图 122，123** 一患有右上颌骨骨纤维异常增殖症的 18 岁男性患者的正、侧面观。

患者右上颌骨的增大不对称首先由病人的父母发现。然而，近期病变的生长加速而导致右面部明显的膨隆。

**Fig. 122, 123** Frontal and lateral views of a 18-year-old young patient with fibrous dysplasia of the right maxilla.

Gradually increasing facial asymmetry of the patient is first noticed by his parents. However, growth of tumor is more rapid and causes marked swelling of the right maxilla.

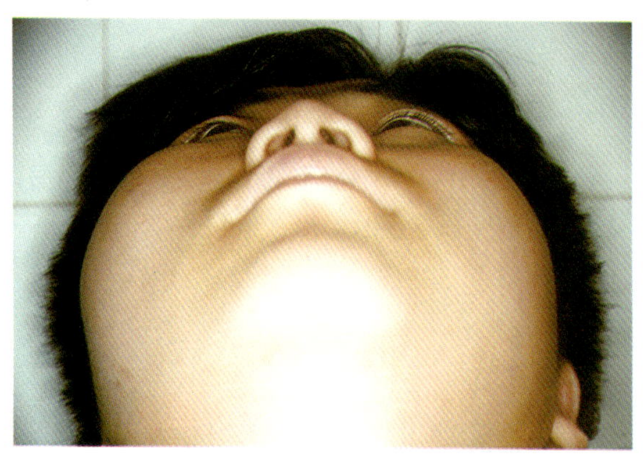

图 124

**图 124** 患者的仰面观显示右侧面部明显不对称。

**Fig. 124** Submental view of the patient shows facial asymmetry of both face, right side obvious expansion.

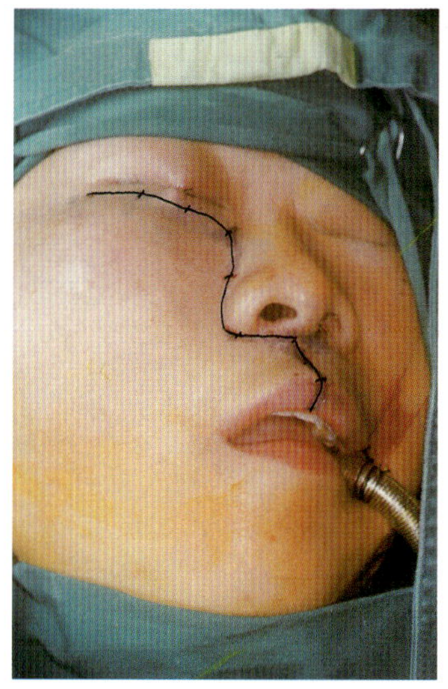

图 125

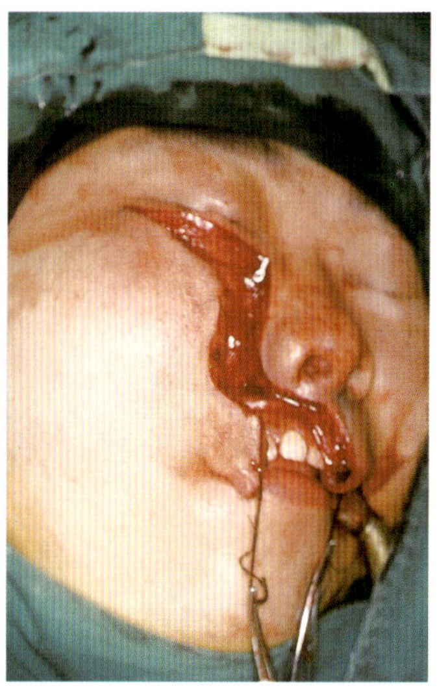

图 126

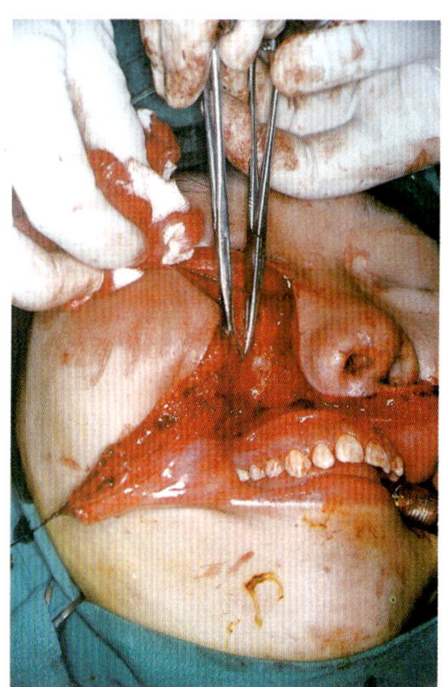

图 127

**图 125** 用美蓝画出右上颌骨部的切口线。

**图 126** 根据已标示的切口线，由上唇正中向上达鼻小柱基部，然后沿鼻小柱基部向外并绕鼻翼外侧，在鼻的外侧面向上达内眦下缘，在下睑下缘约 3mm 向外作横切口，切口可达颧骨。

**图 127** 从上颌正中向后达上颌结节，在龈颊沟内做切口，使颊瓣的下缘游离。用骨膜剥离器钝性分离将颊瓣在骨膜下与骨之间完全掀起，当分离颊瓣达眶下神经血管束处时可用血管钳钳夹后将其切断、丝线结扎。

**Fig. 125** The incision line of the right maxilla was marked out with methylene blue.

**Fig. 126** According to the marked incision line, the Fergusson incision is used to raise a cheek flap, splitting the upper lip in the midline. The incision is carried up to the nasal columella, then curved laterally to skirt the nostril and ala nasi. It is then continued upward along the side of the nose to a point just medial and inferior to the inner canthus. A lateral limb 2 – 3 mm below the lid margin is carried outward as far as the zygoma.

**Fig. 127** The cheek flap is raised by a sharp dissection close to the bone. The inferior margin of the flap is freed by an incision in the gingivobuccal sulcus carried from the midline anteriorly as far laterally as the tuberosity of the maxilla. Dissection superiorly is carried superficially to preserve the orbicularis oculi muscle. During the dissection, suborbital nerve is clamped, divided and ligated.

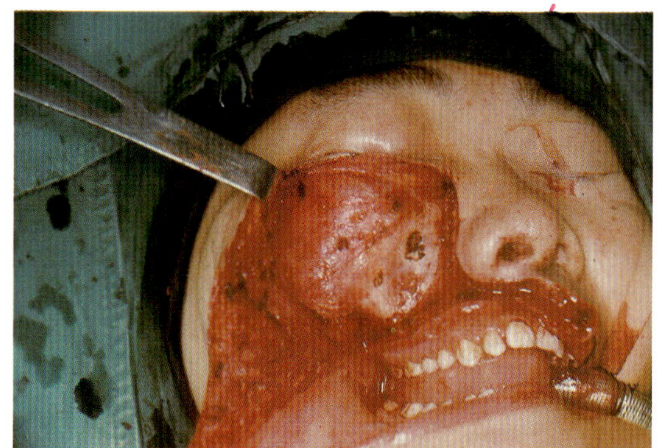

图 128

**图 128** 用骨膜剥离器继续向后分离颊瓣至上颌结节后将肿瘤完全暴露在手术野中。

**Fig. 128** The buccal flap continued to be separated from the bone to backward with elevator and the tumor is completely exposed to the operative field.



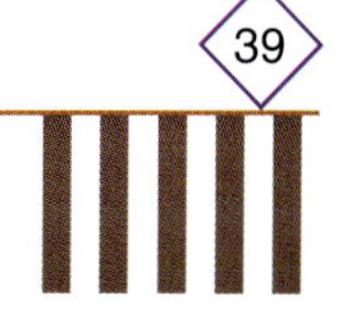

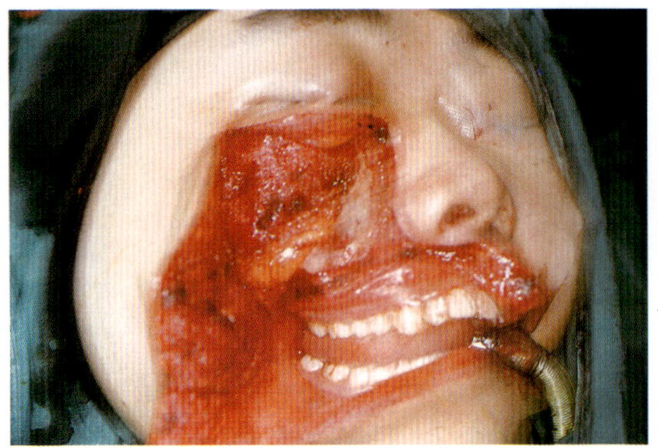

图 129

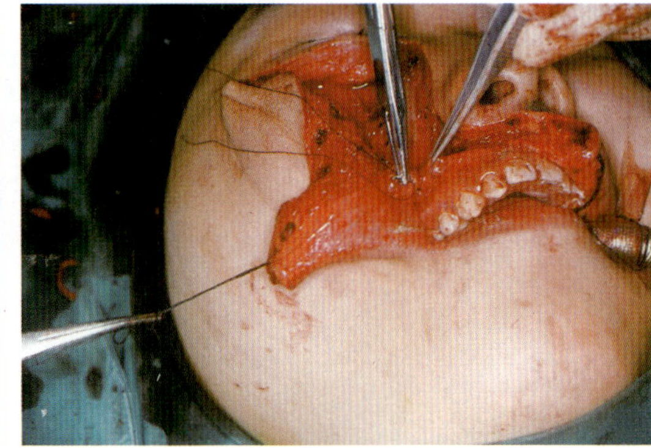

图 130

**图 129** 用骨凿将增生的骨组织完全去除。此时，上颌窦前壁有穿破的可能，如果有穿破的话，可利用同侧的颊脂垫来修复穿破的上颌窦前壁。

**图 130** 将颊部组织瓣还回后，先用细丝线间断缝合龈颊沟粘膜，然后对位缝合骨膜及肌层，此时应特别注意上唇红唇皮肤交界处的对合。

**Fig. 129** The proliferated bony tissue is completely removed with the chisels. At the time, the anterior wall of the maxillary sinus may be perforated, if possible, the perforated anterior wall of the maxillary sinus may be repaired with the ipsilateral buccal fat pad.

**Fig. 130** After the buccal flap is returned in place, the mucoperiosteal flap of the gingivobuccal sulcus is sutured with 4－0 silk with the knots tied in the mouth. The underlying muscles and the orbiculius oris muscle are sutured by numerous sutures of 3－0 chromic catgut. It is important to approximate the vermilion border with accuracy.

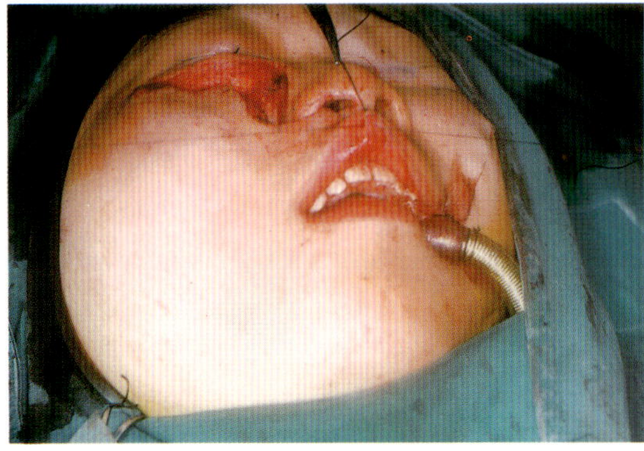

图 131

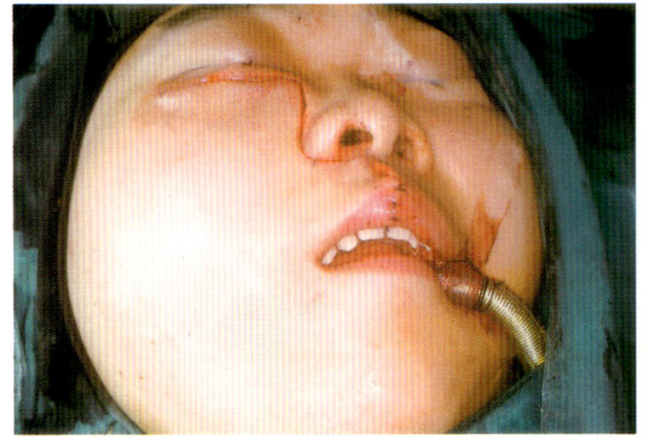

图 132

**图 131** 缝合上唇的口轮匝肌及红唇粘膜。

**图 132** 缝合创缘内的肌肉及皮下组织，使创缘对合良好，皮肤创口用医用粘合胶粘合皮肤，目的是防止面部创口瘢痕。

**Fig. 131** The orbiculius oris muscle and the mucosa of the vermilion of the upper lip are sutured.

**Fig. 132** The muscles in the wound margin and the underdermal soft tissue are sutured with interrupted sutures. After the muscles and underdermal tissue have been approximated, the skin incised is adhered with medical gelatin.

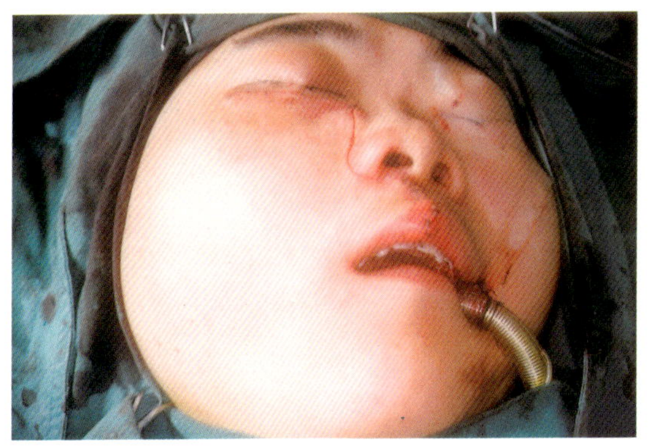

图 133

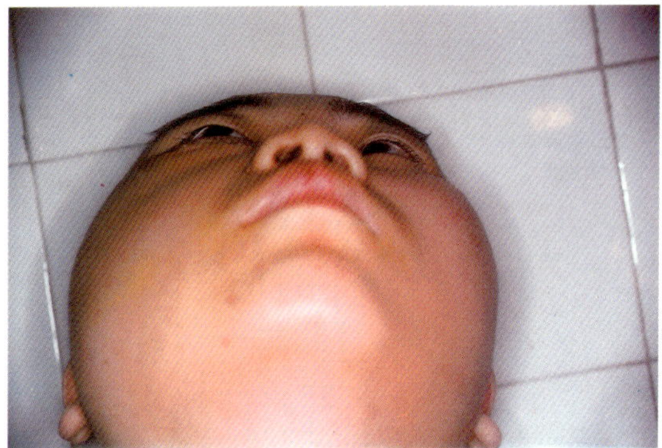

图 134

**图 133** 皮下组织用铬制羊肠线缝合后的情景。
**图 134** 术后 7 天的仰面观见创口愈合良好。

**Fig. 133** The condition after the underdermal tissue and muscles was sutured with fine catgut.
**Fig. 134** Lateral view of the patient 7 days after operation shows wound healing fine.

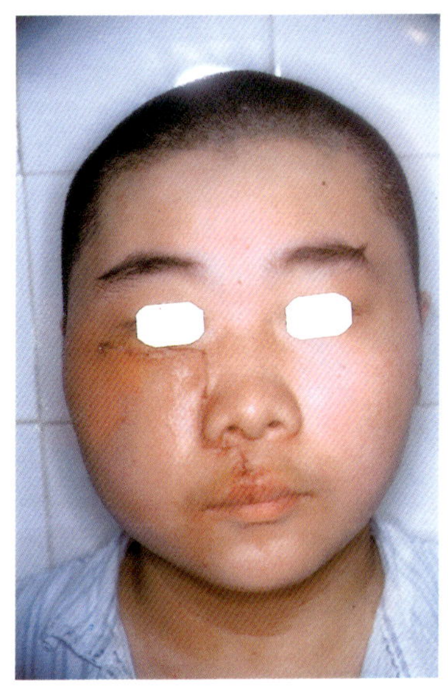

图 135

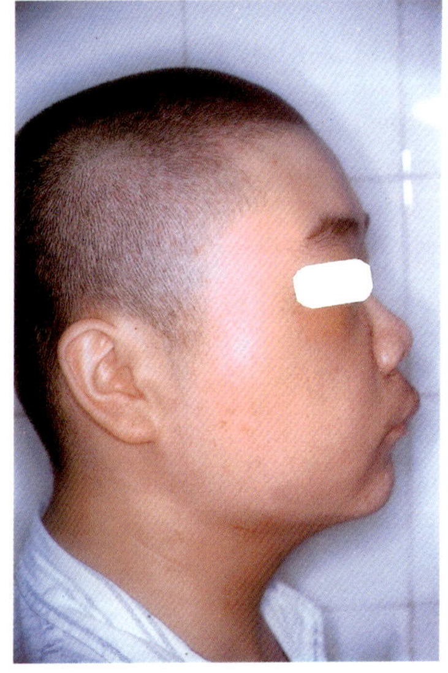

图 136

**图 135, 136** 术后第 7 天患者正面及侧面观。

正面观见创口愈合良好，无裂开及感染存在，眶下及鼻侧缘创面已趋于不明显；侧面观显示右侧面部稍有肿胀。

**Fig. 135, 136** Frontal and lateral views of the patient 7 days after surgery.

Frontal view shows condition of wound healing, no fissure and infection. A incision line of the suborbital rim and along the side of the nose is no obvious. Lateral view shows the right face slight swelling.

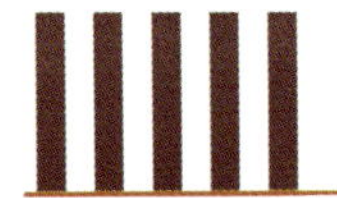



# 9. 上颌骨骨化纤维瘤的外科手术治疗

# 9. Surgical excision of ossifying fibroma in the maxilla

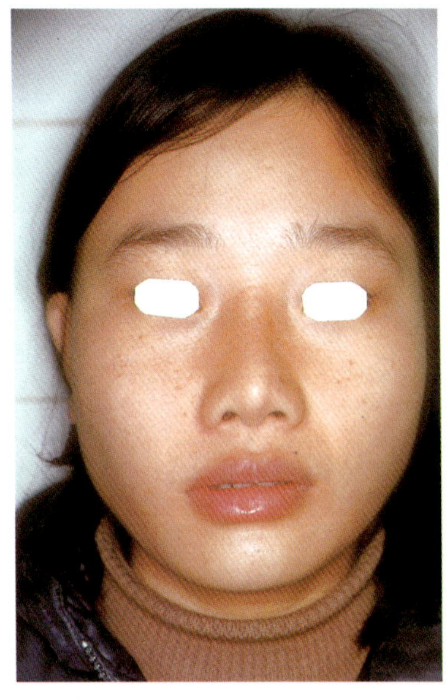

图 137

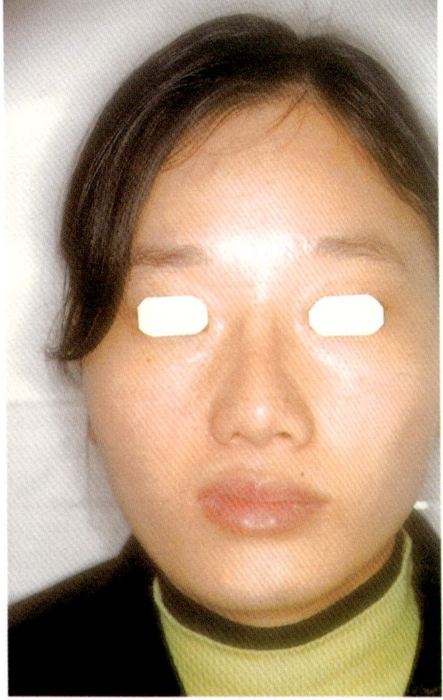

图 138

**图 137** 患有右上颌骨骨化纤维瘤的一 32 岁的女性患者。右上颌骨膨隆逐渐增大已 5 年。上颌骨的病变逐渐累及上颌窦，生长缓慢，逐渐增大，出现右面部畸形。

**图 138** 患者术后 6 个月正面观，美容效果满意。

Fig. 137 Ossifying fibroma of the right maxilla in a woman of 32 years. The swelling has been presented for 5 years, gradually enlarging. Maxillary lesion involves the maxillary sinus. Growth is generally slow, with gradually increasing right facial deformity.

Fig. 138 Postoperative frontal view 6 months. Cosmetic results are satisfactory.

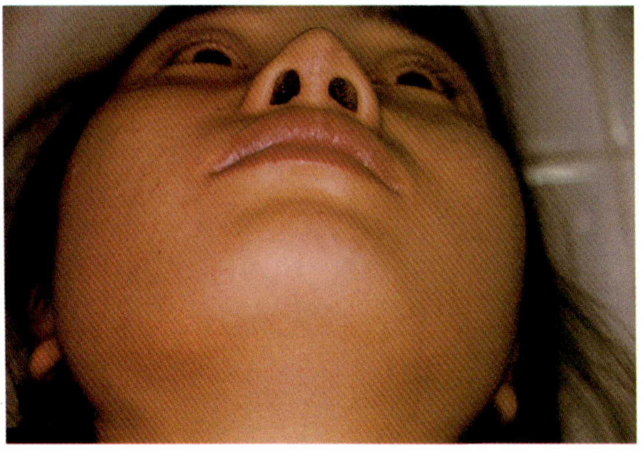

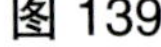

图 139

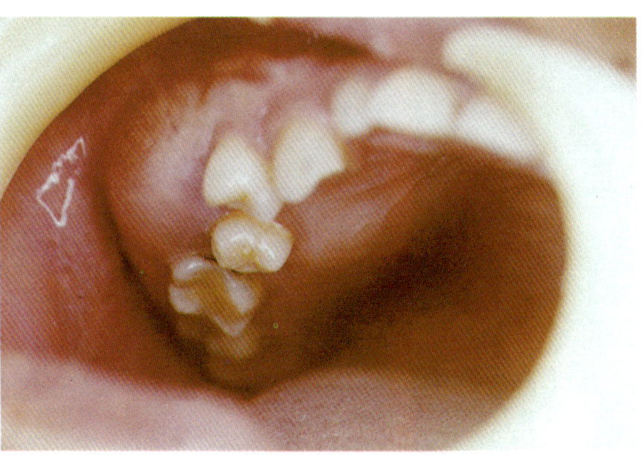

图 140

**图 139** 患右上颌骨骨化纤维瘤的一 32 岁女性患者右面部较左面部大。

**图 140** 患右上颌骨骨化纤维瘤患者口腔内见右侧牙槽骨增大并向颊腭侧膨隆，但表面粘膜正常。

Fig. 139 The right face of a 32-old-year woman patient with ossifying fibroma is larger than the left face.

Fig. 140 There is expansion of the maxilla by a diffuse swelling, which extended into the hard palate and cheek. The mucosa in the oral cavity is normal.

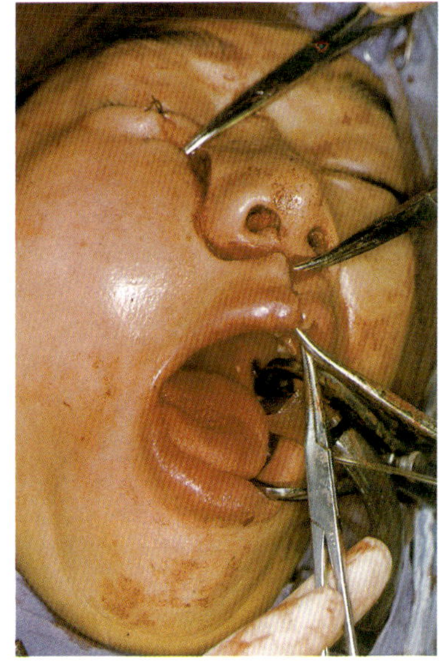

图 141

**图 141** 自上唇正中至鼻小柱基部稍下方，而后沿鼻翼基底，向上沿鼻侧面沟边缘直抵内眦下 1cm，自此向外达颧弓切开。

**Fig. 141** Endotracheal anesthesia is essential. The Fergusson incision is used to raise a cheek flap, splitting the upper lip in the midline. The incision is carried up to the nasal columella, then curved laterally to skirt the nostril and ala nasi. It is then continued upward along the side of the nose to a point just medial and inferior to the inner canthus. A lateral limb 2 to 3mm below the lid margin is carried outward as far as the zygoma.

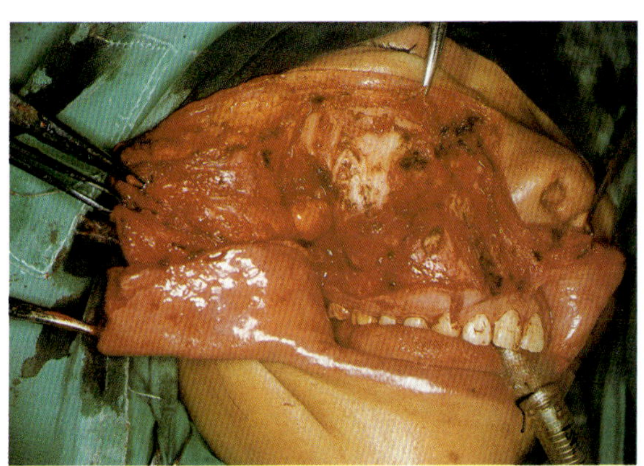

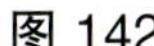

图 142

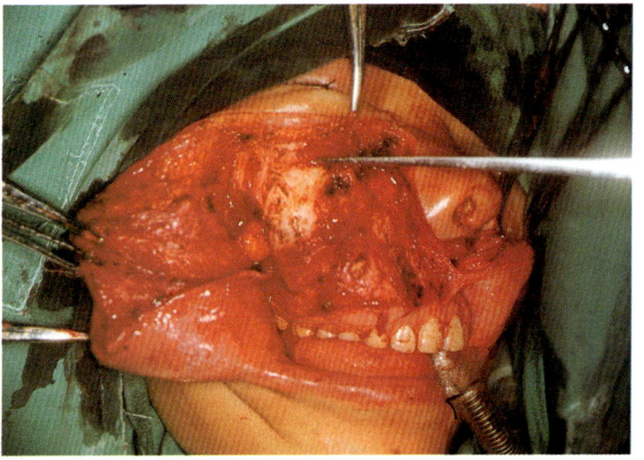

图 143

**图 142** 自龈颊沟的切口中从下面中线向外侧达上颌结节游离瓣的下缘，向上在浅面解剖以保护眼轮匝肌。在解剖时，结扎活跃的出血点。

**图 143** 用切骨钳或骨凿分离上颌骨的鼻突，将鼻软骨与上颌骨的连接分开。暴露眶下缘，用线锯在眶外侧分离颧弓，在颧骨上用骨锯锯开眶外侧缘。

**Fig. 142** The cheek flap is raised by a sharp dissection close to the bone. The inferior margin of the flap is freed by an incision in the gingivobuccal sulcus carried from the midline anteriorly as far laterally as the tuberosity of the maxilla. Dissection superiorly is carried superficially to preserve the orbicularis oculi muscle. During the dissection, numerous bleeding vessels must be secured.

**Fig. 143** The nasal process of the maxilla is divided with bone cutting forceps or osteotome. The nasal cartilages are separated from their junction with the maxilla. The inferior orbital edge is exposed. The zygomatic arch is divided with a Gigli saw just lateral to the orbit, and the lateral edge of the orbit is severed just above the zygoma with a chisel or bone saw.

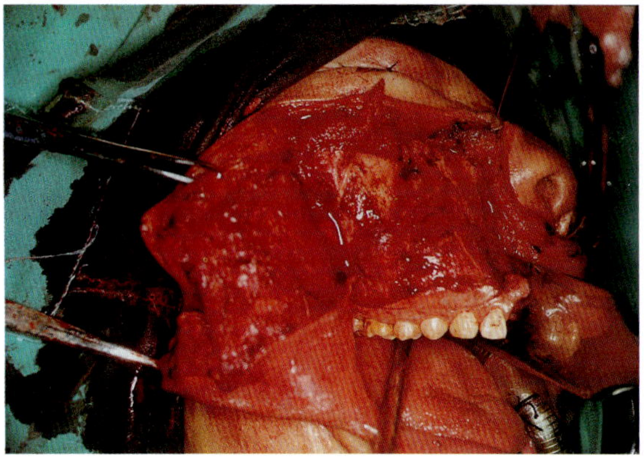
图 144

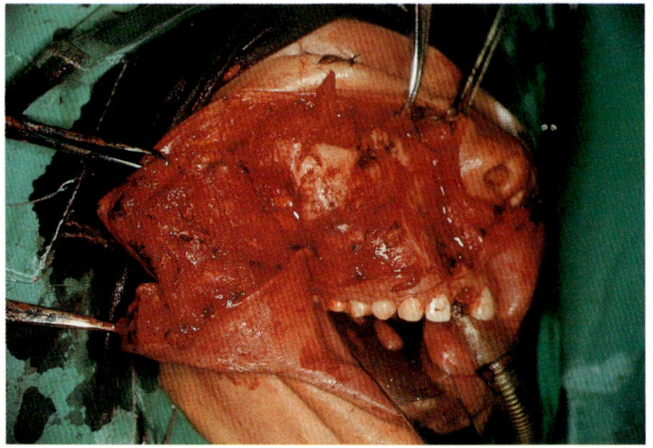
图 145

**图 144** 拔除受累侧的中切牙。在近硬腭粘膜的正中线做切口，向后达硬软腭交界处，然后转向外侧并与以前在龈颊沟做的切口相连。用凿子将患侧硬腭及牙槽突分离。

**图 145** 硬腭分离后，在上颌结节后方翼突与上颌骨附着之间放一个凿子，轻击凿子，使其分开并向外撬动。

**Fig. 144** The central incisor tooth on the involved side is extracted. An incision near the midline of the mucosa of the hard palate is carried from this point posteriorly to the junction of the hard and soft palates. The incision is then directed laterally to meet the incision previously made in the gingivobuccal sulcus. A chisel is used to divide the alveolus and hard palate. This division is carried just far enough from the midline to preserve the nasal septum.

**Fig. 145** Following division of the hard palate, a chisel is placed just behind the tuberosity of the maxilla. The attachments between the pterygoid process and the maxilla are divided by gentle tapping the chisel upward and prying it outward.

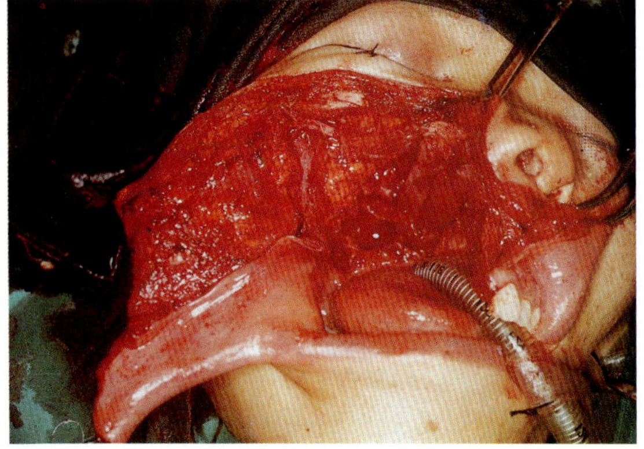
图 146

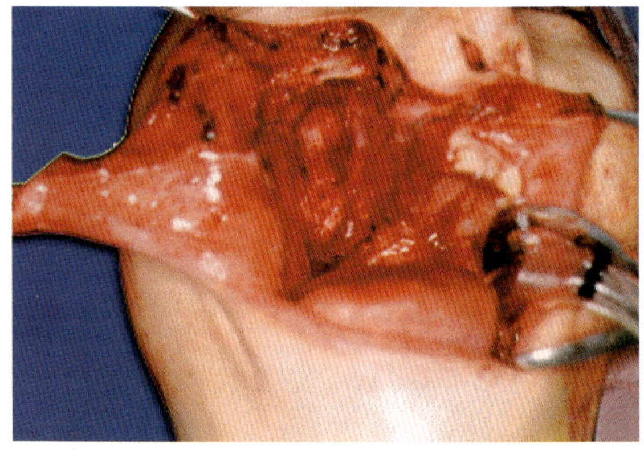
图 147

**图 146** 然后抓住上颌骨，并向两侧摇动以暴露剩余附着。用剪刀或切骨钳分离薄的眶下，分离剩余附着的软组织并去除整个上颌骨。

**图 147** 用纱布团塞入手术缺损区以止血。将创内的颌内动脉分支结扎。

**Fig. 146** The maxilla is then grasped and rocked from side to side to expose its remaining attachments. The thin inferior orbital edge may be divided with scissors or bone cutting forceps. The few remaining soft tissue attachments are then severed and the entire maxilla removed.

**Fig. 147** Application of a gauze pack to the operative defect for a few minutes at this stage aids in hemostasis. Several spurting branches of the internal maxillary artery in the wound are secured.

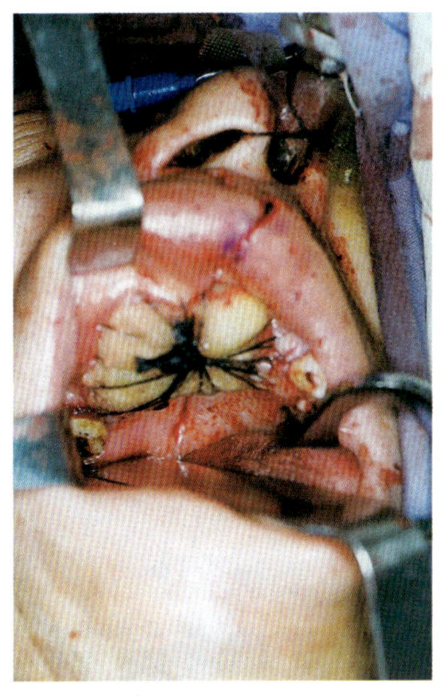

图 148

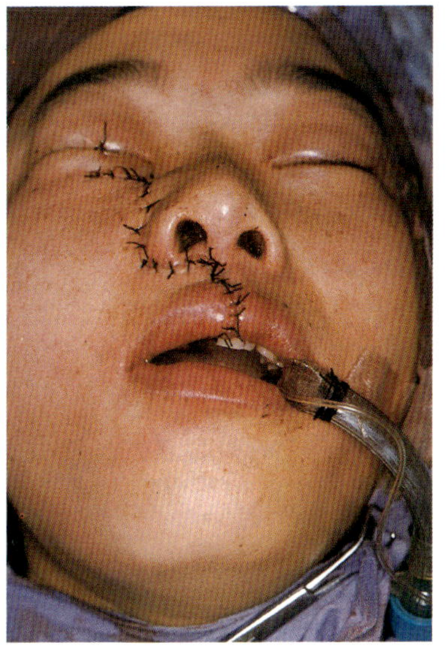

图 149

**图 148** 将创面用断层皮片覆盖，将移植体的边缘与颊瓣的游离缘及粘膜边缘缝合。腔内填入纱布块并固定。

**图 149** 还回颊瓣，用丝线行间断缝合，修整上唇并缝合之。

**Fig. 148** The cheek flap and the operative defect are then lined with a split-thickness skin graft. The graft is sutured near the free edges of the cheek flap and to the incised mucosa, and is held in place in the remainder of the defect with a snug packing of petrolatum gauze.

**Fig. 149** The cheek flap is then sutured back in place with numerous interrupted sutures of fine silk. The upper lip is repaired in the usual manner. Packing in the operative defect is reinforced through the palatal defect below, and the pharyngeal pack removed.

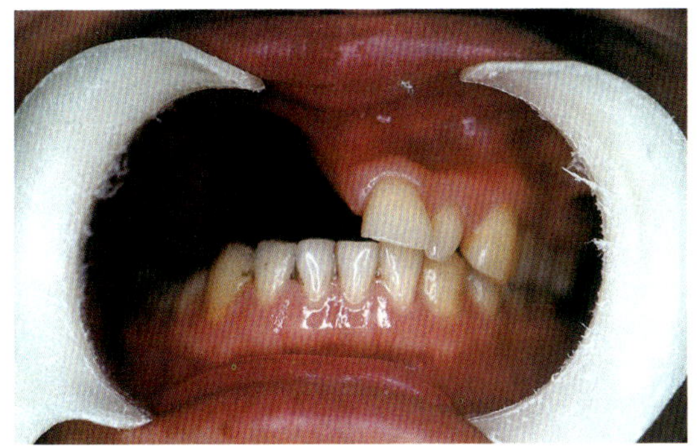

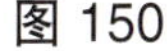

图 150

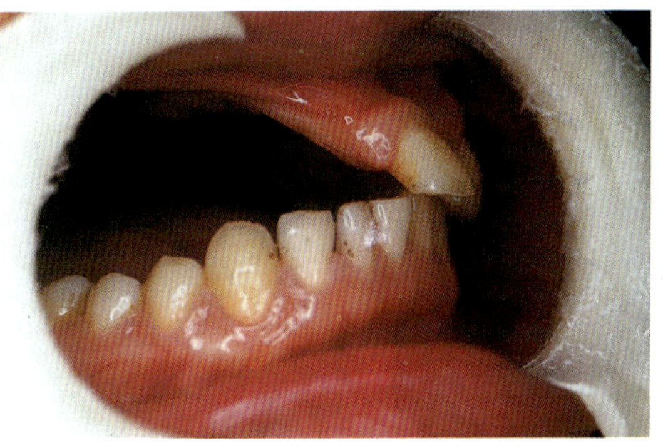

图 151

**图 150, 151** 上颌骨切除后剩余牙的咬𬌗关系正面及侧面观。

**Fig. 150, 151** Frontal and lateral views of the occlusal relationships of remaining teeth after maxillary resection.

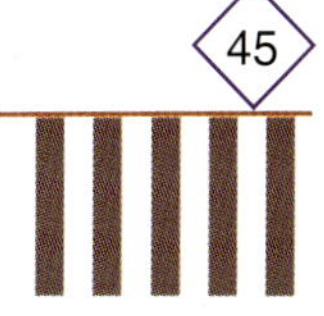

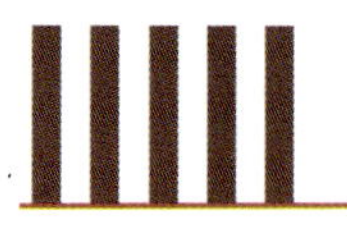



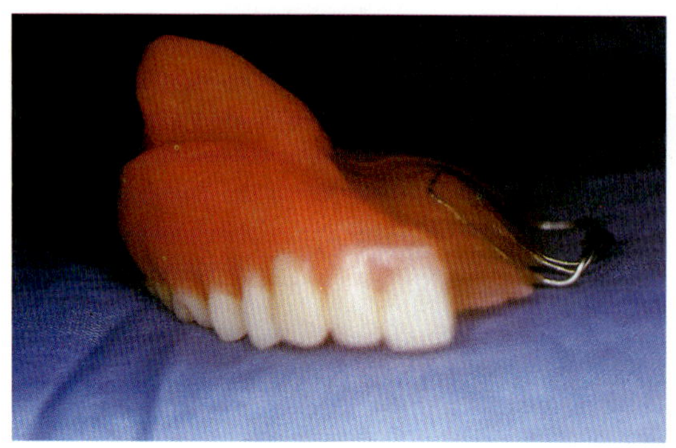

图 152

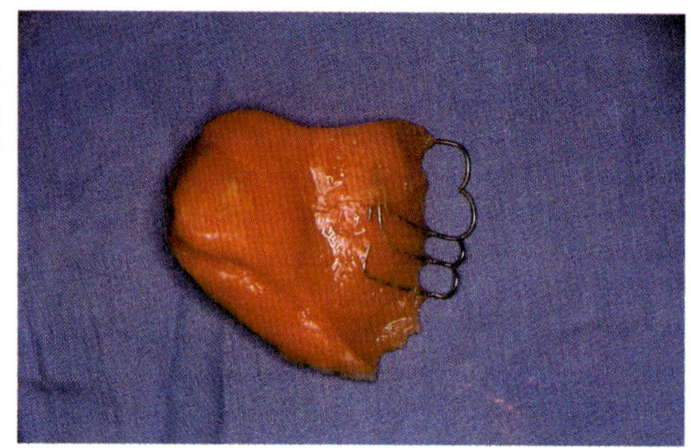

图 153

**图 152, 153** 在术后 9 天或 10 天，去除缺损区的填塞纱包。为了使患者术后说话及吞咽无困难，制作一个暂时性的塑料修复体以封闭腭部缺损。术后 3 个月再制作永久性赝复体。

**Fig. 152, 153** On the 9th or 10th postoperative day, the packing is removed from the operative defect. A temporary plastic prosthesis is constructed to close the palatal defect, allowing the patient to speak and swallow without difficulty. After 3 months, a permanent prosthetic device will be necessary.

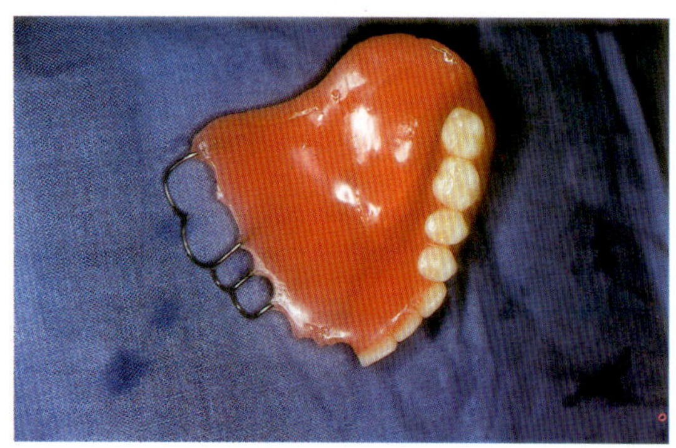

图 154

**图 154** 剩余上颌骨上保留的自然牙被用来接纳赝复的𬌗支托和卡环以帮助防止赝复体的撬动及分布𬌗力。

**Fig. 154** Natural teeth which remain in the residual jaw are clasped with bent stainless-steel wire or wrought metal clasps to help retain and stabilize the prosthesis.

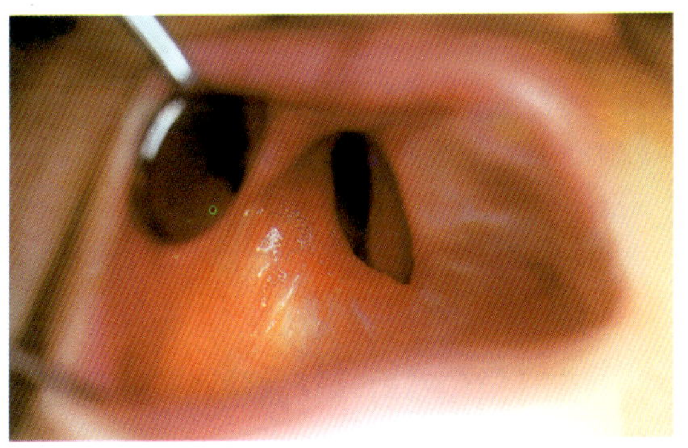

图 155

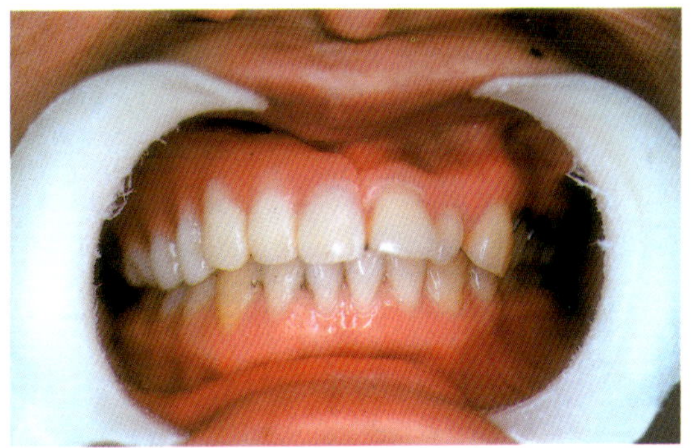

图 156

**图 155** 右上颌骨切除后遗留的腭部缺损，该缺损影响患者的语言与吞咽。
**图 156** 患者戴上永久性赝复体之后的咬殆关系及美容效果。

**Fig. 155** The palatal defect resulting from maxillary resection affects the patient's speaking and swallowing.

**Fig. 156** Particular attention should be given the occlusal relationships of the teeth. The use of acrylic-resin artificial teeth will temper harsh occlusal contacts.

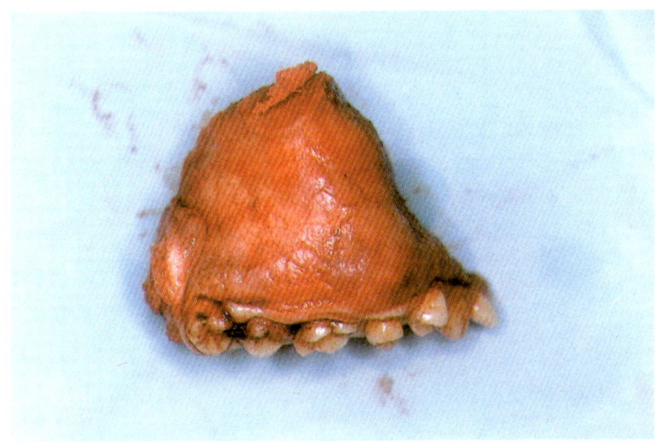

图 157

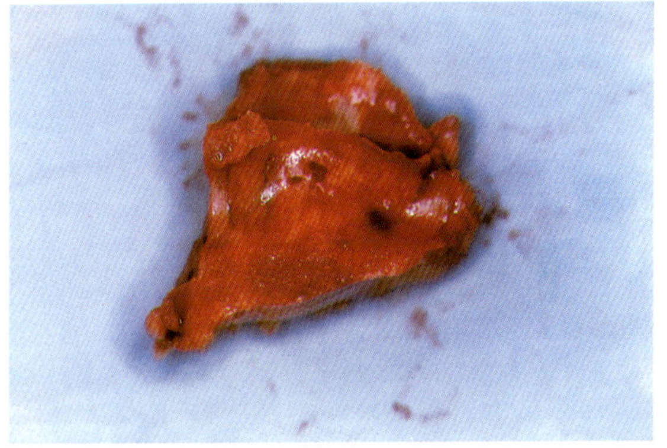

图 158

**图 157** 被切除的右上颌骨，上颌骨被破坏，代之以肿瘤组织。
**图 158** 被切除的肿瘤上部扩展进入眶下缘，切除的标本显示肿瘤的上面。

**Fig. 157** The maxilla was excised. It was largely destroyed and replaced by a tumor, and there was extension of growth toward the right maxillary sinus.

**Fig. 158** The upper part of the tumor extending into and displacing the infraorbital margin was ill-defined. The resected specimen shows the upper surface of the tumor.

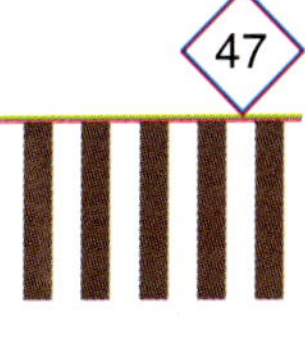

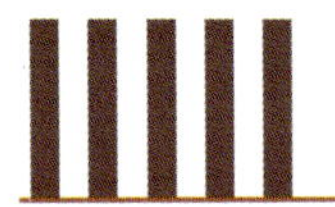



# 10. 上颌骨恶性纤维组织细胞瘤的外科治疗

# 10. Surgical excision of the malignant fibrohystoblastoma in the maxilla

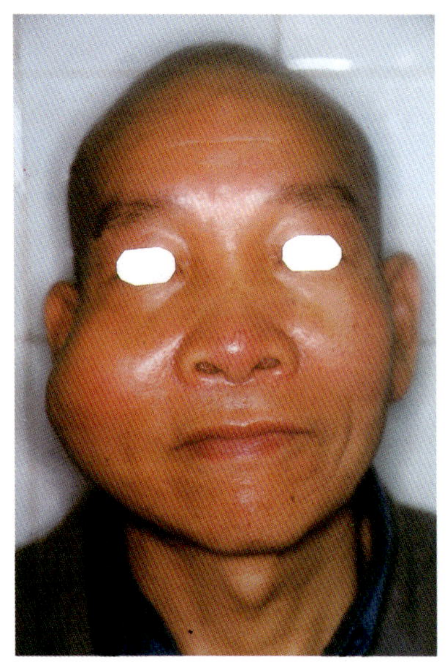

图 159

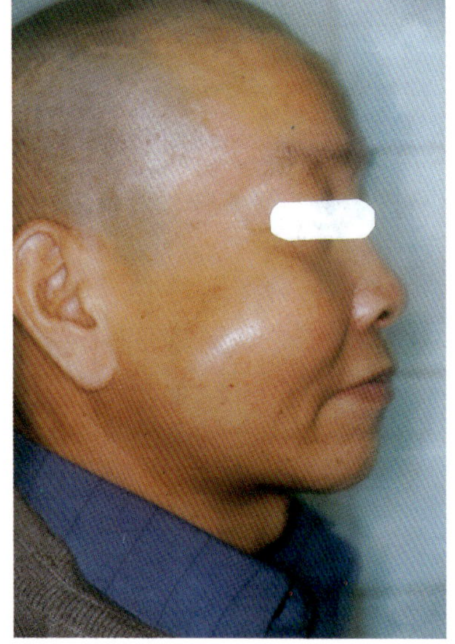

图 160

**图 159, 160** 患右上颌窦恶性纤维组织细胞瘤的 61 岁男性患者正、侧面观。正面观显示两侧面部不对称，右侧面部明显膨隆。侧面观显示右上颌膨隆,表面皮肤正常。

**Fig. 159, 160** A 61-year-old male patient's frontal and lateral views with the malignant fibrohystoblastoma on the right maxillae. The bilateral faces are asymmetrical on the frontal view, the right face is expansive. The right maxillae is expansive and the surfacial skin is normal on the lateral view.

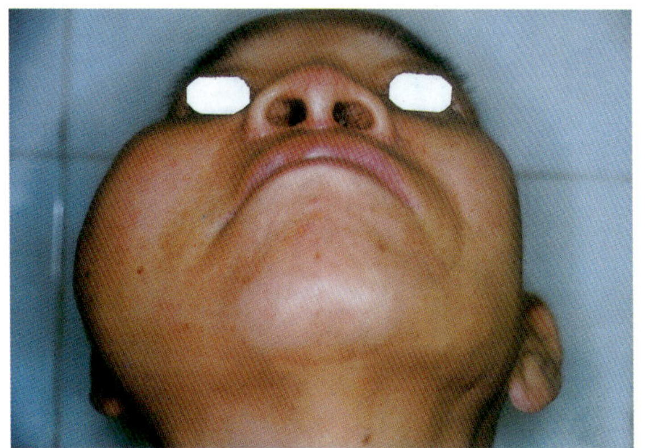

图 161

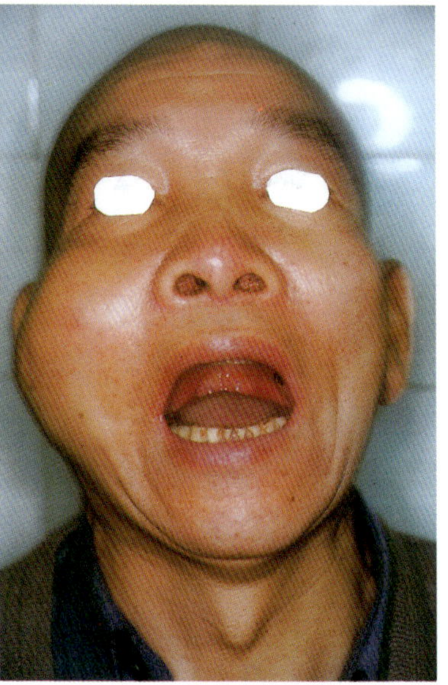

图 162

**图 161, 162** 仰面观右上颌骨膨隆明显。正面观张口度无明显改变。

**Fig. 161, 162** The right maxillary expansion is obvious on the submental view. The change of opening size is not obvious on the frontal view.

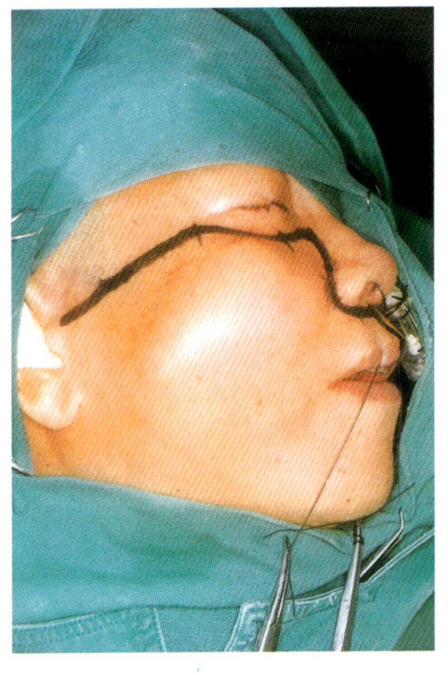

图 163

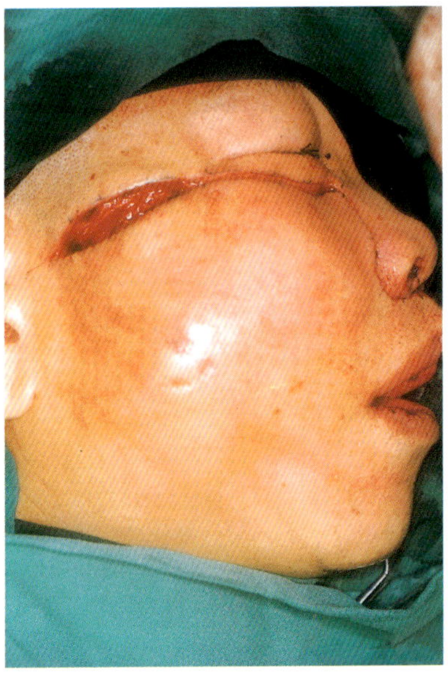

图 164

**图 163, 164** 病人仰卧，头偏健侧。健侧鼻腔气管插管静脉麻醉。按图 163 进行切口。首先在上唇正中做切口，经鼻梨状孔下，然后向外侧延伸达颞颌关节。另一切口在受累侧的上颌龈颊沟从正中向后达磨牙后区，沿受累侧下颌龈颊沟从尖牙至磨牙后区做切口。

**Fig. 163, 164** The patient is placed in a recumbent position with the head rotated 45° to the uninvolved side. Intravenous anesthesia with endotracheal intubation via the opposite nasal cavity is used. The first incision divides the upper lip in the midline, passes under the nasal pyramid and extends laterally, reaching the level of the temporomandibular joint. An incision is then made along the maxillary buccogingival fold on the involved side, running from the midline to the retromolar area. Another incision is made along the mandibular buccogingival fold on the involved side, running from canine to retromolar area.

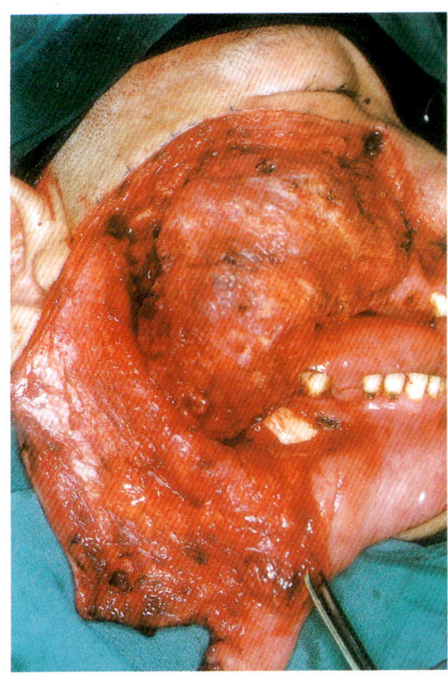

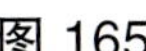

图 165

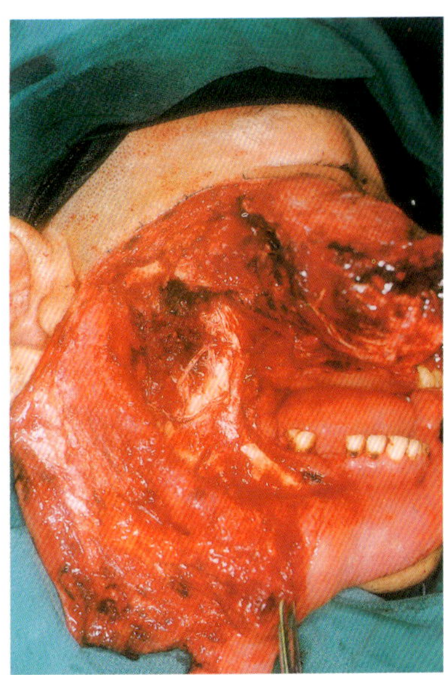

图 166

**图 165, 166** 在表情肌的表面用电刀掀起并翻转以暴露上颌前面、眶缘下部、颞肌下部、颧骨和颧弓、颞下颌关节外侧、嚼肌和下颌升支。暴露下颌升支后缘，向前牵拉下颌骨，向后牵拉腮腺，此时出现一个间隙，颌内动脉横行经过此间隙，将其结扎后切断。

在颧弓之上用电刀切断颞肌，用骨剪剪断颧弓两端不将其去除，而使其与嚼肌相连。在下颌角之上用线锯锯断下颌升支，用电刀使颞颌关节断离。

将外科标本部分向前移，翻起附着在髁状突的翼外肌，保留该肌的前附着。该步骤对肿瘤的外侧面、颞窝的下面、眼眶至眶下裂的外面、翼突的外侧面、翼腭窝和翼内肌的外侧面提供了足够多的暴露。

拔除受累侧的中切牙，从该点向后达硬软腭交界硬腭正中线切开，切口相接与以前在龈颊沟做的切口相连。用咬骨钳切断上颌骨的鼻突，在鼻软骨与上颌骨相连处分离鼻软骨。用钝骨膜下分离掀起眶内容物，暴露眶下缘。在颧骨之上切断眶外侧缘，用骨凿凿开牙槽突与硬腭，根据肿瘤的内容，翼突可包括在外科标本之中。

为了移去标本，切断附着在突上的翼内肌。

骨切开完成后，向前移动标本。夹住上颌骨，向侧面摇动上颌骨以决定剩余的附着，用剪刀或骨钳分离薄的眶下缘，切断剩余的软组织附着，移去整个标本。结扎出血的小血管。

**Fig. 165, 166** A large flap is raised at the level of the mimetic muscles with an electrosurgical knife. This flap is reflected to yield adequate exposure of the anterior aspect of the maxilla, the inferior half of the orbital rim, the inferior portion of the temporalis muscle, the zygomatic bone and zygomatic arch, the external aspect of the temporomandibular joint, and the masseter and the mandibular ramus.

The posterior border of the mandibular ramus is well exposed, the mandible is retracted anteriorly, and the parotid gland is retracted posteriorly. A space is thus created where it is possible to isolate the internal maxillary artery. The vessel is tied and severed.

Temporalis muscle is sectioned with an electrosurgical knife a little above the zygomatic arch. The zygomatic arch is cut at both ends with a bone-cutting forceps but not removed. It remains attached to the stumps of the masseter. The mandibular ramus is sectioned transversely with a Gigli saw above the angle of the mandible, and disarticulation of the temporomandibular joint is done using the electrosurgical knife.

The portion of the surgical specimen so delineated is turned forward. The lateral pterygoid muscle, which is inserted on the condyle, is raised and remains attached by its anterior insertions. This maneuver provides adequate exposure of the external aspect of the tumor, the inferior portion of the temporal fossa, the external aspect of the orbital cavity to the inferior orbital fissure, the lateral surface of the lateral pterygoid process, the pterygopalatine fossa, and the lateral surface of the internal pterygoid muscle, allowing an adequate margin around the posterior limit of the tumor.

The central incisor tooth on the involved side is now extracted. An incision near the midline of the hard palate is carried from this point posteriorly to the junction of the hard and soft palates. The incision is then directed laterally to meet the incision previously made in the buccogingival sulcus. The nasal process of the maxilla is then divided with a bone-cutting forceps and the nasal cartilages are separated from their junction with the maxilla. The orbital contents are elevated by blunt subperiosteal dissection, exposing the inferior orbital plate. The zygomatic arch has already been divided. The lateral edge of the orbit is severed just above the zygoma with a chisel. A chisel is also used to divide the alveolus and hard palate. This division is made just far enough from the midline to preserve the nasal septum. Depending on the extent of the tumor, the pterygoid process may be included in the surgical specimen. To remove the surgical specimen, the fibers of the medial pterygoid muscle attached to the process are cut.

After all the bone cuts are completed, the surgical specimen is easily mobilized anteriorly. The maxilla is then grasped and rocked from side to side to determine the remaining attachments. The thin inferior orbital plate may be divided with a scissors or a bone-cutting forceps. The few remaining soft tissue attachments are then severed, and the entire specimen is removed. This technique allows removal of the surgical specimen without significant bleeding and with adequate margins. Small bleeding vessels are tied or electrocoagulated.

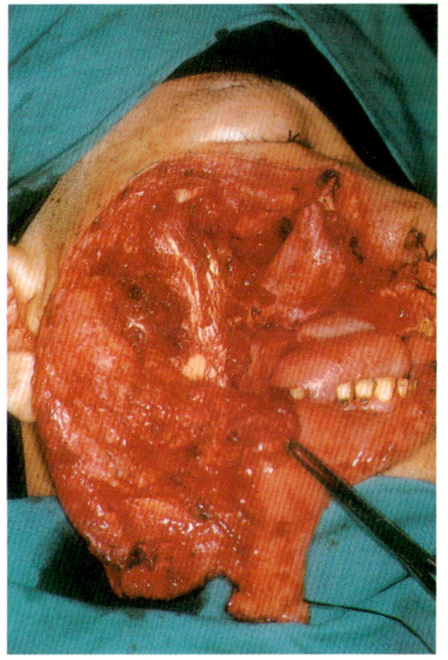

图 167

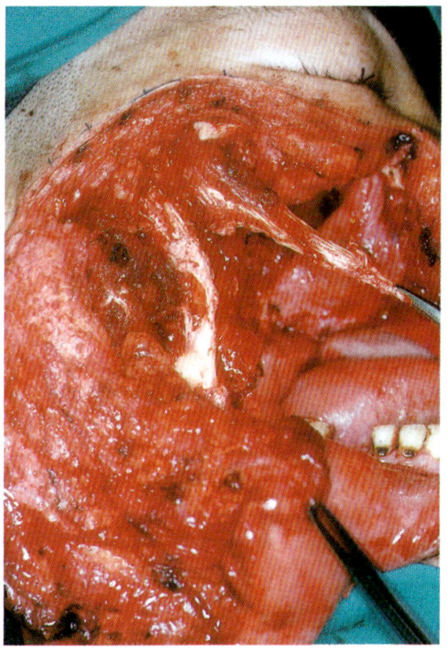

图 168

**图 167，168** 眶板的大部分被去除后，采用部分颞肌将眶内容物悬吊起来以防眶内容物的下移。其方法是将附着在下颌骨上前部的部分颞肌分离达眶外侧缘平面，然后将其游离的末端缝合在鼻骨的骨膜上。

**Fig. 167, 168** After most of the inferior orbital plate has been removed, the orbital contents are suspended by a sling of temporalis muscle. The muscle is divided at its point of insertion on the mandible beneath the orbit and sutured to the periosteum of the nasal bone.

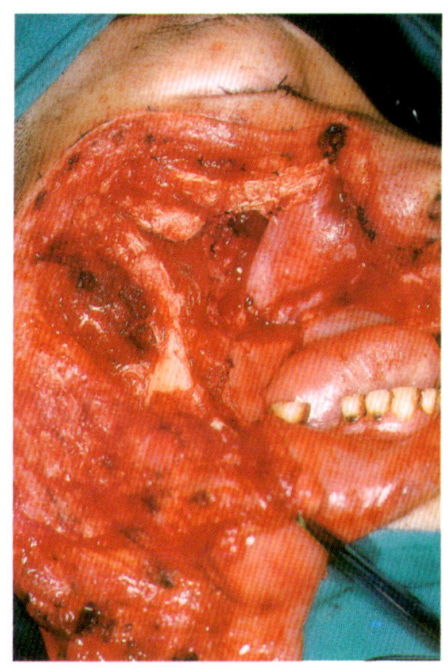

图 169

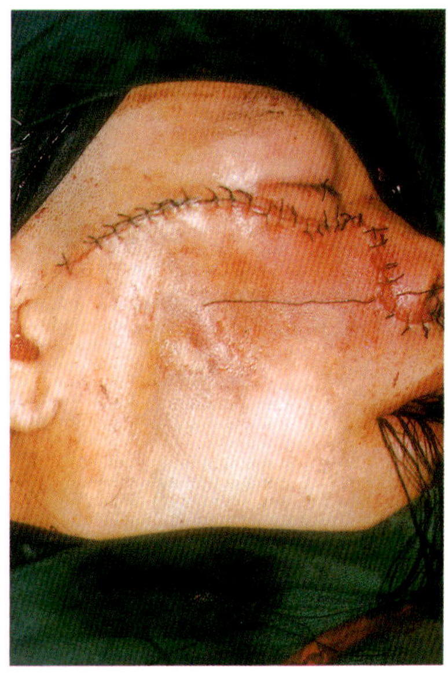

图 170

**图 169, 170** 手术缺损区的颊部行刃厚皮片移植，皮片的边缘与颊瓣的游离缘的粘膜相缝合。将颊瓣还回原处，用细丝线行间断缝合。用常用的方法修复上唇。

**Fig. 169, 170** The cheek flap and the operative defect are then lined with a split-thickness skin graft. The graft is sutured near the free edges of the cheek flap and to the incised mucosa. The cheek flap is then sutured back in place with numerous interrupted sutures of fine silk. The upper lip is repaired in the usual manner.

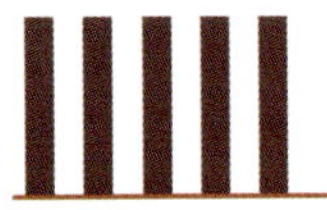



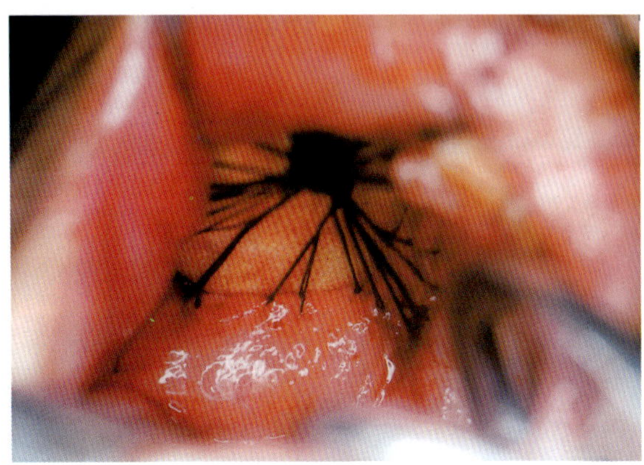

图 171

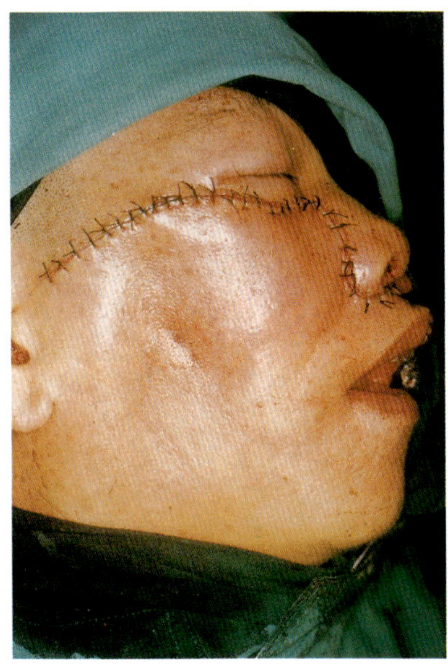

图 172

**图 171, 172** 缺损区用凡士林纱布填塞，用缝合后留的丝线将纱布固定。在术后的第 10 或 12 天，去除填塞纱布，制作暂时性的塑料假体以封闭腭部缺损使其语言及吞咽无困难，术后 3 个月再行永久性修复。

**Fig. 171, 172** The place in the remainder of the defect helds a snug packing of petrolatum gauze. Packing in the operative defect is reinforced through the palatal defect below.

On the 10th or 12th postoperative day, the packing is removed from the operative defect. A temporary plastic prosthesis is constructed to close the palatal defect, allowing the patient to speak and swallow without difficulty. After 3 months, shrinking of the tissues will necessitate a new and permanent prosthetic device.

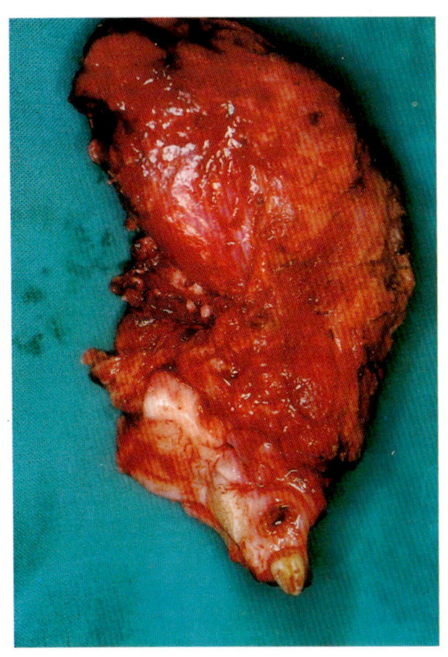

图 173

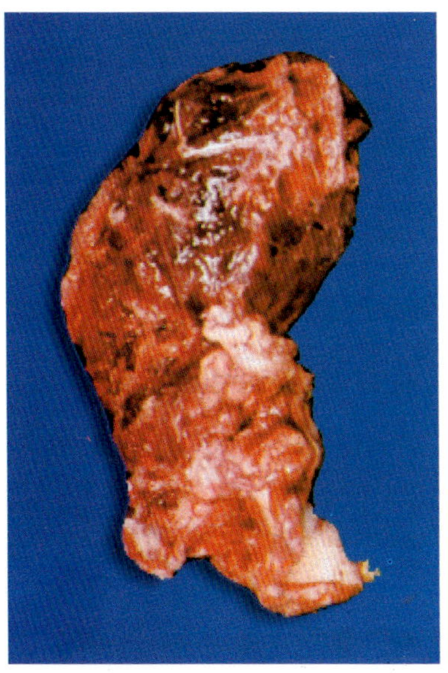

图 174

**图 173, 174** 手术后标本的外面及内侧面观。

**Fig. 173, 174** The external and internal views of the postoperative specimen.

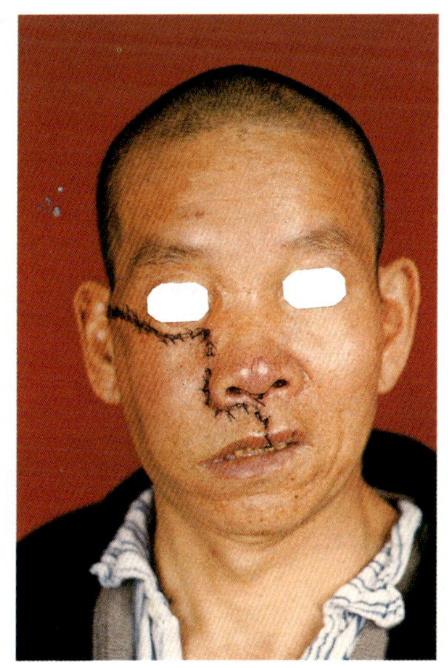
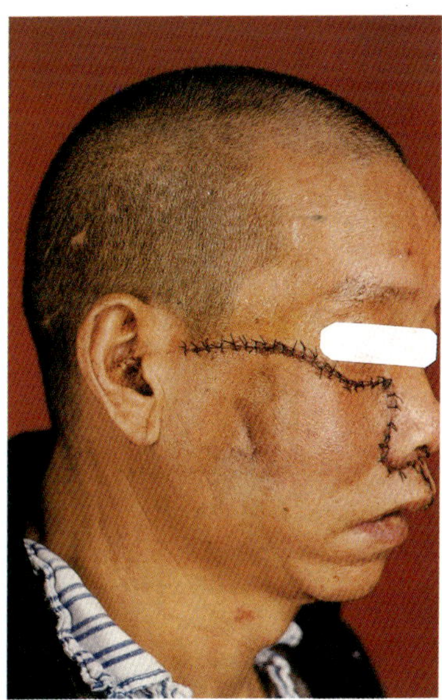

**图 175, 176** 患者术后 5 天的正、侧面观。

**Fig. 175, 176** The Patient's frontal and lateral views 5 days postoperatively.

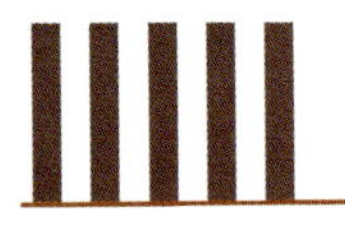



# Ⅲ. 上唇部肿瘤

11. 上唇癌切除 Abbé 瓣转移修复治疗

# Ⅲ. Upper lip tumors

11. The Abbé flap used to reconstruct a central defect of the upper lip

# 11. 上唇癌切除 Abbé 瓣转移修复治疗

# 11. The use of Abbé flap reconstructing a central defect of the upper lip

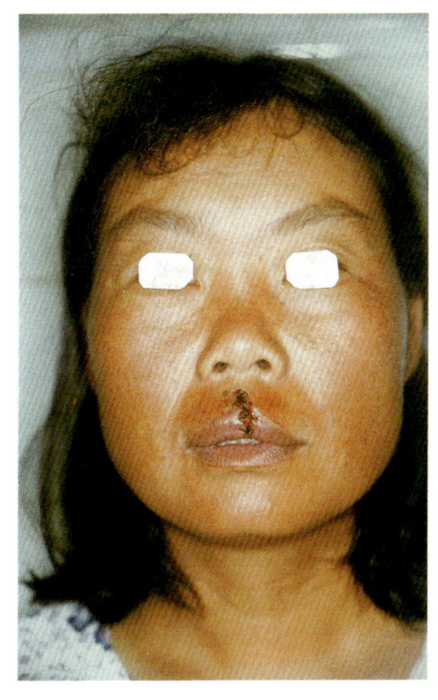

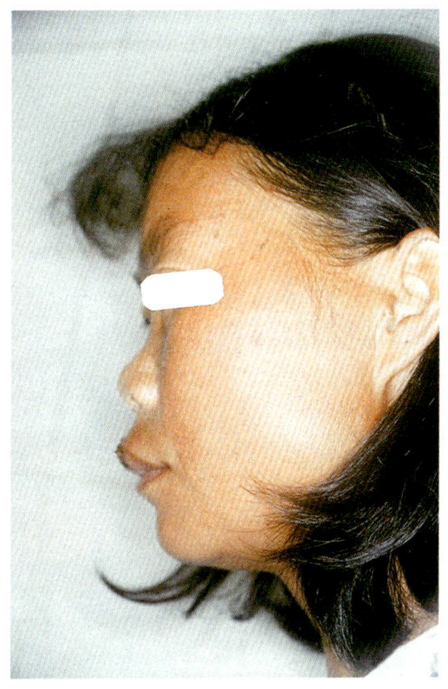

图 177, 178 一 44 岁患有上唇鳞状细胞癌的女性患者的正面观及侧面观。

Fig. 177, 178 Frontal and lateral views of a woman patient with squamous cell carcinoma of the upper lip.

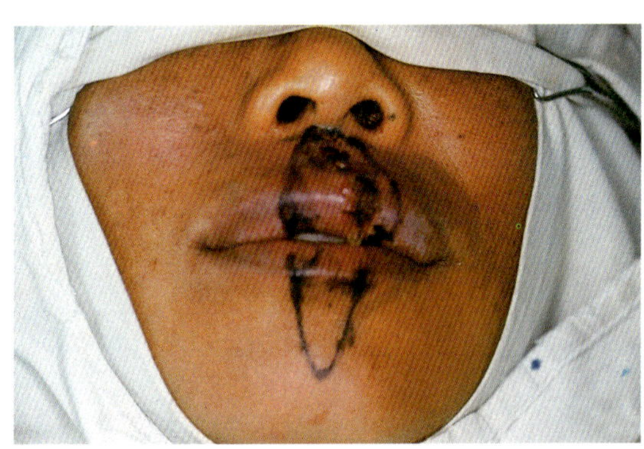

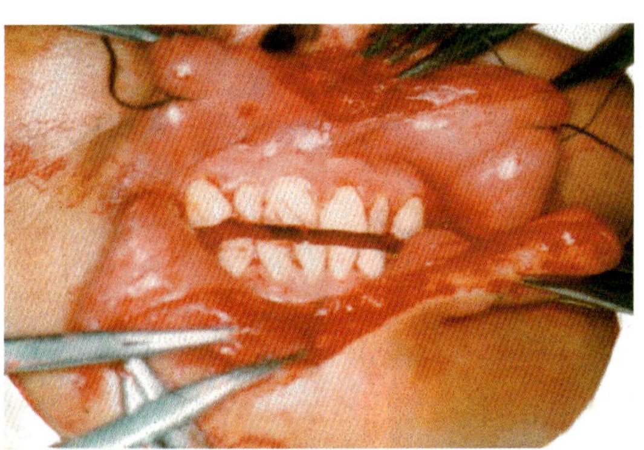

图 179, 180 在 Abbé 氏手术中，不到全上唇宽度 1/3 的癌可以通过楔形切除进行治疗，这种切除必需是在肿瘤周围 1cm 正常内进行。预计切除的组织用美蓝画线。切除病变组织，掀起对侧全层唇组织三角瓣。

Fig. 179, 180 In Abbé-type procedure, cancer occupying less than one third of the length of the upper lip may be treated by wedge excision, in which the full thickness of the lip and adjacent skin is removed with the lesion. All points of the incision should be carried through normal-appearing tissue at least 1 cm from the margin of the tumor. The proposed excision is outlined around the lesion with methylene blue. The lesion is excised. The triangular flap consisting of the full thickness of the opposite lip is elevated.

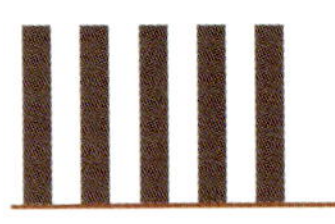



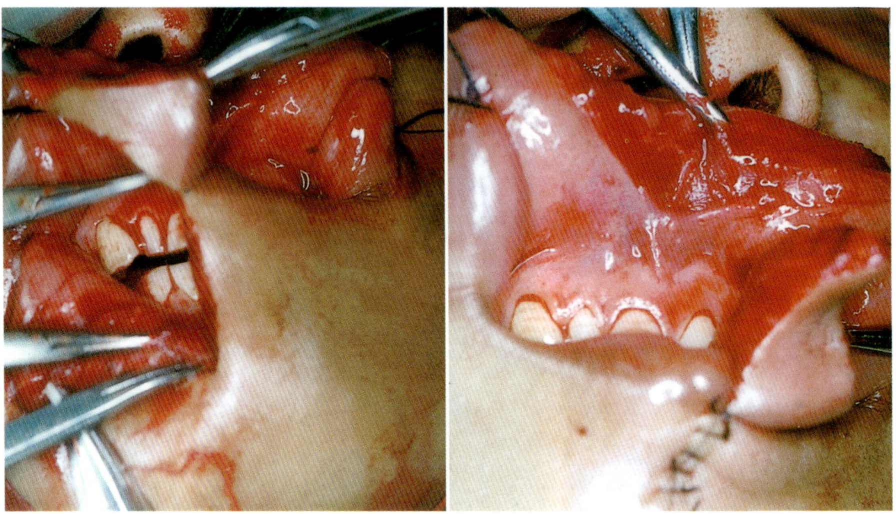

图 181

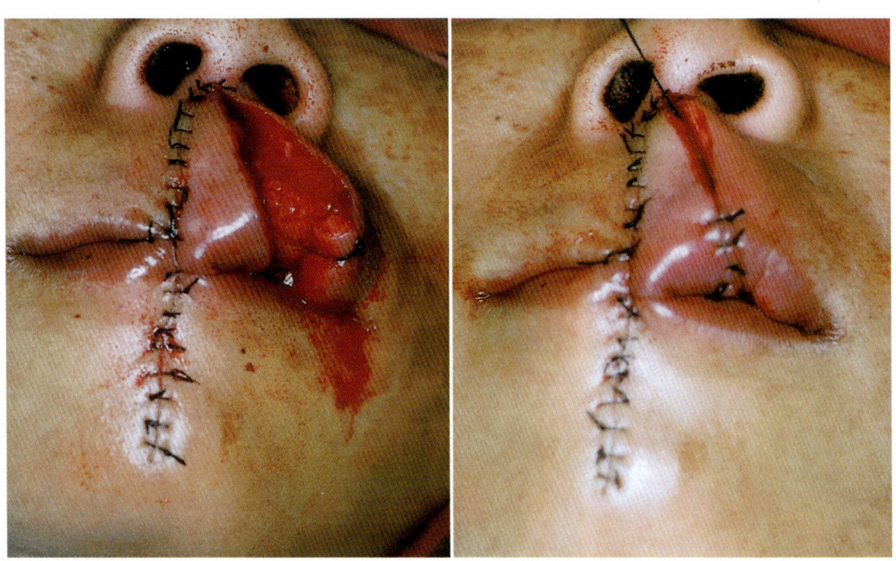

图 181

**图 181** 将其三角组织由下向上旋转进入上唇的手术缺损区。将下唇互相对合缝合粘膜、肌层和皮肤。将下唇的三角组织瓣旋转进入上唇的缺损区后分粘膜、肌层和皮肤缝合。应注意的是缝合不应太靠近狭窄的瓣蒂部以免三角瓣的血供中断。

**Fig. 181** The triangular flap is rotated into an operative defect of the upper lip. The lower lip defect is directly closed. The triangular flap of the lower lip is rotated 180° and sutured into the upper lip defect. Suturing is carried out in the usual way, the most important point is to make sure that sutures in the vicinity of the pedicle are placed to avoid constricting the labial vessels.

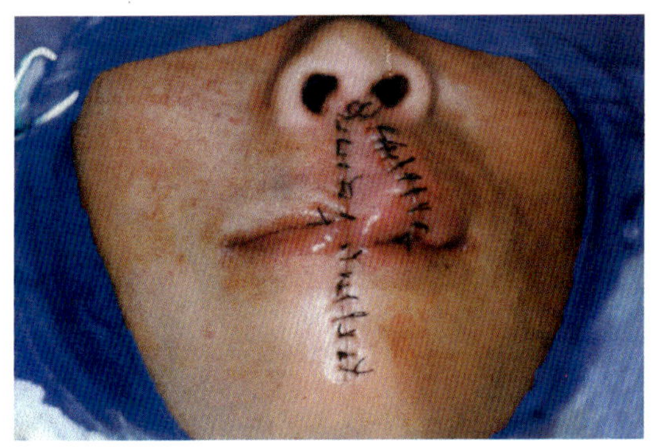

图 182

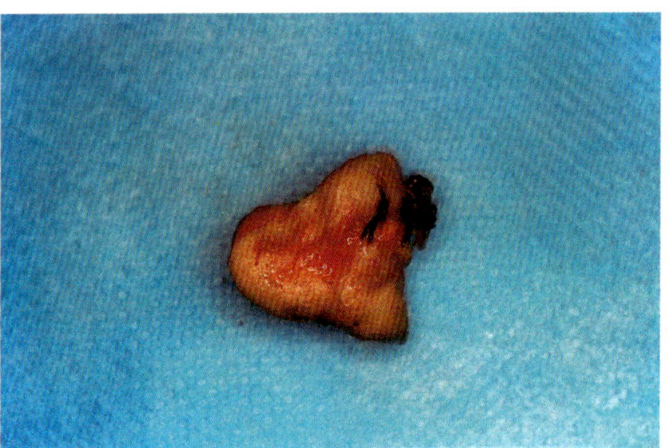

图 183

图 182 缝合后的情景，注意唇红缘的匹配。
图 183 为术后的标本。

Fig. 182 Sutured in position. Note the matching of all vermilion margins at this stage of the transfer.

Fig. 183 shows postoperative specimen.

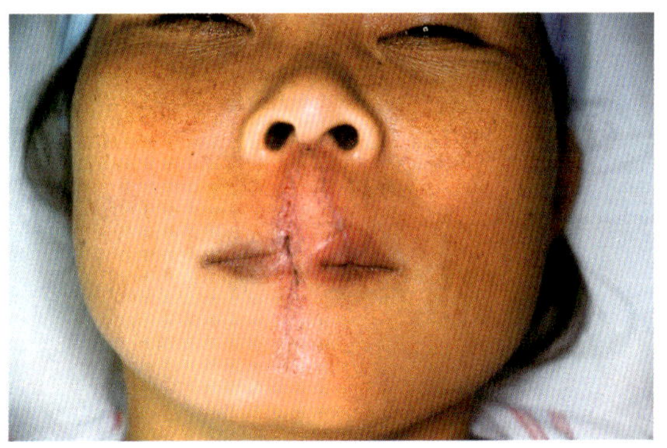

图 184

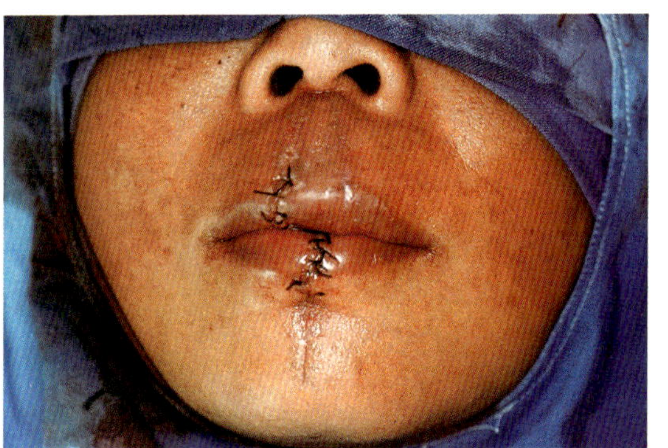

图 185

图 184, 185 第一次术后 2 周，在局麻下断蒂。调整上唇的红唇缘。在下唇的蒂处创面做一个小的楔形切除后修整唇红缘以形成正常的红唇外形。

Fig. 184, 185 After a waiting period of 2 weeks, the pedicle is divided. The vermilion immediately adjacent to the site of the pedicle on the upper and lower lip is incised a short distance. Small wedges of the exposed raw surface of the pedicle are excised, allowing repair of the vermilion and reestablishment of normal lip contour.

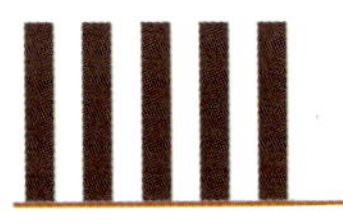

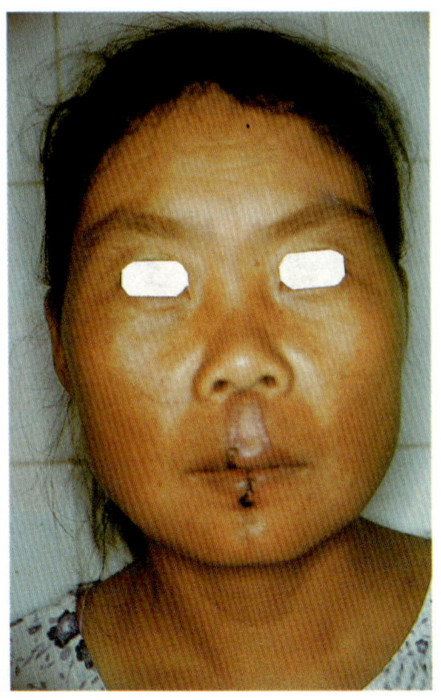

图 186

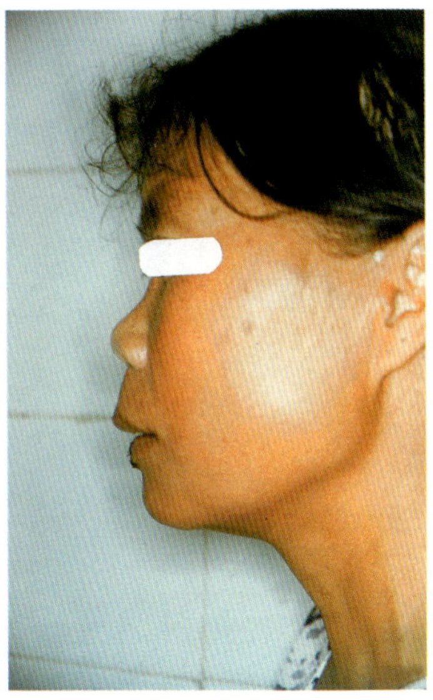

图 187

图 186, 187 断蒂后的正、侧面观。

Fig. 186, 187 Frontal and lateral views after the pedicle was divided.

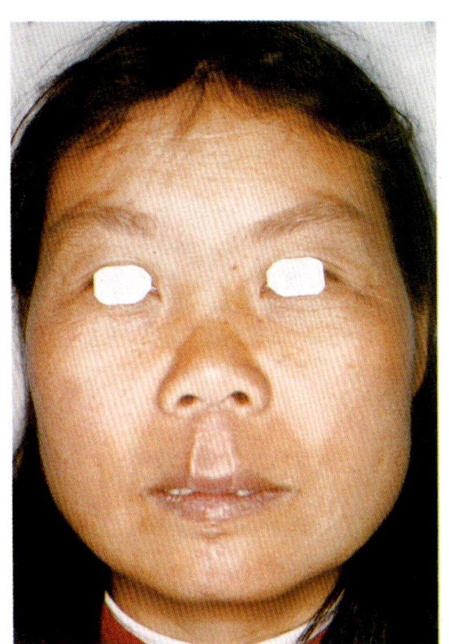

图 188

图 188 手术后 1 年的正面观。

Fig. 188 Frontal view 1 year postoperatively.

# Ⅳ. 面颊部肿瘤



# Ⅳ. Facial and buccal region tumors

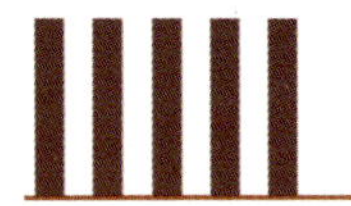



# 12. 嚼肌内海绵状血管瘤摘除术

# 12. Excision of cavernous haemangioma in the masseter

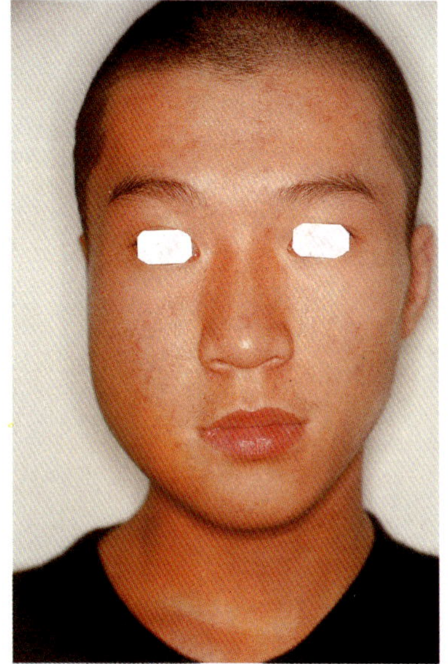

图 189

图 189，190 一患右嚼肌内海绵状血管瘤的 18 岁男性患者的正面及仰面观。

正面观显示双侧面部不对称，右侧嚼肌区明显膨隆，仰面观右侧嚼肌区较左侧为大。

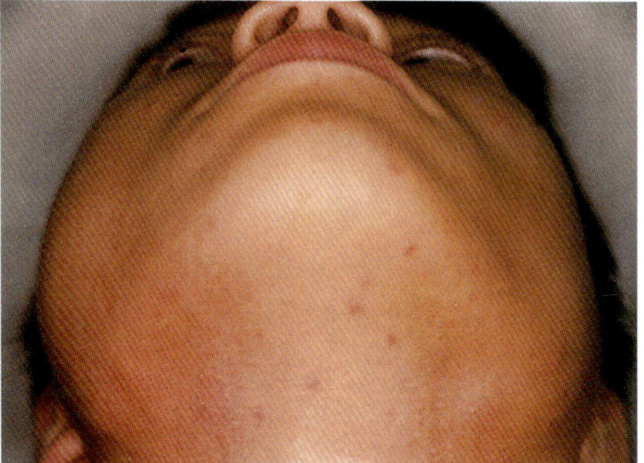

图 190

Fig. 189 Frontal and submental views of a 18- year-old male patient with cavernous haemangioma in the masseter.

Frontal view shows both facial asymmetry, right masseter region obvious expansion.

Fig. 190 Submental view shows that the right masseter region is larger than the left masseter region.

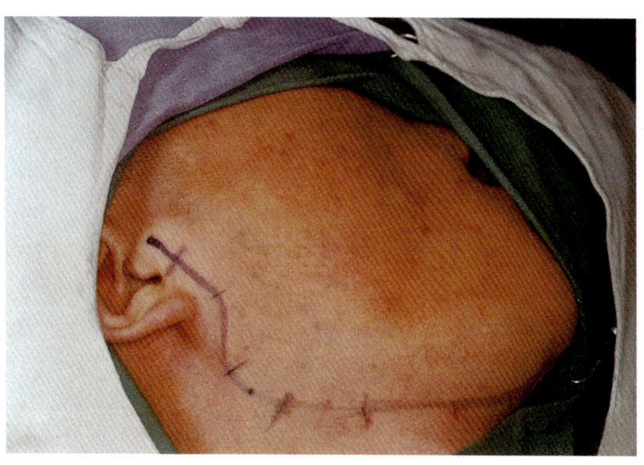

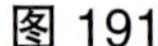

图 191

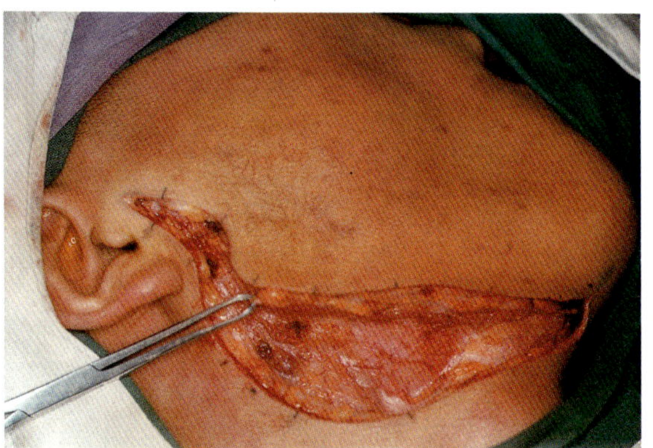

图 192

图 191 按腮腺切除术的切口画出切口线。
图 192 根据已标出的切口线切开皮肤、皮下组织及颈阔肌。

Fig. 191 The incision line is marked out with methylene blue.
Fig. 192 According to be marked line, an incision is made.

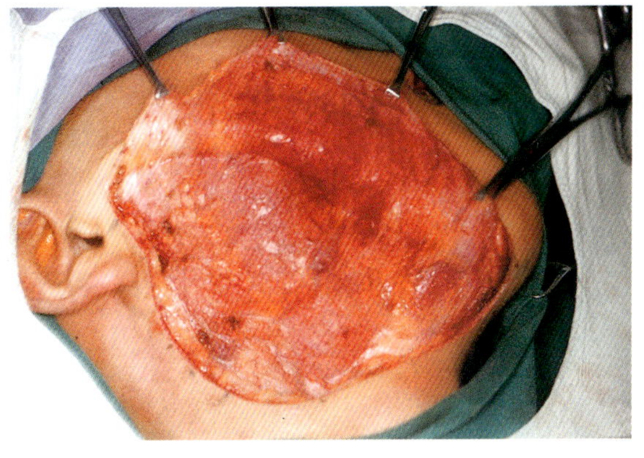

图 193

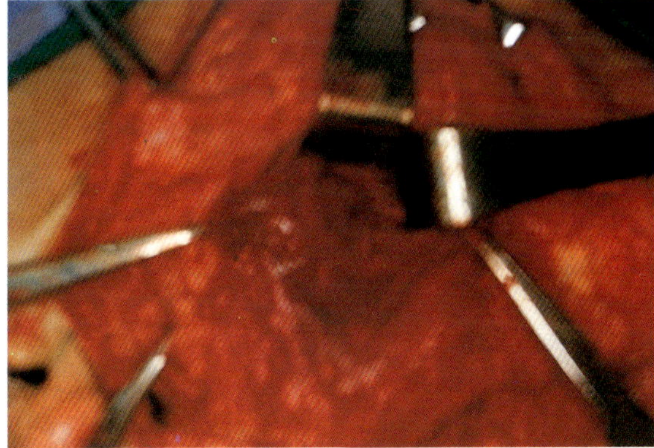

图 194

**图 193** 在腮腺嚼肌筋膜的浅面掀起皮肤肌瓣，此时，可见血管瘤的浅面。横行切开腮腺嚼肌筋膜后，纵行分离嚼肌肌纤维，嚼肌内血管瘤暴露于手术野中。

**图 194** 用小拉钩牵开嚼肌肌纤维，钝分离血管瘤的上极、前界、下界及后界，最后分离深层组织并钳夹后切断结扎。

**Fig. 193** The skin flap is now elevated, exposing the entire superficial surface of the parotid gland and the masseter region. The superficial surface of cavernous haemangioma is exposed in the operative field. A parallel incision is made along the orientation of the branches of facial nerve on the thin parotid and masseter fascia. After the fibers of the masseter are separated with the sharp dissection, haemangioma in the masseter is exposed in the operative field.

**Fig. 194** The blunt dissection arounding haemangioma is performed and deep tissue is clamped、divided and ligated with fine silk finally.

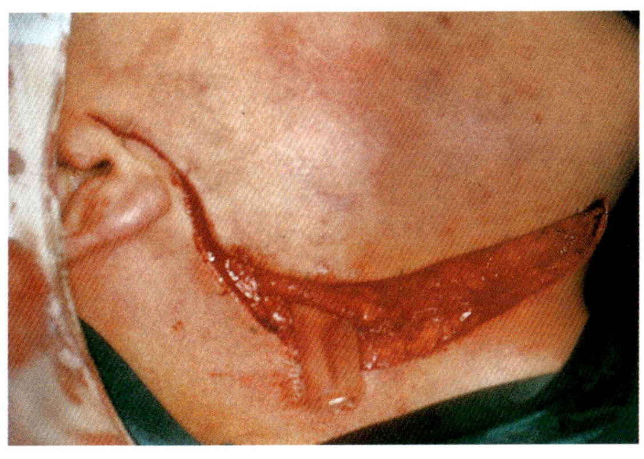

图 195

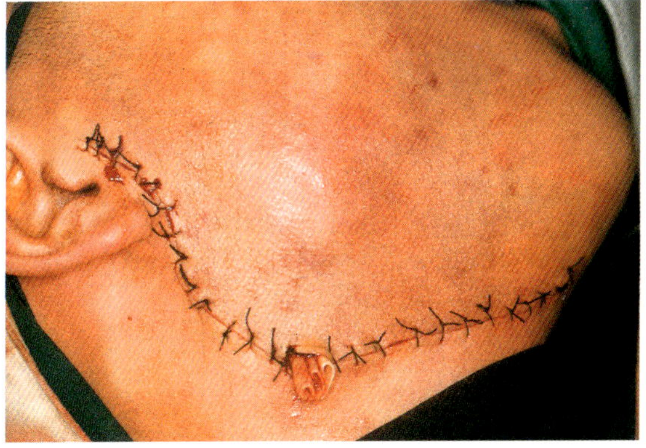

图 196

**图 195** 用生理盐水冲洗创口，彻底止血后间断缝合嚼肌。放橡皮条一根。

**图 196** 还回颊部肌皮瓣，分别缝合颈阔肌、皮下组织及皮肤。局部纱布轻压包扎。

**Fig. 195** After the wound is irrigated with saline solution, the masseter is sutured with interrupted sutures.

**Fig. 196** The wound is closed using catgut sutures for the platysma in the neck and superficial fascia on the face and interrupted silk for the skin. A small drain is inserted and a slight pressure dressing applied.

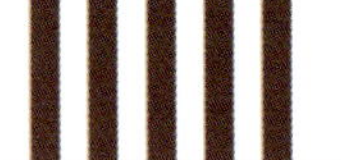



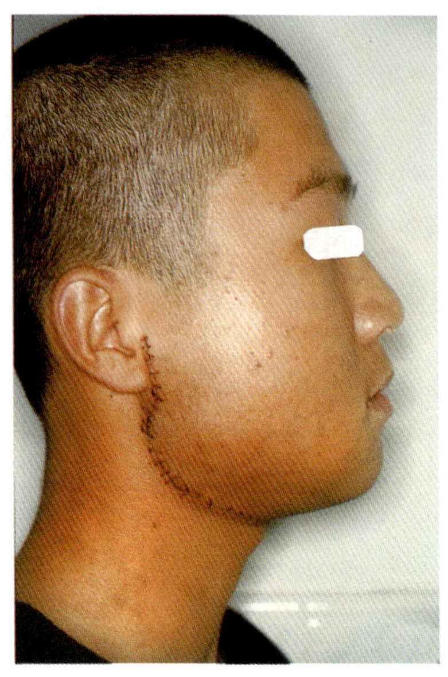

图 197

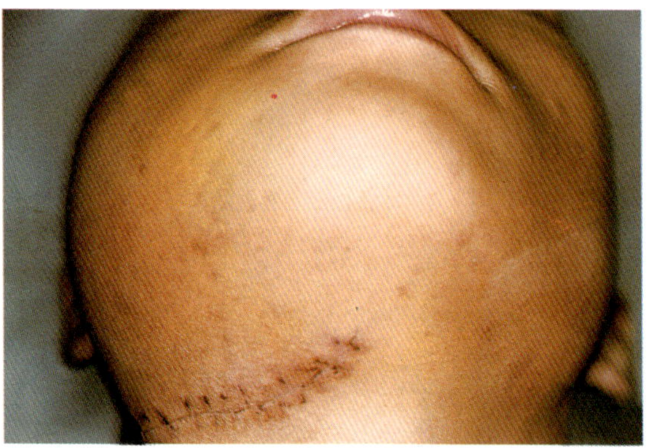

图 198

图 197, 198 术后第七天，缝线拆除后的侧面及仰面观显示创口愈合正常。

Fig. 197, 198 Lateral and submental views after suture lines have been removed 7 days after surgery show that the wound healing is normal.

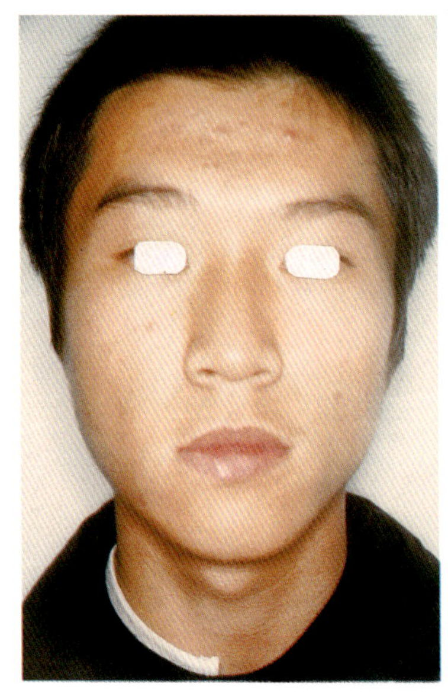

图 199

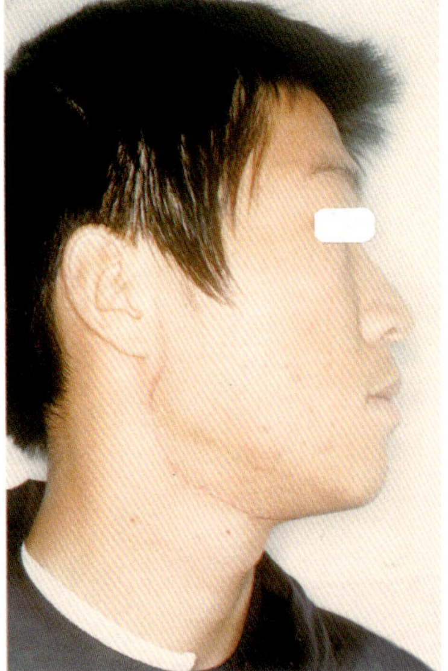

图 200

图 199, 200 术后 6 个月患者正侧面观显示两侧面部对称，血管瘤无复发。

Fig. 199, 200 Frontal and lateral views of the patient 6 mouths after surgery show that the both faces are symmetry and haemangioma no recurrence.

# 13. 颊部巨细胞瘤的外科手术治疗

# 13. Surgical excision of giant cell tumor in cheek

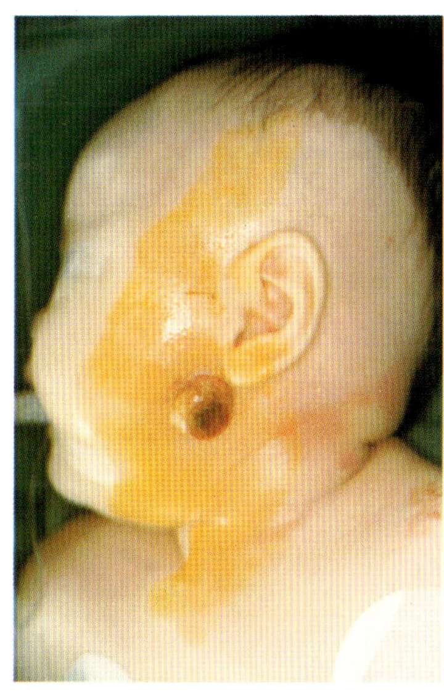

图 201

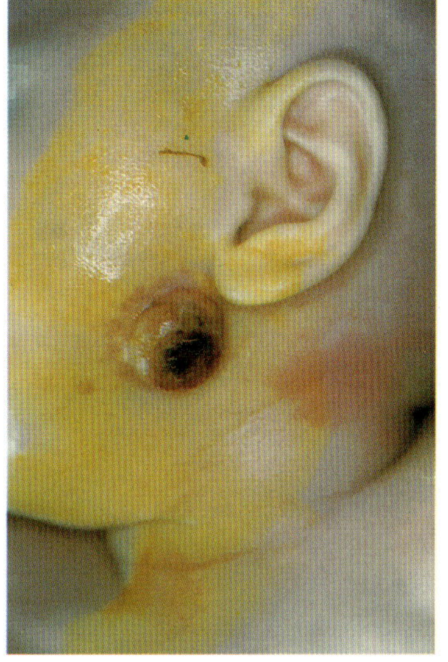

图 202

图 201，202 一患有左耳垂下巨细胞瘤的 3 个月男性患者的侧面观。

Fig. 201, 202 Lateral view of a 3 months male patient with giant cell tumor under the left ear pinna.

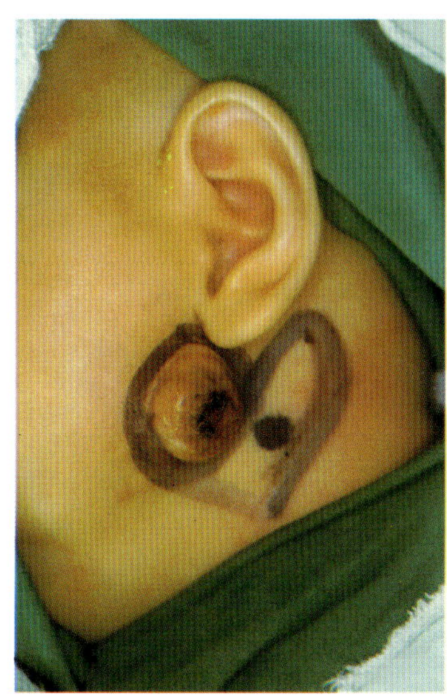

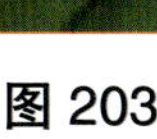

图 203

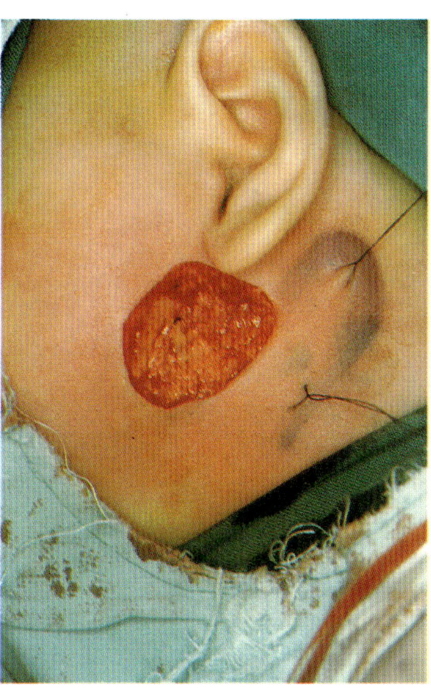

图 204

图 203 肿瘤切除及局部旋转瓣修复缺损切口设计。

图 204 肿瘤切除之后遗留的缺损区。

Fig. 203 Incision design of excision of the tumor and local rotative flap is marked out with methylene blue.

Fig. 204 Defective area after the tumor has been excised.

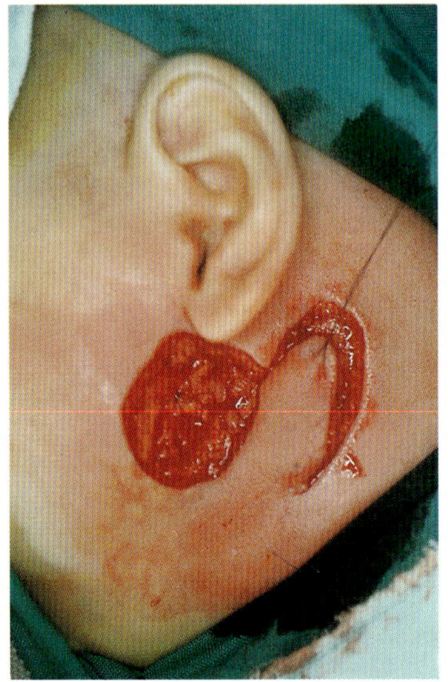

图 205

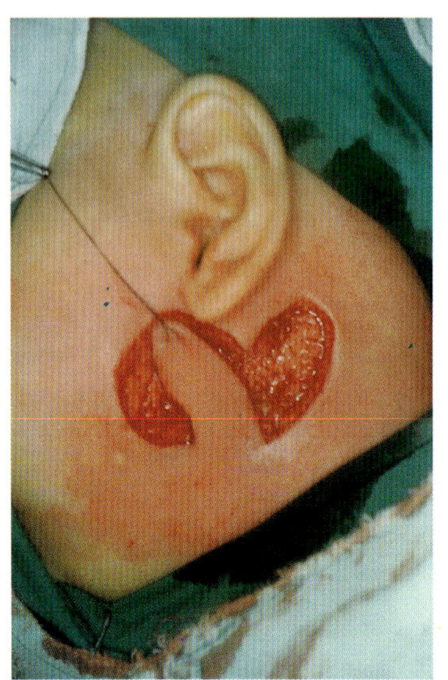

图 206

图 205　按设计的切口线切开局部旋转组织瓣，在颈阔肌上分离皮瓣。

图 206　将皮瓣转移到缺损区后行分层间断缝合。

Fig. 205　According to incision line, local rotative flap is incised and dissected from platysma.

Fig. 206　The local flap is rotated to the defective area and sutured to the defective all edges with interrupted sutures with fine silk.

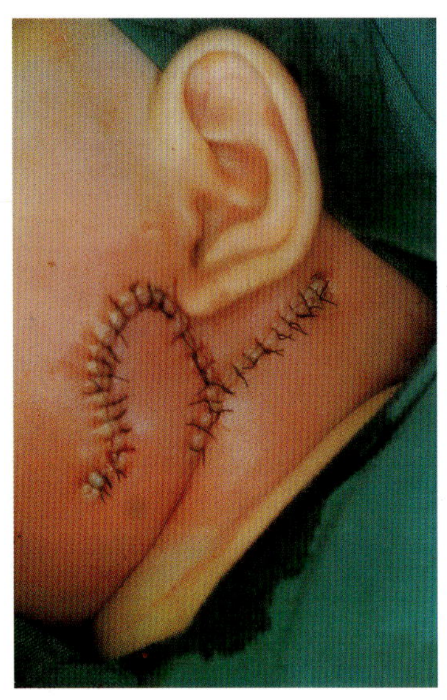

图 207

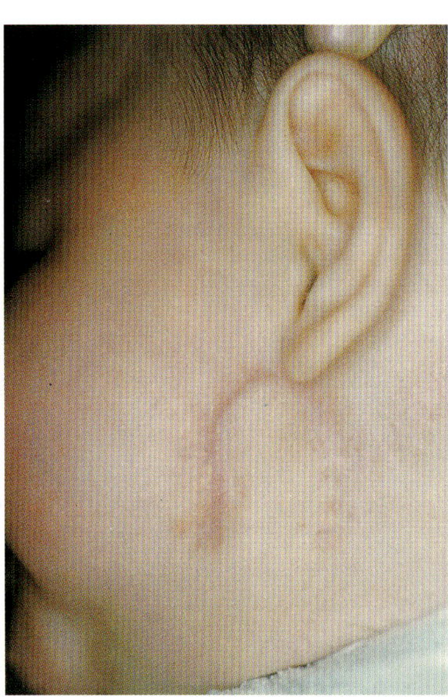

图 208

图 207　局部旋转组织瓣被缝合后的情景。

图 208　术后 8 天拆线后的情景，创口愈合良好。

Fig. 207　The condition after the local tissue flap has been sutured.

Fig. 208　The condition after the suture lines have been removed 8 days after surgery. The wound healing is fine.

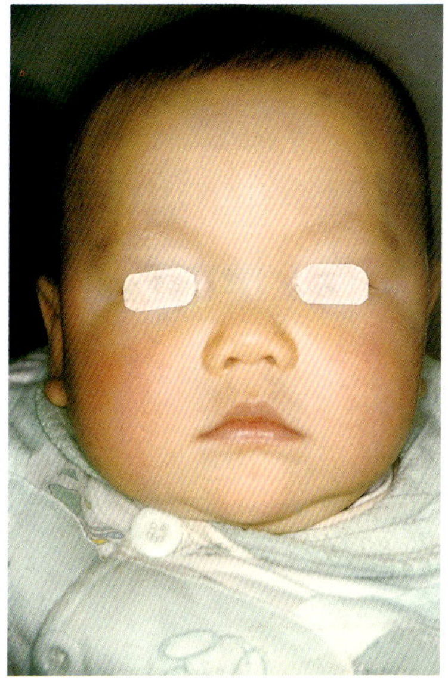

图 209

图 209 患者术后 8 天拆线后正面观。

Fig. 209 Frontal view of the patient 8 days after surgery.

# 14. 腮腺及颈上部区域血管瘤摘除术

# 14. Excision of haemangioma in the regions of parotid gland and upper neck

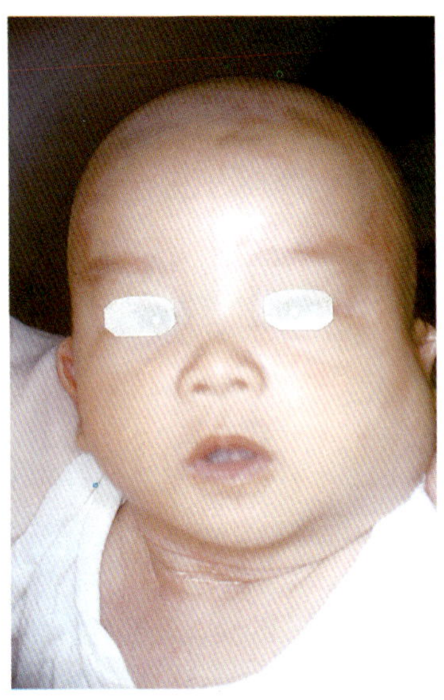

图 210

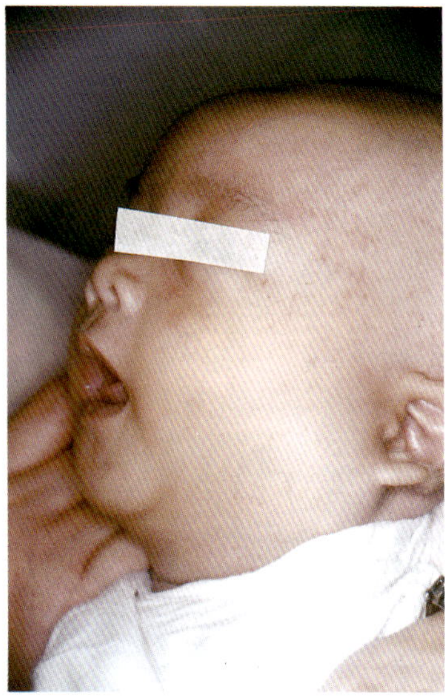

图 211

**图 210，211** 一患左腮腺及颈上部区血管瘤 53 天的男性婴儿患者正、侧面观。

正面观显示双侧腮腺区不对称，左侧明显膨隆；侧面观显示左侧颈部也明显膨隆。

**Fig. 210，211** Frontal and lateral views of a 53-day-old male infant with haemangioma in the left regions of parotid gland and upper neck.

Frontal view shows both the regions of parotid gland and upper neck asymmetry, the left regions of parotid gland and upper neck obvious expansion. Lateral view shows that the left neck region is also obvious expansion.

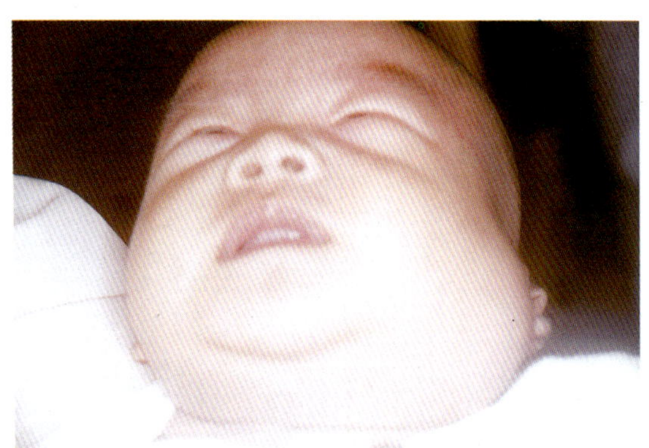

图 212

**图 212** 仰面示左侧面颈部区域明显大于右侧。

**Fig. 212** Submental view shows that the left facial and neck region is larger than the right facial and neck region.

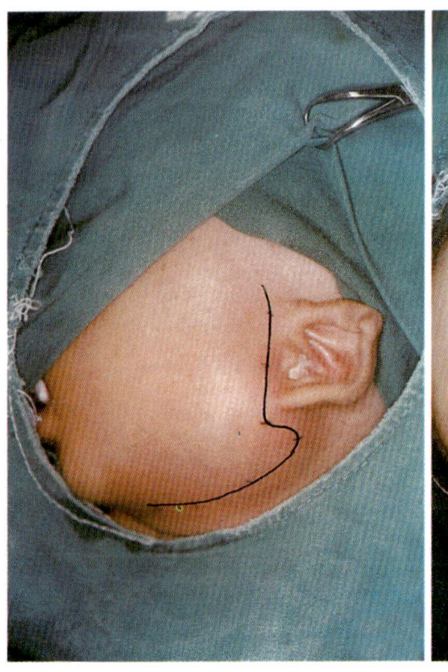

图 213

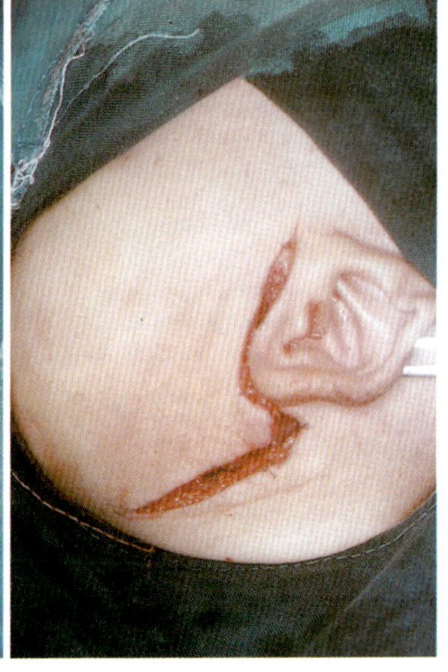

图 214

**图 213，214** 按腮腺切除术的手术术式做切口。切口从颧骨后角开始，于耳屏前向下绕耳垂向后达乳突之上，作轻度的弯曲至颈部，于下颌骨下缘并与之平行继续向前达嚼肌前缘，切开皮肤、皮下组织和颈阔肌。

**Fig. 213, 214** The skin incision for parotidectomy is made. The incision begins at the posterior angle of the zygoma and extends downward just in front of the tragus of the ear. It continues behind the lobule of the ear backward over the mastoid process. Following a gentle curve, it continues downward and forward on the neck, parallel to and below the body of the mandible. The skin and platysma is incised.

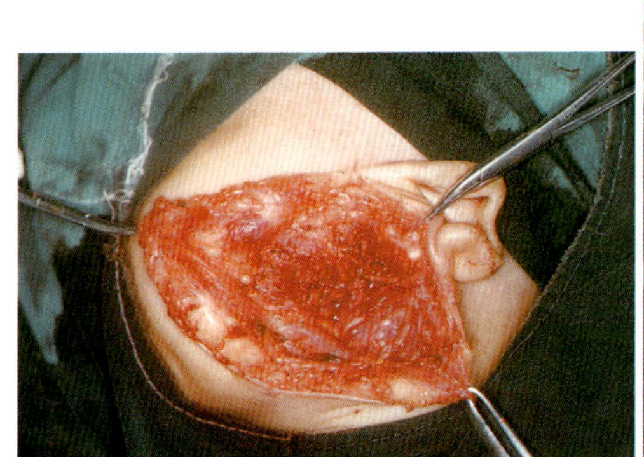

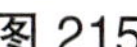

图 215

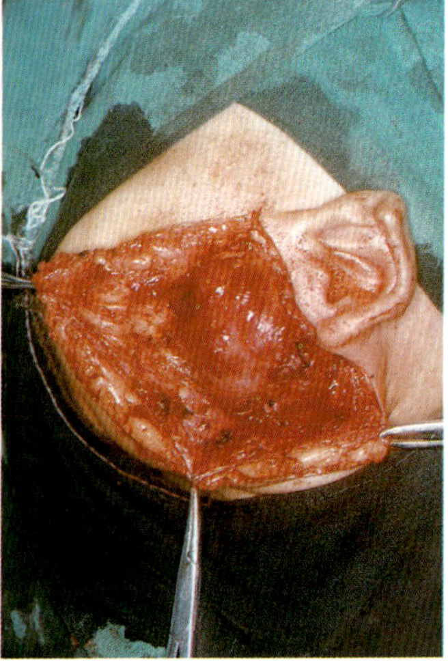

图 216

**图 215** 由后向前掀起肌皮瓣，暴露腮腺的浅面。在腮腺下极的后部切开颈深筋膜浅层并暴露胸锁乳突肌的前缘。将胸锁乳突肌向后，腮腺向前牵开，在腮腺的尾部下方鉴别二腹肌的后腹并将其向后牵开。

**图 216** 二腹肌后腹和外耳道软骨为寻找面神经的基本标志。当将二腹肌向后牵开后，沿其前缘向上解剖，将腮腺下极与肌肉分离。面神经平分了由外耳道软骨和二腹肌后腹形成的角。当分离到达此处时，继续向前分离腮腺组织见面神经。一旦神经被暴露，并在其浅面解剖腮腺下极浅叶及肿瘤，并将其结扎去除。

**Fig. 215** The skin flap is elevated, exposing the superficial portion of the parotid gland. The superficial layer of the deep cervical fascia is incised just posterior to the lower pole of the parotid and the anterior margin of the sternocleidomastoid muscle is exposed. The sternocleidomastoid is retracted posteriorly and the parotid gland pull forward, allowing the posterior belly of the digastric muscle to be identified in its location beneath the tail of the parotid. This muscle is also retracted posteriorly.

**Fig. 216** The posterior belly of the digastric muscle and the cartilage of the external auditory canal form the essential landmarks for identification of the facial nerve. As the digastric is retracted posteriorly, dissection is carried upward along its anterior margin, separating deep portions of the parotid from the muscle. The facial nerve bisects the angle formed by the cartilage of the external auditory canal and the posterior belly of the digastric. As this angle is approached, the parotid gland is dissected forward with care until the nerve is identified. Once the nerve has been exposed, dissection is carried forward immediately on its surface and the haemangioma and lower pole superficial portion of the parotid gland removed.

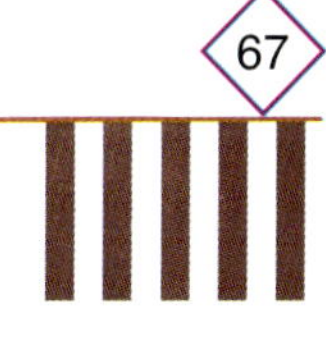

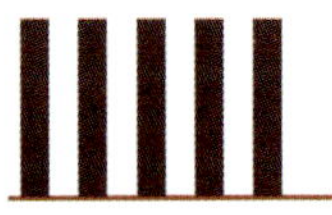



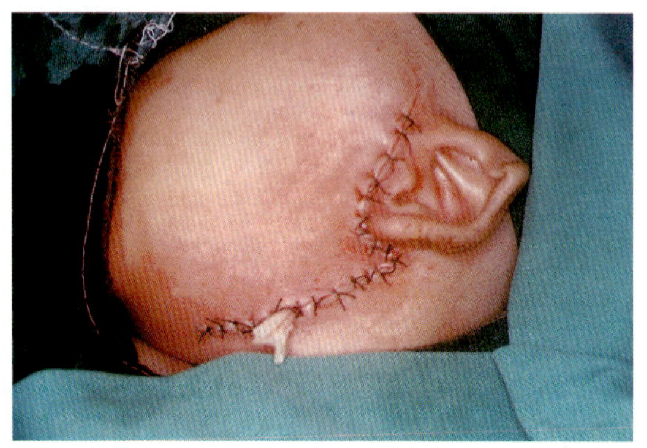

图 217

**图 217** 将皮瓣还回，使用细羊肠线缝合颈部的颈阔肌和面部的浅筋膜，间断缝合皮肤。将皮瓣还回前，将橡皮引流条放入创口中，缝合后局部加压包扎。

**Fig. 217** The wound is closed, using fine catgut sutures for the platysma in the neck and superficial fascia on the face and interrupted silk for the skin. A small drain is inserted and a large pressure dressing applied.

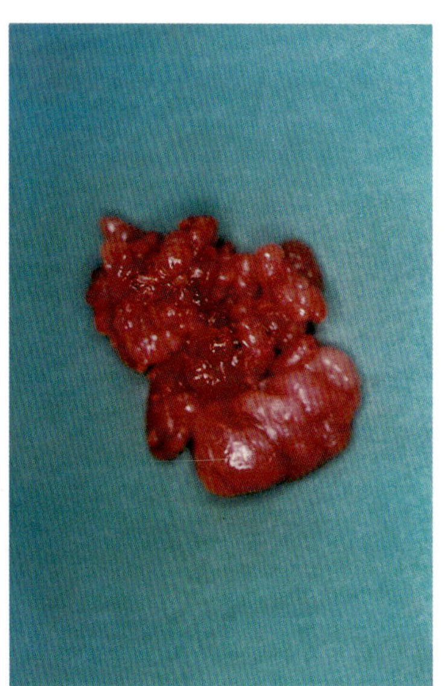

图 218

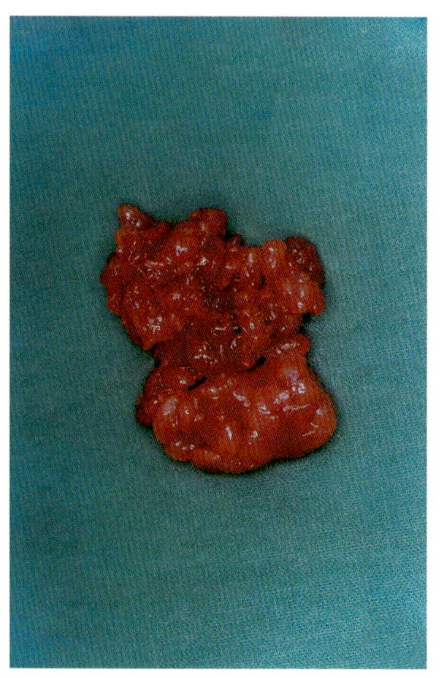

图 219

**图 218, 219** 术后标本的外及内侧面观。

**Fig. 218, 219** External and internal views of the specimen postoperatively.

# 15. 根治性颈淋巴清扫术

# 15. Radical neck dissection

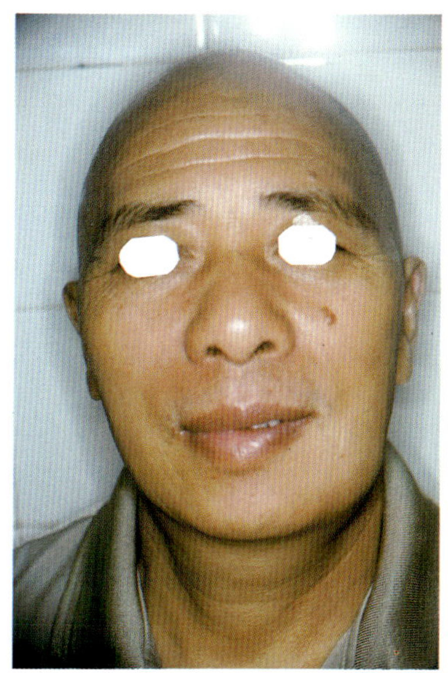

图 220

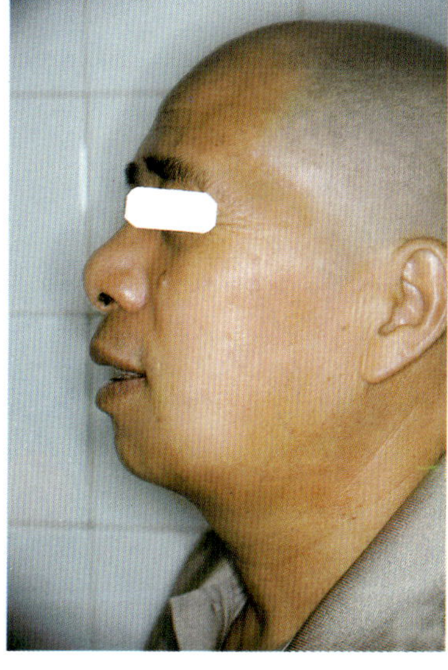

图 221

**图 220，221** 患左下颌骨中央性癌的58岁患者术前正面及侧面观。

正面观示双侧颊部不对称，左侧大于右侧。左侧颌下淋巴结增大变硬；侧面观示左颊部膨隆，下颌缘下移，颌下区膨隆。

**Fig. 220, 221** Frontal and lateral views of a 58-year-old male patient with central carcinoma of the left mandible.

Frontal view shows the cheek asymmetry, the left cheek is larger than the right cheek. The left submandibular lymphadenectasis. Lateral view shows expansion of the left cheek, the inferior border of the mandible removes downward, the submandibular region is expansive.

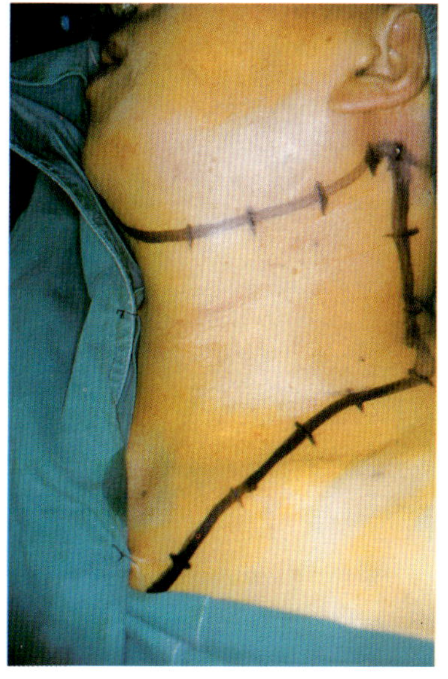

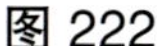

图 222

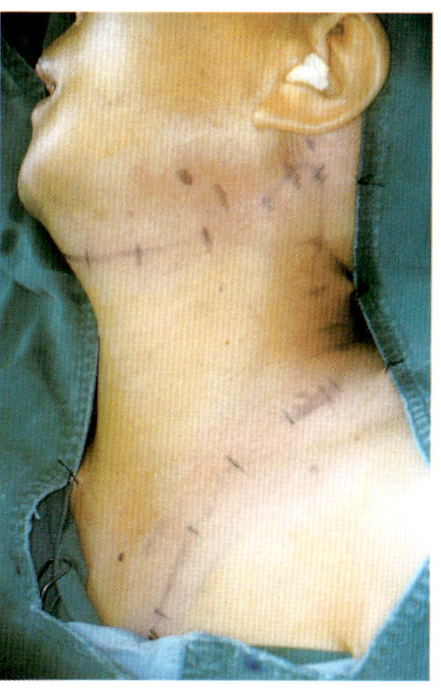

图 223

**图 222，223** 用美蓝标出颈根治性淋巴清扫术切口线。

**Fig. 222, 223** The incision line of the radical neck dissection has been marked out with methylene blue.

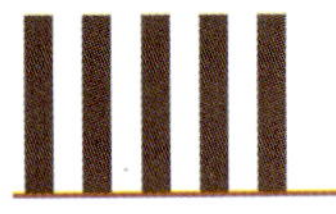



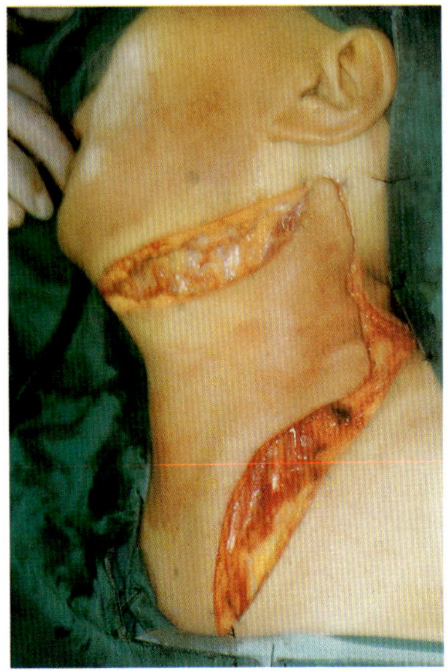

图 224

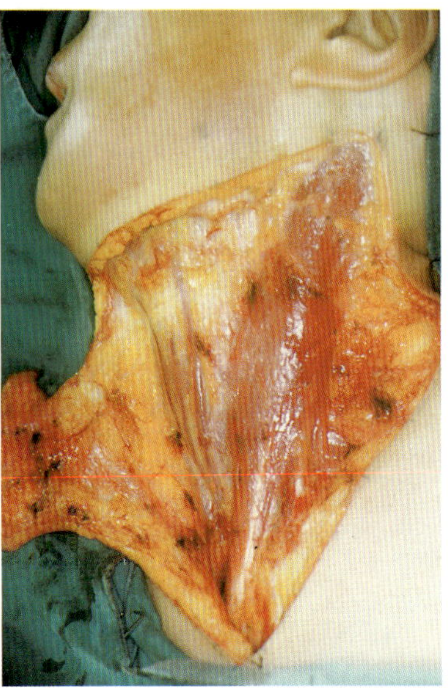

图 225

**图 224，225** 切开皮肤、皮下组织和颈阔肌，在颈阔肌深面自上而下，由后向前掀起皮肤－颈阔肌瓣，上至下颌骨下缘，前至颈中线，后至斜方肌前缘，下至锁骨下。

**Fig. 224，225** The upper curved incision is made through the skin and platysma. The vertical portion of the incision is made and flaps of skin and platysma are reflected anteriorly and posteriorly to expose the entire lateral region of the neck and the clavicle below. As the upper skin flap is retracted, the ramus marginalis mandibulae of the facial nerve is identified lying on the deep fascia. It is most easily found at the point where it crosses the facial vessels, just below the edge of the mandible. If no gross cancer is present along its course, the nerve is preserved by reflecting it upward with flap of skin and platysma. The flap is dissected a distance of 2 cm above the inferior border of the mandible. The upper limit of the dissection may be defined by incising the fascia on the lower edge of the mandible, dividing the facial vessels, and transecting the tail of the parotid gland. The anterior flap is raised until the anterior midline of the neck is reached. Posteriorly, the platysma thins out and disappears, and fibers of the upper portion of the sternocleidomastoid muscle are attached to the skin. Dissection is continued just beneath the skin until the anterior margion of the trapezius muscle is exposed. As the flaps are raised, branches of the anterior and external jugular veins are severed, the veins themselves left in situ to be removed with the block excision.

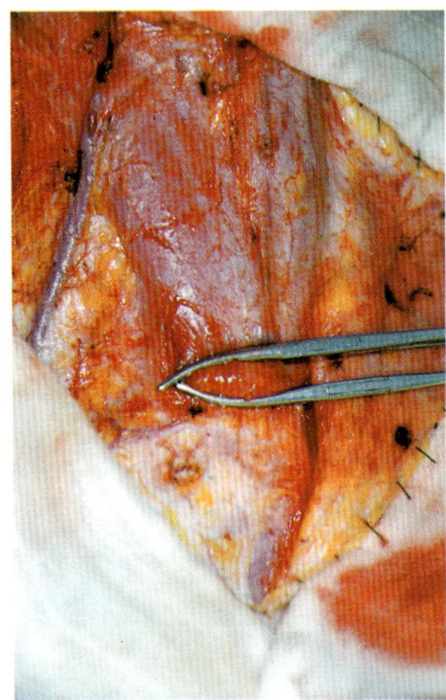

图 226

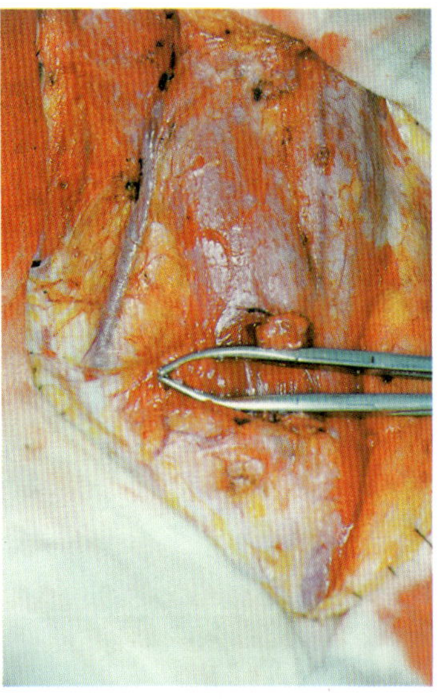

图 227

**图 226，227** 在锁骨上方约 2cm 处，用弯止血钳将胸锁乳突肌与深层组织分离，于锁骨上约 1cm 分别钳夹、切断胸锁乳突肌胸骨头和锁骨头，且缝扎其残端。

**Fig. 226，227** Block dissection of the deep structures of the neck is now commenced. The sternal and clavicular attachments of the sternocleidomastoid muscle are severed at a point 1 cm above the clavicle, care being taken to protect the underlying carotid sheath. Dissection is then carried posteriorly along the clavicle by incising the superficial layer of the deep fascia.

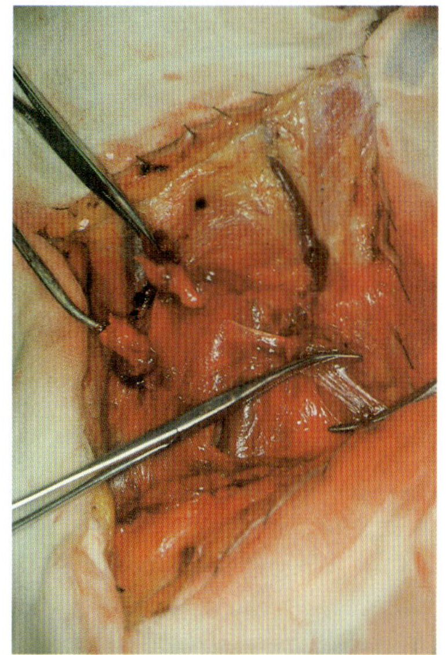

图 228

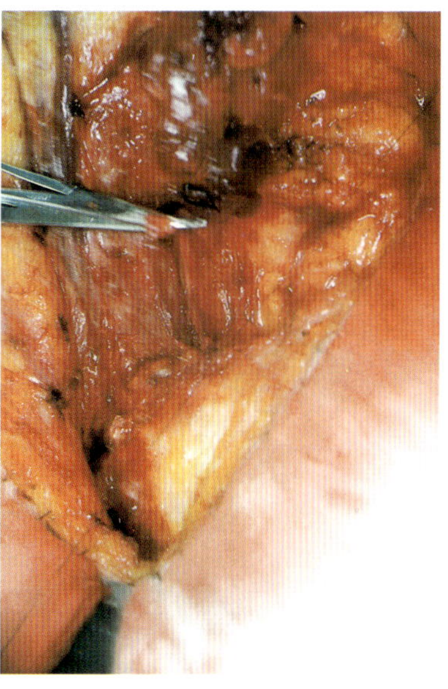

图 229

**图 228, 229** 向上翻起切断的胸锁乳突肌下端，即可见到斜行于血管鞘浅层的肩胛舌骨肌，切断其肩胛端并顺其方向游离。细心分层切开颈血管鞘，显露颈内静脉、颈总动脉和迷走神经。小心分离颈内静脉，保护其内后侧的迷走神经和颈总动脉，分别用 7 号、4 号丝线结扎颈内静脉，然后切断，再用 1 号丝线结扎其近心断端并将其固定在胸锁乳突肌的残端深面以保护。

**Fig. 228, 229** The external jugular vein is exposed and divided near the midpoint of this incision. Laterally, the omohyoid muscle is encountered and is severed just above its scapular attachment where it meets the anterior edge of the trapezius muscle. This point is the posterior corner of the block dissection. The carotid sheath is entered about 1 cm above the clavicle. The internal jugular vein is isolated at this point by careful blunt dissection. The vein is divided between ligatures, care being taken to avoid injury to the vagus nerve, which lies immediately adjacent to its posteromedial surface. After division of the vein, its lower end is additionally secured with a transfixion suture. The thoracic duct often may be identified just lateral and inferior to the point of division of jugular vein on the left side of the neck.

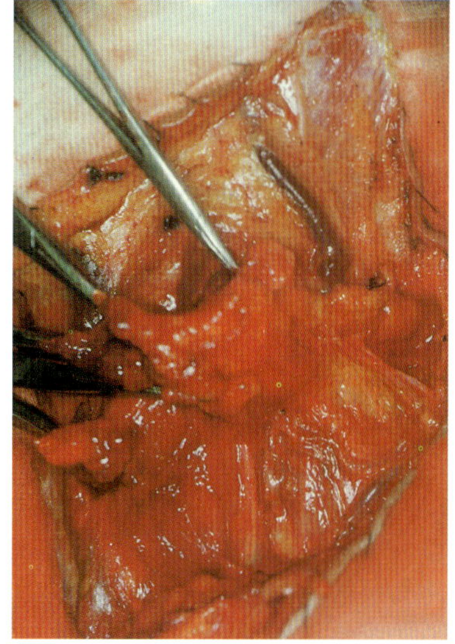

图 230

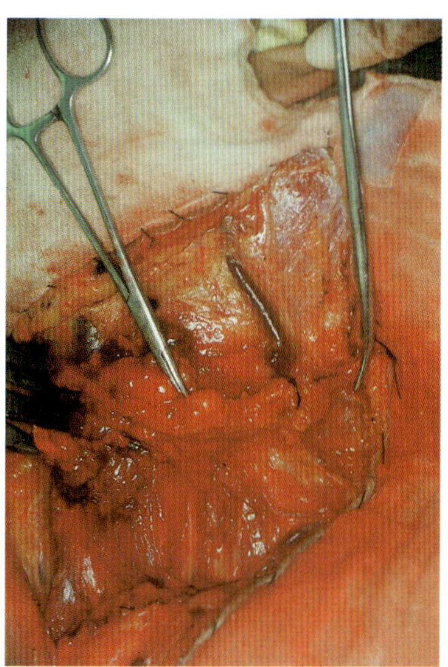

图 231

**图 230, 231** 从颈内静脉近心断端平面向斜方肌前缘作横形切口，切开颈深筋膜和脂肪，切断锁骨上皮神经分支。结扎、切断颈外静脉近心端。在脂肪组织内显露出颈横动脉、静脉，切断其分支后予以保留。继续向下解剖分离至斜角肌浅面，显露在斜角肌表面、椎前筋膜下的由外上方向内下方越过的膈神经和该肌外侧的臂丛神经，均予以保护。此平面即为手术区的底界。最后再横断斜方肌前缘处的脂肪和蜂窝组织。至此，整个手术区的下界已全部被解剖游离。

**Fig. 230, 231** The common carotid artery and vagus nerve are identified within the carotid sheath. The anterior portion of the sheath is elevated a short distance. Dissection is once again carried laterally through the fatty areolar tissue of this deep plane to outline the lower limits of the block excision. As dissection proceeds from the carotid artery outward, three important structures are encountered. The thyrocervical artery trunk or its transverse cervical branch must be divided and ligated just lateral to the carotid sheath. The phrenic nerve is noted coursing downward in an oblique direction from the posterior toward the anterior edge of the scalenus anterior muscle and is preserved. Near the outer third of the clavicle, the brachial plexus is seen in the same plane as the scalene muscles. The fatty and areolar tissue overlying the brachial plexus is continuous with the contents of the axilla. This tissue is transected at the lower outer corner of the operative field, branches of the transverse cervical vessels encountered being clamped and ligated.

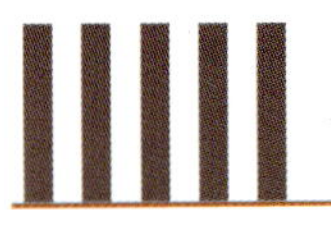



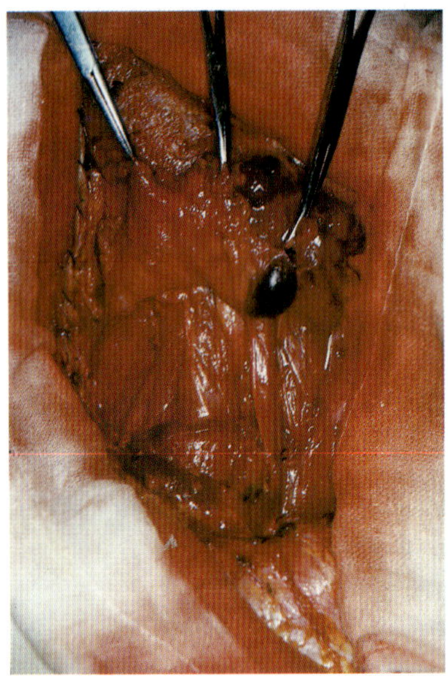

图 232

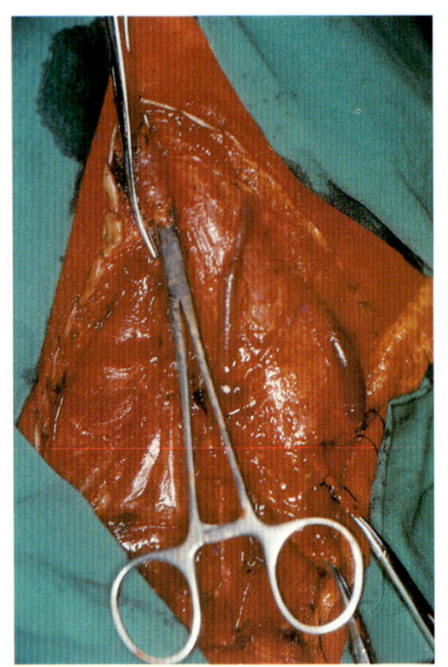

图 233

**图 232, 233** 沿斜方肌前缘及臂丛、提肩胛肌、斜角肌浅面向上解剖游离蜂窝组织和淋巴组织。沿斜方肌前缘由下向上解剖。切断并结扎斜方肌前缘的脂肪结缔组织及颈横及肩胛横动、静脉的分支。约在斜方肌前缘的中、下 1/3 交界处剪断副神经，继续向上清扫，直至胸锁乳突肌后缘。在此过程中，必须切断由椎前筋膜穿出的颈丛神经各支，但需保留膈神经，防止损伤。

**Fig. 232, 233** Once of the lower limit of the operative field has been delineated, attention is directed to the posterior triangle of the neck. Dissection commences at the anterior margin of the trapezius muscle and this is cleared upward. From this landmark, dissection is continued medially just superficial to the brachial plexus and the levator scapulae, and the scalene muscles. Numerous anastomatic branches of the transverse cervical and suprascapular arteries are encountered in this region and must be secured. No attempt is made to preserve the spinal accessory nerve. To do so would necessitate entering a plane potentially containing cancer. As the nerve is severed, one notes a sudden contraction of the trapezius and levator scapulae. As dissection proceeds medially in the excellent fascial plane forming the floor of the posterior triangle, branches of the cervical nerves are encountered emerging from the deep structures of the neck and curving superficially into the tissue being removed. Care should be taken to sever the branches of the 5th and 6th cervical nerves peripheral to the origin of the phrenic nerve from them.

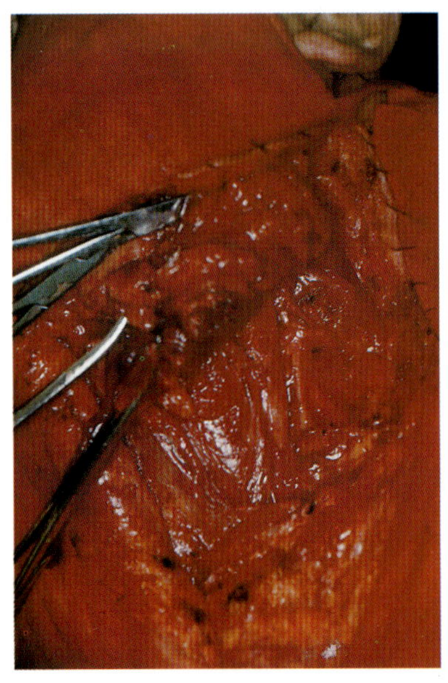

图 234

**图 234** 将已解剖游离的胸锁乳突肌、颈内静脉、肩胛舌骨肌及脂肪结缔组织在椎前筋膜、颈动脉和迷走神经浅面向上分离，直至颈动脉分叉部。

**Fig. 234** Dissection passes over the phrenic nerve, the carotid artery and vagus nerve are again exposed. The anterior and lateral portions of the carotid sheath are dissected upward with the sternocleidomastoid, the internal jugular vein, surrounding lymphatic and areolar tissue. The cervical sympathetic trunk is identified in its position just lateral and posterior to the common carotid artery.

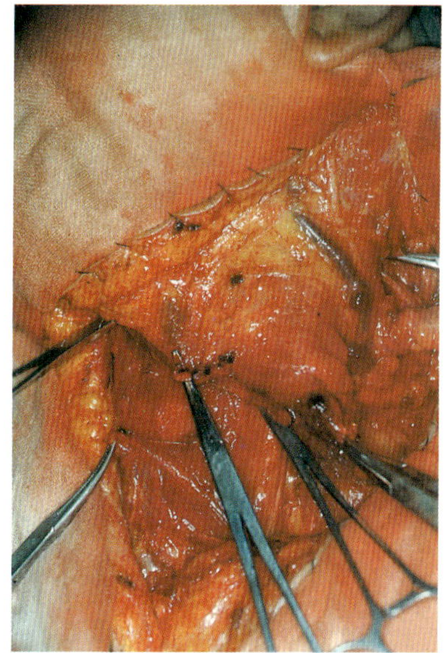

图 235

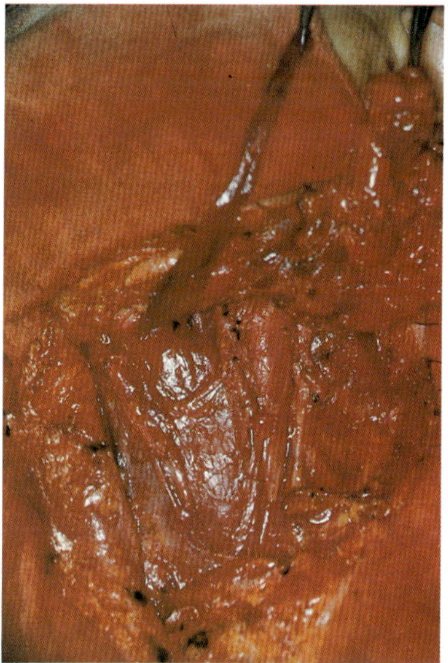

图 236

**图 235，236** 沿胸骨舌骨肌内侧切开颈深筋膜浅层，由前向后解剖游离胸骨舌骨肌浅面组织，并在肩胛舌骨肌的舌骨附着处剪断该肌。

**Fig. 235，236** The anterior portion of the block dissection may now be completed rapidly by incising the superficial layer of the deep cervical fascia just lateral to the sternohyoid muscle. The anterior margin of the anterior belly of the omohyoid muscle forms an excellent landmark for this incision. The muscle is followed upward and is finally severed at its attachment to the hyoid bone. It is advisable at this point to review the entire field, ligate bleeding vesseles, remove all hemostats, and cover the dissected area with fresh warm pads.

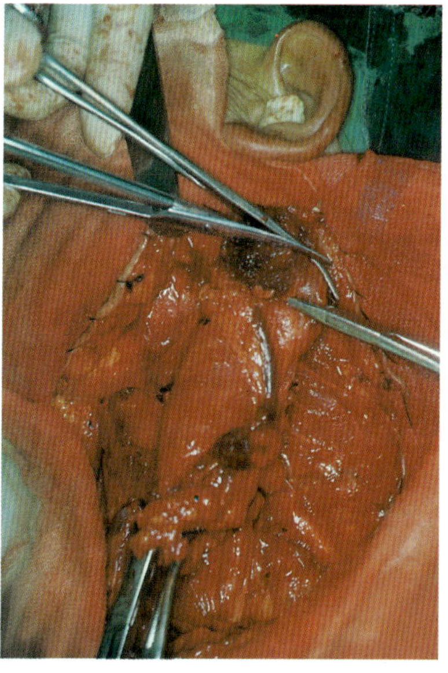

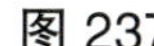

图 237

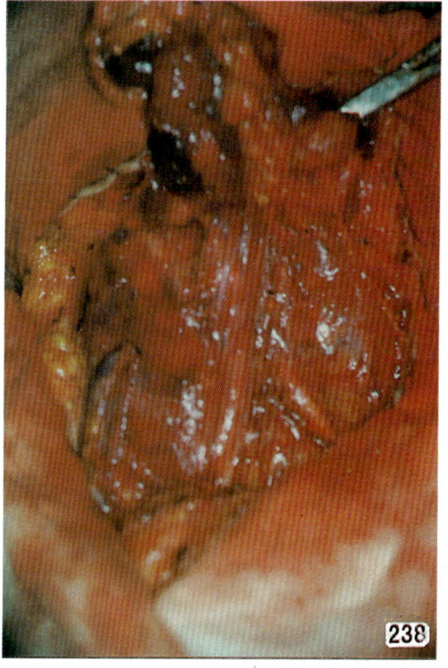


图 238

**图 237, 238** 继续向上解剖分离胸锁乳突肌直至该肌上端，在乳突尖下约 1cm 处切断胸锁乳突肌上端的附着。将游离组织上提，显露颈动脉分支。同时应注意保护舌下神经。

**Fig. 237, 238** Dissection proceeds cephalad and the sternocleidomastoid muscle is severed at the mastoid process and retracted anteriorly. This allows further upward exposure of the carotid artery and its bifurcation. Dissection of the sheath over the bifurcation of the artery may in same patients incite a carotid sinus reflex evidenced by bradycardia and hypotention. The reflex effects can be controlled by infiltration of the adventitia of the artery at its bifurcation with 1% Procaine. The hypoglossal nerve is identified as it crosses the external and internal carotid arteries curving forward beneath the posterior belly of the digastric muscles.

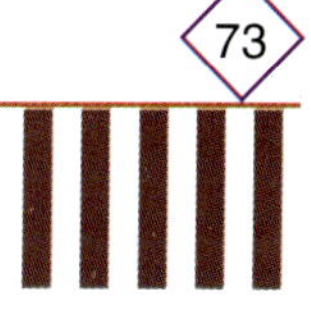

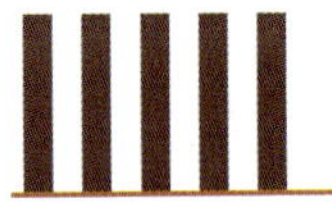



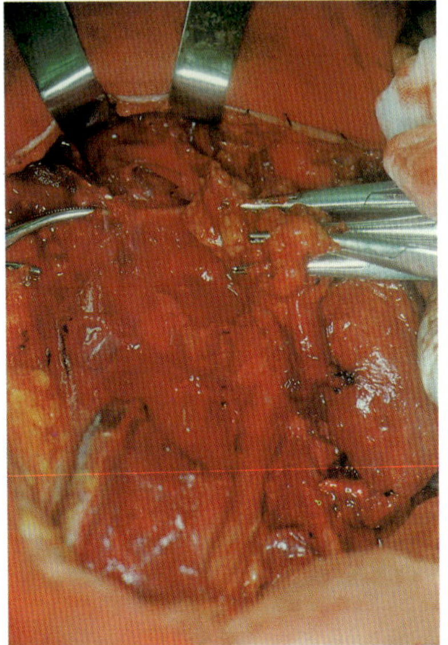

图 239

图 239 沿两侧二腹肌前腹间的下颌舌骨肌浅面由对侧向患侧的颌下方清扫颏下三角区的蜂窝组织和淋巴结。

Fig. 239 The submental space is then cleared from above downward. Dissection is carried between the two anterior bellies of the digastric muscles and directly on the surface of the mylohyoid muscle. The fatty-areolar tissue and lymph nodes forming the contents of the submental space are dissected downward to the hyoid bone and laterally to the side of the operative specimen.

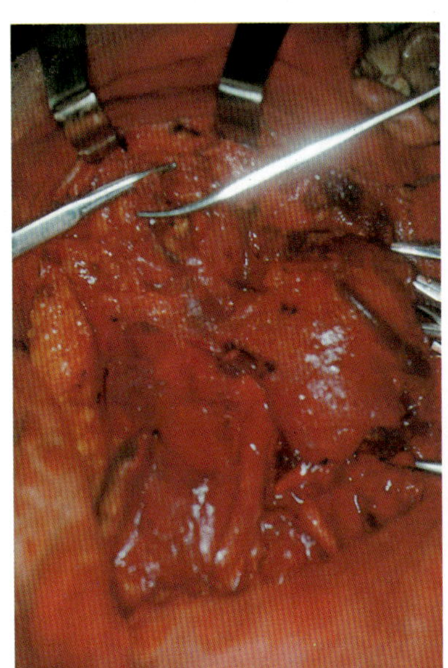

图 240

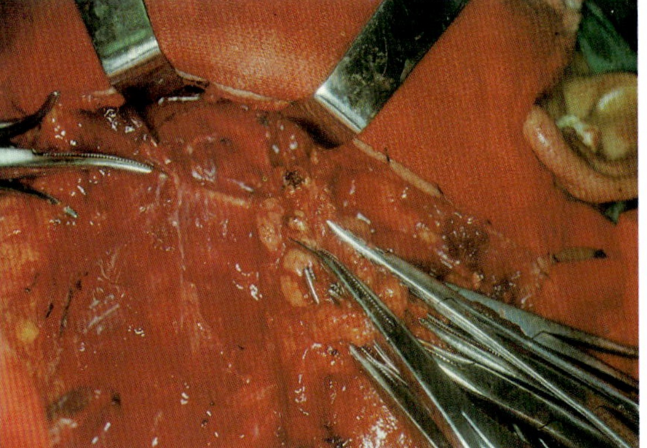

图 241

图 240, 241 自二腹肌前腹至乳突切开颈深筋膜浅层，在下颌角平面切开腮腺尾叶下极，缝扎残端于二腹肌后腹上，以免术后形成涎瘘。在处理腮腺尾部时应注意结扎面后静脉及颈外静脉上端。双重结扎后切断颌外动脉和面前静脉。分离颌下腺并向后下牵拉，将下颌舌骨肌向前上方拉开，即可显露颌下腺、与颌下腺相连的舌神经鼓索支和舌神经。剪断鼓索支，保护舌神经。

Fig. 240, 241 The upper limit of the dissection to be performed is now defined by incising the deep fascia directly on the lower free edge of the mandible. This incision commences anteriorly at the insertion of the digastric muscle. At the midpoint of the mandible, the facial vessels are divided and ligated. As the angle of the mandible is approached, the tail of the parotid gland is encountered. The incision is carried directly across this portion of the parotid to the mastoid process. The external jugular vein and the anterior division of the posterior facial vein are divided within the parotid. The submaxillary triangle is next entered, commencing dissection along the anterior belly of the digastric muscle and proceeding posteriorly on the surface of the mylohyoid muscle. When the free posterior border of the mylohyoid muscle is reached, it is retracted anteriorly to expose the submaxillary salivary gland lying on the hyoglossus muscle. The hypoglossal nerve surrounded by the two lingual veins is seen crossing the hyoglossus beneath the gland. The gland is gently retracted downward away from the mandible, exposing the lingual nerve. The small branch from the lingual nerve to the submaxillary gland is divided.

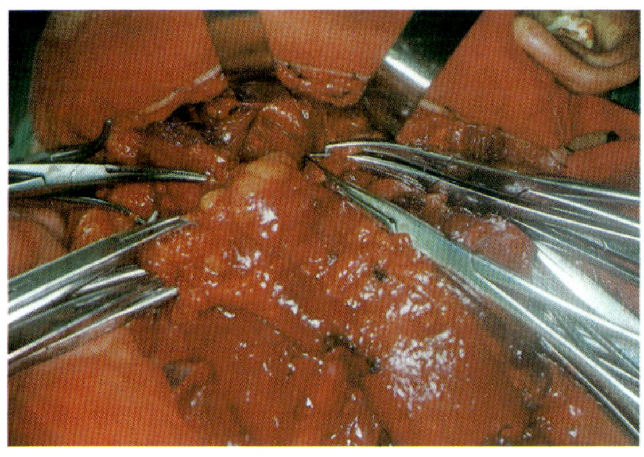

图 242

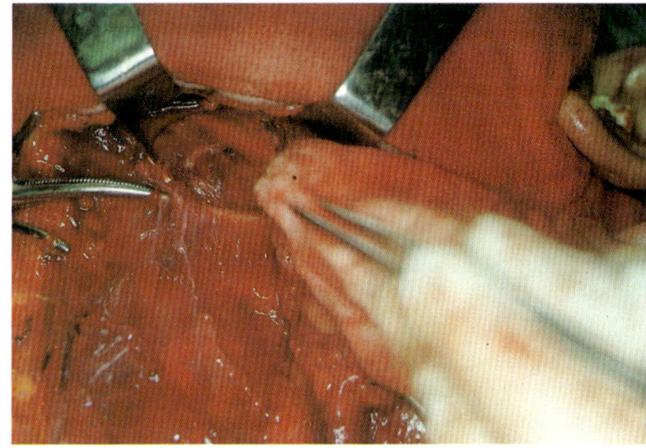

图 243

**图 242，243** 切断并结扎颌下腺导管，将颌下腺及颌下三角区的蜂窝组织、淋巴结解剖分离，在颌下腺外侧、二腹肌后腹上缘处双重结扎后切断颌外动脉近心端。切断二腹肌后腹和茎突舌骨肌在舌骨上的附着，清扫完整个颌下三角区。

**Fig. 242, 243** The submaxillary duct is identified coursing inferior to the lingual nerve. The lingual nerve must be seen before division of the duct to avoid section of the nerve by error. The duct is divided and ligated. The gland, with surrounding fatty－areolar tissue and lymph nodes, is dissected posteriorly and inferiorly toward the posterior belly of the digastric muscle. As the dissection of the submaxillary triangle is completed, the last structure encountered is the facial branch of the external carotid artery. This vessel enters the triangle beneath the posterior belly of the digastric muscle and is applied closely to the posterior surface of the submaxillary gland. The vessel is divided just above the edge of the digastric muscle. For the best exposure of the digastric area, it is advisable to divide the posterior belly of the digastric and stylohyoid muscles at the hyoid bone and reflect them backward to their attachments on the mastoid where they are again divided.

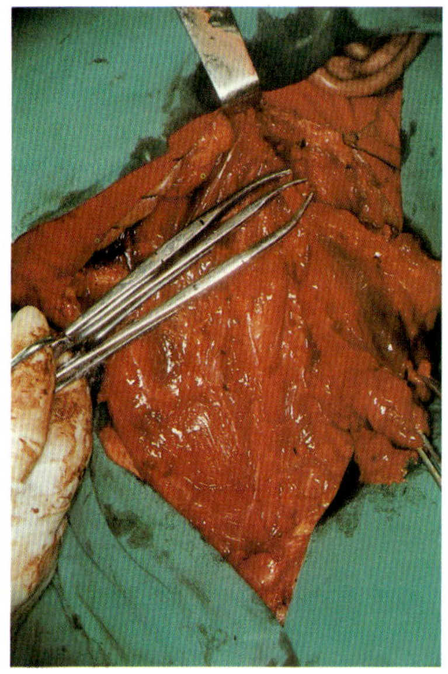

图 244

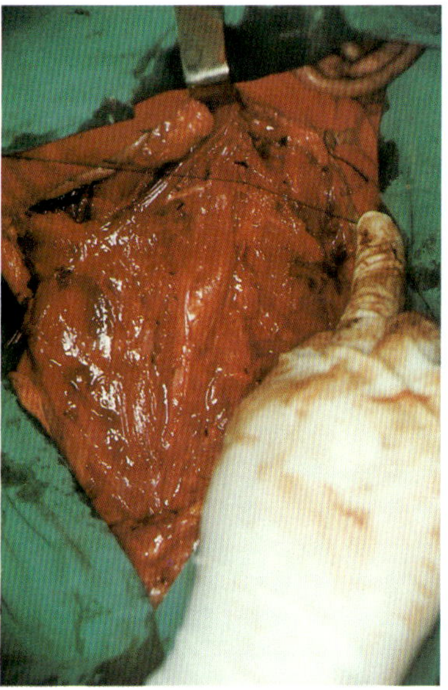

图 245

**图 244，245** 将已解剖游离的各区组织继续向上游离至茎突，最大限度地、仔细分离颈内静脉上端，结扎其分支，最后双重结扎颈内静脉远心端，并缝扎固定其残端，以防结扎线松脱出血。在此过程中，应注意清除二腹肌深面近颅底处的颈深上淋巴结，并避免损伤迷走神经和舌下神经。至此，一侧颈淋巴清扫全部完毕，整块组织即可完整取下。

**Fig. 244, 245** The upper end of the internal jugular vein must now be divided. The vein is exposed by elevating or reflecting the posterior belly of the digastric muscle and carefully dividing the loose facial envelope surrounding the vein beneath the muscle. The proximal portions of the hypoglossal and vagus nerves are once more identified and protected. The vein is divided opposite the palpable prominence of the transverse process of the atlas. As the vein is divided and ligated, the upper portion of the spinal accessory nerve is visualized and severed, thus removing the last attachment of the operative specimen.

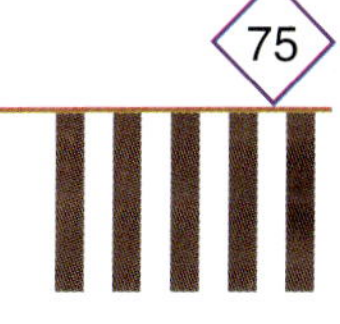

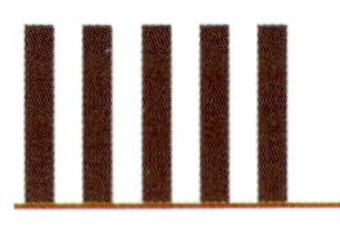



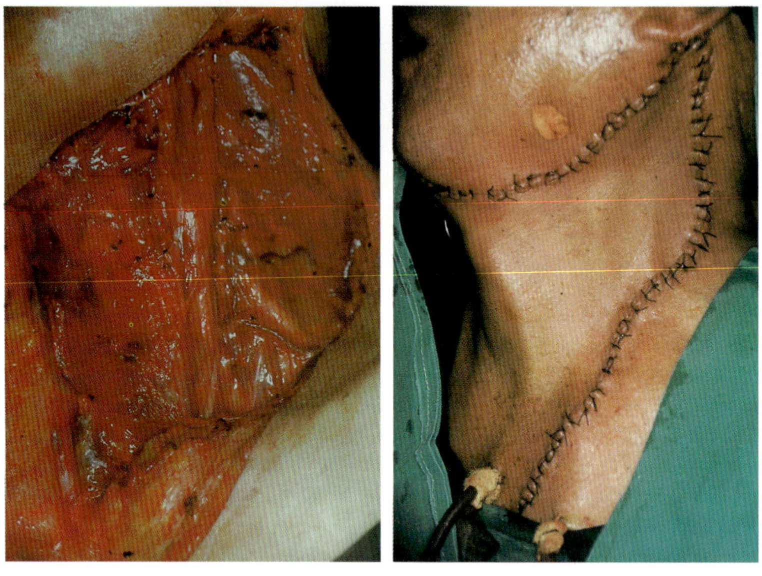

图 246　　图 247

**图 246, 247** 大量生理盐水反复冲洗术创，彻底止血，并用 1% 的氮芥湿敷创面；安置双管负压引流管，并予以固定，将皮肤－颈阔肌瓣复位，分层间断缝合，以消毒纱布覆盖创口。

**Fig. 246, 247** The entire wound is inspected for hemostasis, after which it is irrigated with saline solution. Two penrose drains are placed in the wound, one directed anteriorly and the other posteriorly. The drains may be brought out through the lower angle of the wound or through a stab wound in the lateral skin flap. The flaps are then approximated with buried sutures in the platysma and interrupted sutures of fine silk in the skin. A bulky pressure dressing is applied to the neck.

# 16. 颊癌切除后额岛状瓣颊部缺损修复术

# 16. Island forehead flap repair in resection for buccal cancer

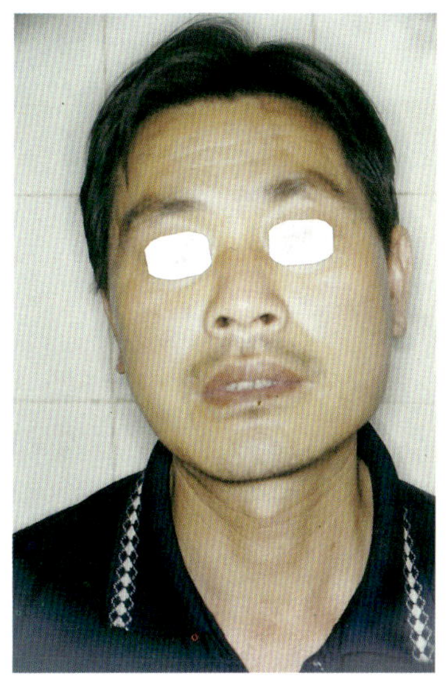
图 248

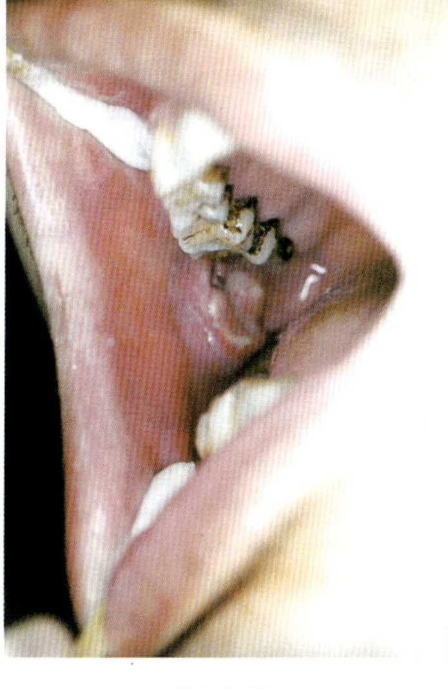
图 249

**图 248** 患右侧颊部鳞状细胞癌患者术前正面观。

**图 249** 显示向深层组织浸润的颊部鳞状细胞癌，但癌未侵犯颊部皮肤。

**Fig. 248** Preoperative frontal view of a patient with a squamous cell carcinoma of the right buccal mucosa.

**Fig. 249** View of a squamous cell carcinoma with a degree of deep inflatration into muscle but not to skin.

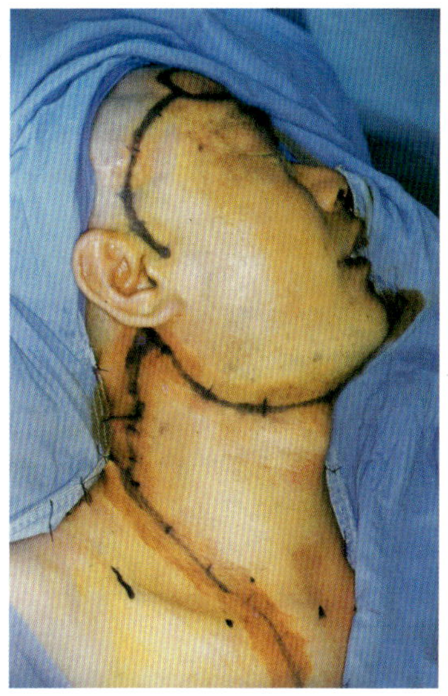
图 250

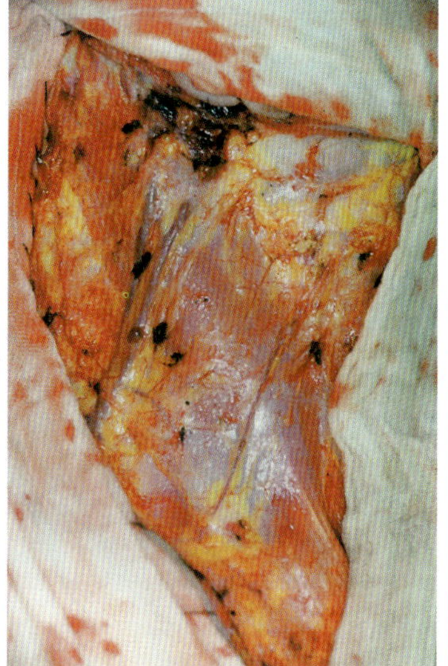
图 251

**图250** 设计手术切口并用美蓝画出切口线。

**图251** 按切口线先切开颈清扫术的颈部皮肤、皮下组织和颈阔肌，在颈阔肌深面自上而下，由后向前掀起皮肤－颈阔肌瓣，上至下颌下缘，前至颈中线，后至斜方肌前缘，下至锁骨下。

**Fig. 250** Incision line is designed with methylene blue.

**Fig. 251** After incision line has been marked out, the upper curved incision of the radical neck dissection is made through the skin and platysma. The vertical portion of the incision is made and flaps of skin and platysma are reflected anteriorly and posteriorly to expose the entire lateral region of the neck and the clavicle below. As the flaps are raised, branches of the anterior and external jugular veins and sternocleidomastoid muscle are exposed within the operative field.

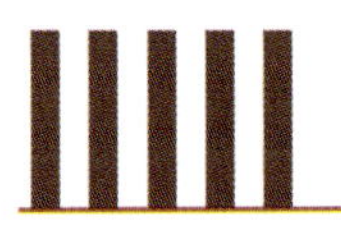



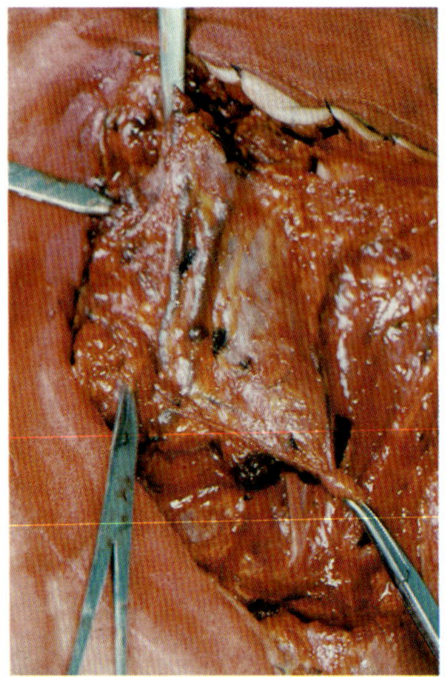

图 252

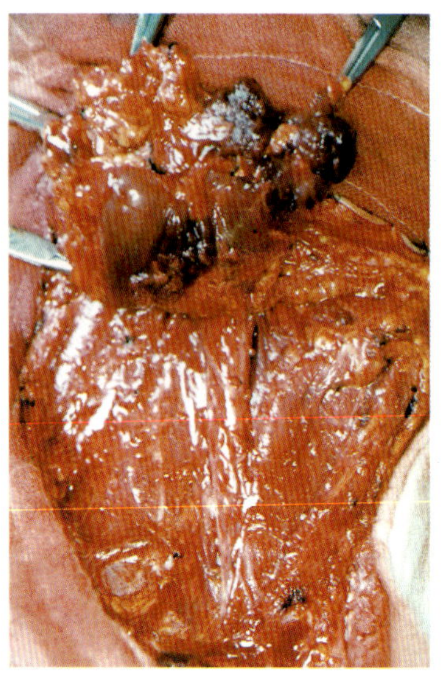

图 253

**图 252** 向上翻起切断的胸锁乳突肌下端，即可见到斜行于血管鞘浅层的肩胛舌骨肌，切断其肩胛端并顺其方向游离。细心分层切开颈血管鞘，显露颈内静脉、颈总动脉和迷走神经。小心分离颈内静脉，保护其内后侧的迷走神经和颈总动脉，分别用 7 号、4 号丝线结扎颈内静脉，然后切断，再用 1 号丝线结扎其近心端并将其固定在胸锁乳突肌的残端深面以保护。

从颈内静脉近心端平面向斜方肌前缘作横形切口，切开颈深筋膜和脂肪，切断锁骨上皮神经分支。结扎切断颈外静脉近心端。在脂肪组织内显露出颈横动脉、静脉，切断其分支后予以保留。继续向下分离至斜角肌浅面，显露在斜角肌表面、椎前筋膜下的由外上方向内下方越过的膈神经和该肌外侧的臂丛神经，均予以保护。此平面即手术区的底界。最后再横断斜方肌前缘处的脂肪和蜂窝组织。至此，整个手术区的下界已全部被解剖游离。

沿斜方肌前缘及臂丛、提肩胛肌、斜角肌浅面向上解剖游离蜂窝组织和淋巴组织。沿斜方肌前缘由下向上解剖。切断并结扎斜方肌前缘的脂肪结缔组织及颈横及肩胛横动、静脉的分支。约在斜方肌前缘的中、下 1/3 交界处剪断副神经，继续向上清扫，直至胸锁乳突肌后缘。在此过程中，必须切断由椎前筋膜穿出的颈丛神经各支，但需保留膈神经，防止损伤。

**图 253** 将已解剖游离的胸锁乳突肌、颈内静脉、肩胛舌骨肌及脂肪结缔组织在椎前筋膜、颈动脉和迷走神经浅面向上分离，直至颈动脉分叉部。

**Fig. 252** The external jugular vein is exposed and divided near the midpoint of this incision. Laterally, the omohyoid muscle is encountered and is severed just above its scapular attachment where it meets the anterior edge of the trapezius muscle. This point is the posterior corner of the block dissection. The carotid sheath is entered about 1 cm above the clavicle. The internal jugular vein is isolated at this point by careful blunt dissection. The vein is divided between ligatures, care being taken to avoid injury to the vagus nerve, which lies immediately adjacent to its posteromedial surface. After division of the vein, its lower end is additionally secured with a transfixion suture. The thoracic duct often may be identified just lateral and inferior to the point of division of jugular vein on the left side of the neck.

The common carotid artery and vagus nerve are identified within the carotid sheath. The anterior portion of the sheath is elevated a short distance. Dissection is once again carried laterally through the fatty areolar tissue of this deep plane to outline the lower limits of the block excision. As dissection proceeds from the carotid artery outward, three important structures are encountered. The thyrocervical artery trunk or its transverse cervical branch must be divided and ligated just lateral to the carotid sheath. The phrenic nerve is noted coursing downward in an oblique direction from the posterior toward the anterior edge of the scalenus anterior muscle and is preserved. Near the outer third of the clavicle, the brachial plexus is seen in the same plane as the scalene muscles. The fatty and areolar tissue overlying the brachial plexus is continous with the contents of the axilla. The tissue is transected at the lower outer corner of the operative field, branches of the transverse cervical vessels encountered being clamped and ligated.

Once of the lower limit of the operative field has been delineated, attention is directed to the posterior triangle of the neck. Dissection commences at the anterior margin of the trapezius muscle and this is cleared upward. From this landmark, dissection is continued medially just superficial to the brachial plexus and the levator scapulae, and the scalene muscles. Numerous anastomatic branches of the transverse cervical and suprascapular arteries are encountered in this region and must be secured. No attempt is made to preserve the spinal accessory nerve. To do so would necessitate entering a plane potentially containing cancer. As the nerve is severed, one notes a sudden contraction of the trapezius and levator scapulae. As dissection proceeds medially in the excellent fascial plane forming the floor of the posterior triangle, branches of the cervical nerve are encountered emerging from the deep structures of the neck and curving superficially into the tissue being removed. Care should be taken to sever the branches of the 5th and 6th cervical nerve peripheral to the origin of the phrenic nerve from them.

Fig. 253 Dissection passes over the phrenic nerve, and the carotid artery and vagus nerve are again exposed. The anterior and lateral portions of the carotid sheath are dissected upward with the sternocleidomastoid, the internal jugular vein an surrounding lymphatic and areolar tissue. The cervical sympathetic trunk is identified in its position just lateral and posterior to the common carotid artery.

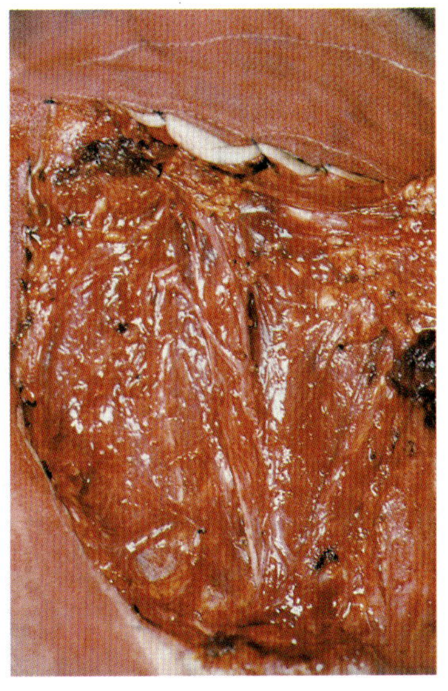

图 254

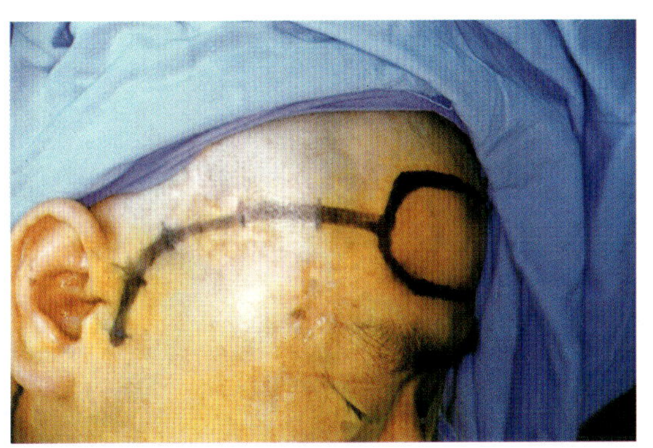

图 255

**图 254** 沿胸骨舌骨肌内侧切开颈深筋膜浅层，由前向后解剖游离胸骨舌骨肌浅面组织，并在肩胛舌骨肌的舌骨附着处剪断该肌。继续向上解剖分离胸锁乳突肌直至该肌上端，在乳突尖下约 1cm 处切断胸锁乳突肌上端的附着。将游离组织上提，显露颈动脉分支。同时应注意保护舌下神经。沿两侧二腹肌前腹间的下颌舌骨肌浅面由对侧向患侧的颌下方清扫颏下三角区的蜂窝组织和淋巴结，最后清扫颌下三角区。颈清被完成。

**图 255** 按全额岛状瓣设计画出切口线，其范围为两侧至眼外眦角，上界为发际，下界为眉弓之上，皮下蒂达患侧耳屏前区。

Fig. 254 The anterior portion of the block dissection may now be completed rapidly by incising the superficial layer of the deep cervical fascia just lateral to the sternohyoid muscle. The anterior margin of the anterior belly of the omohyoid muscle forms an excellent landmark for this incision. The muscle is followed upward and is finally severed at its attachment to the hyoid bone. It is advisable at this point to review the entire field, ligate bleeding vesseles, remove all hemostats, and cover the dissected area with fresh warm pads.

Dissection proceeds cephalad and the sternocleidomastoid muscle is severed at the mastoid process and retracted anteriorly. This allows further upward exposure of the carotid artery and its bifurcation. Dissection of the sheath over the bifurcation of the artery may in same patients incite a carotid sinus reflex evidenced by bradycardia and hypotention. The reflex effects can be controlled by infiltration of the adventitia of the artery at its bifurcation with 1% Procaine. The hypoglossal nerve is identified as it cross the external and internal carotid arteries are curves forward beneath the posterior belly of the digastric muscles.

The submental space is then cleared from above downward. Dissection is carried between the two anterior bellies of the digastric muscles and directly on the surface of the mylohyoid muscle. The fatty-areolar tissue and lymph nodes forming the contents of the submental space are dissected downward to the hyoid bone and laterally to the side of the operative specimen. Finally, the dissection of the submaxillary triangle is completed. The radical neck dissection is completed.

Fig. 255 The forehead flap used in intraoral reconstruction is laterally based, its base extending from the lateral border of the eyebrow to the anterior border of the pinna at approximately the level of the zygomatic arch, the flap itself curving across the hairless forehead. Its breadth is generally that of the forehead from eyebrow to hairline; Its length is variable but most often extends to the hair-line on the opposite temple. The flap design is outlined with methylene blue.

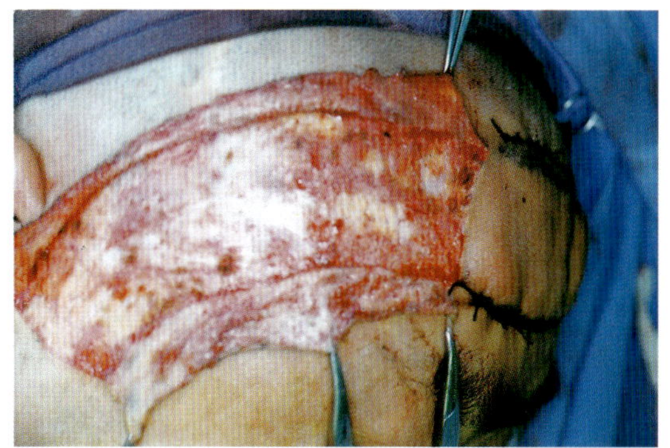

图 256

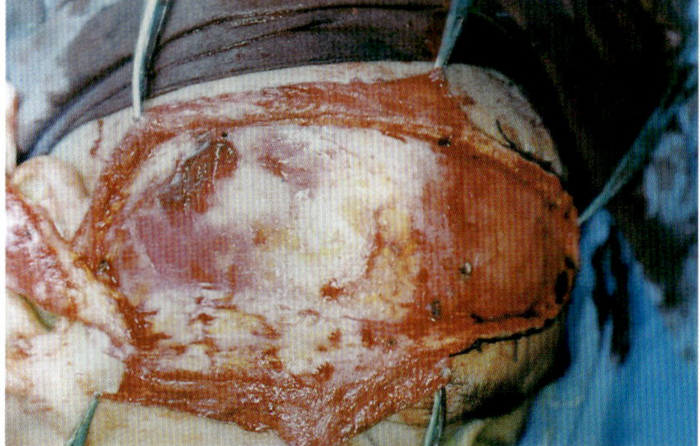

图 257

**图 256** 制备岛状额瓣：在制备岛状额瓣时，应使蒂部的血管保存完整，剥离表皮时应尽量在毛囊下进行，不宜过深。去表皮可见蒂部有一套动、静脉血管沿耳前颧弓上方向上向前直达岛状皮瓣内。

**图 257** 岛状额瓣被制备好后，由岛状额瓣远端向颧弓方向分离至颧弓上缘为止。将岛状额瓣用生理盐水纱布保护好，此时应特别注意不要使蒂部扭转，以避免岛状额瓣远端血供中断。

Fig. 256 The preparation of the island forehead flap: During preparation of the island forehead flap, the vessels of the pedicle of the island forehead flap should be perfectly preserved. The flap pedicle to the island is developed in the subfollicular plane through a curve temporal incision.

Fig. 257 The whole of the forehead is raised on a unilateral pedicle thereby including a symmetrical cosmetic unit. The base of the flap lies between the lateral end of the eyebrow and the upper pole of the ear and is situated just above the zygomatic arch. The lower incision runs along the upper edge of the eyebrows and the superior incision passes just anterior to the hairline. The incisions can be bevelled, which allows a better insetting of the subsequent skin graft on the donor defect. The island and pedicle are then bluntly separated from the pericranium and galea. Elevation of flap continues until the line joining the lateral corner of the eyebrow and the superior pole of the ear is reached. The island forehead flap is preserved with saline solution gauzes.

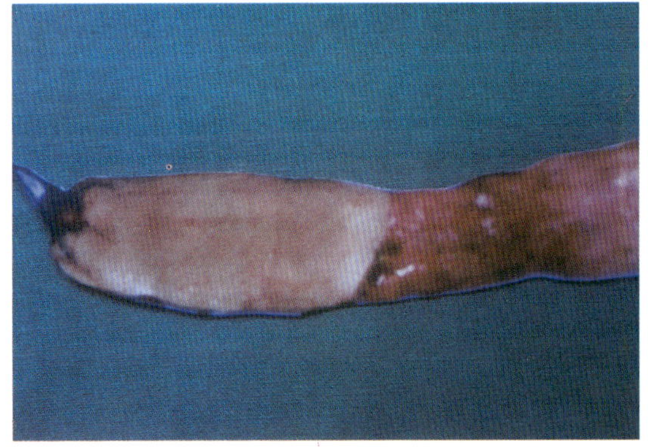
图 258

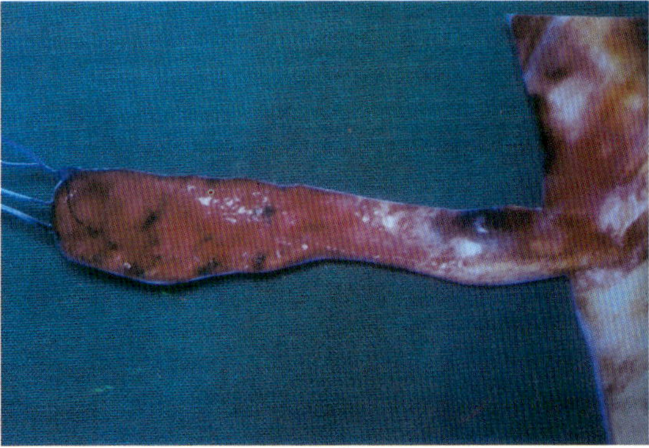
图 259

**图258，259** 额部岛状瓣的外表面及内面观。

**Fig. 258，259** The external surface and internal surface views of the island forehead flap.

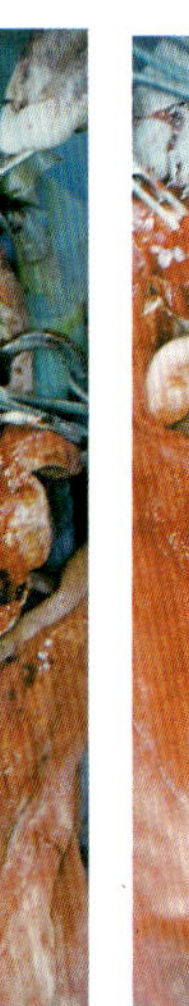
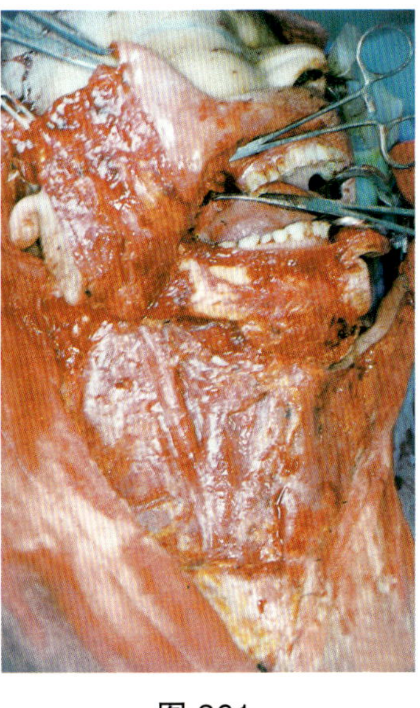
图 260　　图 261

**图 260** 沿下唇正中切开达颏部并与颈淋巴清扫术的颌下切口线相连。然后在靠颊粘膜侧沿下颌骨体切开龈颊沟粘骨膜并将颊瓣翻开。在行下颌龈颊沟粘膜切口时，应注意靠牙龈侧多保留些粘膜组织以便于在关闭龈颊沟创口时颊粘膜的对合。

在肿瘤边界外 1cm 处切除颊部肿瘤，结扎腮腺导管并标记，以备导管再通。

**图 261** 沿额瓣蒂部切口之下缘向下内分离，切断颧弓上缘颞筋膜附着，继续向下分离至颧弓深面的翼颌间隙，直至喙突深面上颌龈颊沟，并从此穿通，充分钝剥离，尽量扩大间隙，必要时由口腔侧分离显露喙突，沿喙突表面切断颞肌附着，咬除喙突。

**Fig. 260** The anterior arm of the incision for a neck dissection is continued vertically across the midline of the chin and the lower lip. The cheek flap is then reflected laterally by incision of the mucosa in the gingivobuccal gutter and subperiosteal dissection along the body of the mandible. During the incision of the mucosa in the gingivobuccal gutter, a narrow strip of mucosa must be preserved along the gingiva for approximation to the buccal mucosa at the close of the operation.

An incision is outlined around the tumor, leaving at least 1. 0 cm of normal mucosa on all its edges. The incision is carried through the deep musculature of the cheek and the tumor is removed. The main duct of the parotid gland should be management and be marked for reconstruction.

**Fig. 261** With the flap elevated, the region of the pedicle can be undermined so that the flap is turned inwards. A separate incision can be made in front of the ear and the flap gain entry into the oral cavity through a separate incision. The length of the incision should be at least two-third of the width of the temporal flap so that there is no possibility of constriction. By using blunt dissection and spreading the tissue with scissors, a safe passage can be made to the oral cavity and yet avoid damage to the facial nerve. If a cheek flap has been elevated, as during many of our composite resections, the coronoid process of the mandible is removed after severing the inserting ligament of the temporalis muscle. This will allow the flap to seat neatly medial to the mandible without the added pressure of the coronoid process.

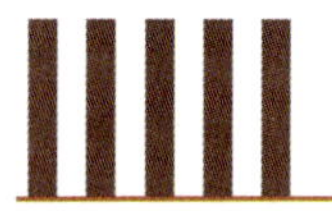



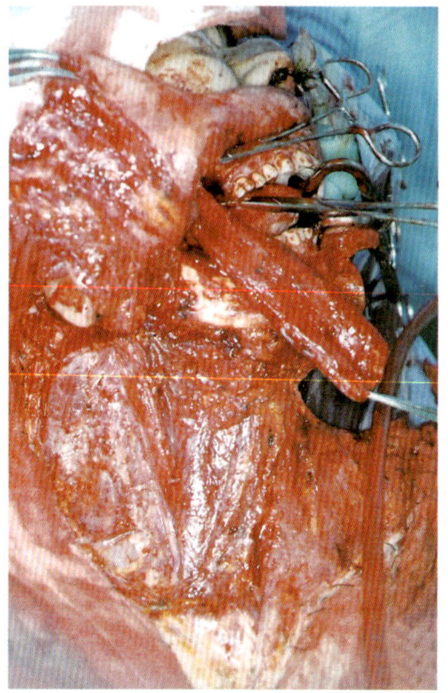

图 262

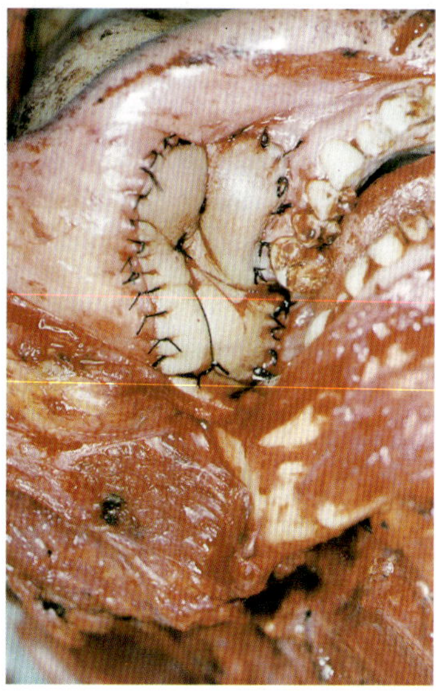

图 263

**图 262** 将岛状额瓣通过隧道转移至颊部缺损区，并于皮瓣上相当于腮腺导管口内开口处制作洞孔，以备导管植入。从口内将硅胶管通过额瓣洞孔穿出至额瓣创面，将腮腺导管的断端分别在 12、6、3、9 处缝合 4 针，并将硅胶管固定于额瓣上。

**图 263** 将穿入口内的额瓣与缺损周围粘膜缝合。将翻转之颊瓣还回原处后缝合下颌龈颊沟粘膜。

**Fig. 262** After the island forehead flap has reached the oral cavity through a tunnel, a hole is made on the island forehead flap, resected end of the duct of the parotid gland is fixed in the point 12、6、3、9 with fine silk line.

**Fig. 263** The flap is then maneuvered into its bed and sutured to the surrounding mucosa with interrupted suture. The cheek flap is returned in place, and closure is completed anteriorly by approximating the mucosa in the gingivobuccal gutter with fine silk.

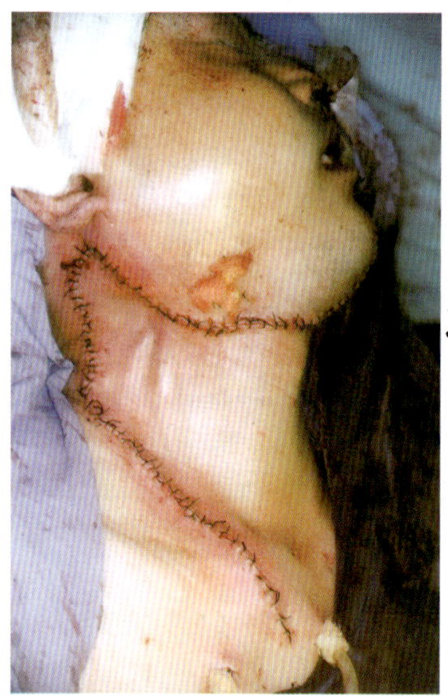

图 264

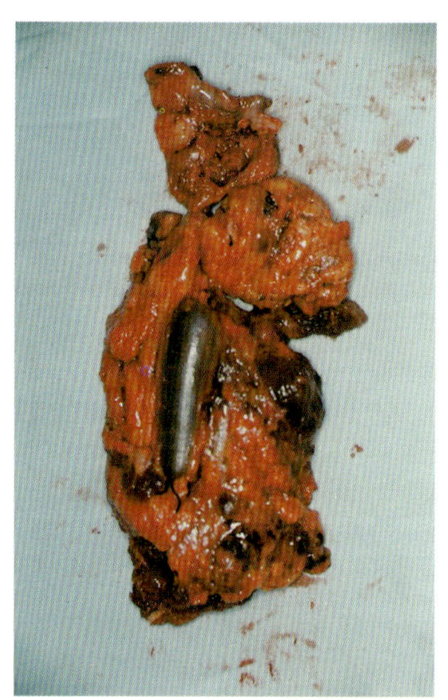

图 265

**图 264** 将额瓣蒂部的上皮组织还回原处后对位缝合，缺损区植前臂全厚皮片以覆盖额部缺损区。分层缝合下唇及颏部。生理盐水冲洗颈部创面后，植橡胶引流管 2 根，将颈部肌皮瓣还回原处后分层缝合，局部稍加压包扎。

**图 265** 术后组织标本。

**Fig. 264** The dermal layer of the forehead portion of the pedide of the island is returned in place and is sutured each other. A thick split thickness skin graft is tightly applied to the donor area and secured with flutted gauzes.

The lip is reconstructed with buried chromic sutures in the orbicularis muscle and fine silk sutures in the skin and mucosa. Care is taken to align accurately the vermilion-skin junction. The neck wound is drained and closed in the usual manner.

**Fig. 265** The surgical specimen postoperatively.

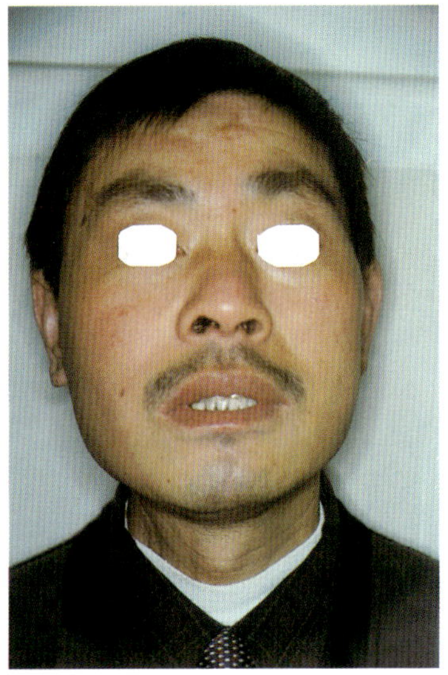

图 266

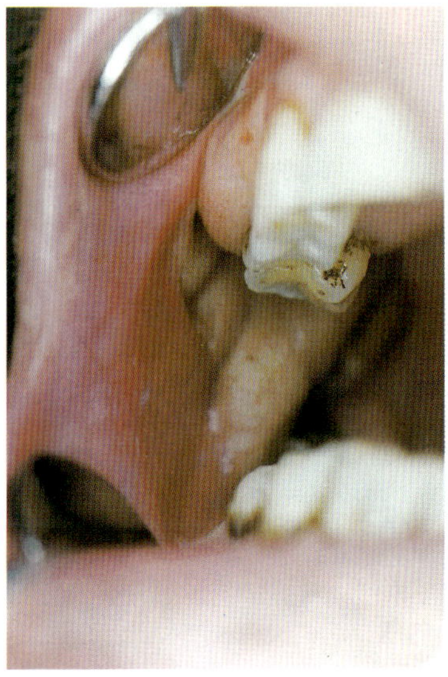

图 267

**图 266** 患者手术后 1 年正面观。
**图 267** 患者手术后 1 年张口及移植瓣区情况。

**Fig. 266** This patient underwent composite resection of a squamous cell carcinoma of the right buccal mucosa with immediate island forehead flap reconstruction and is now 1 year after operation.
**Fig. 267** The condition of patient's opening mouth 1 year after surgery.

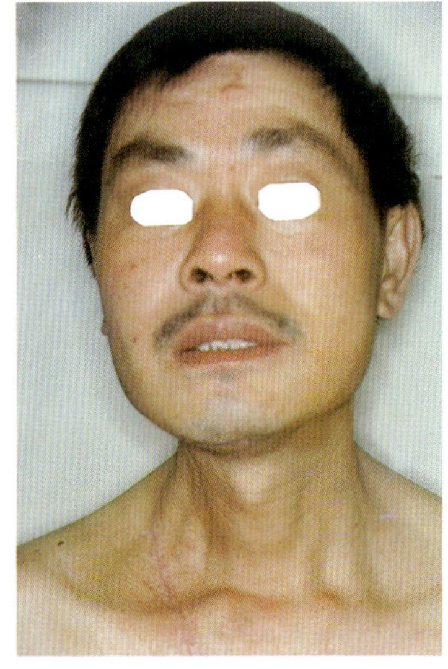

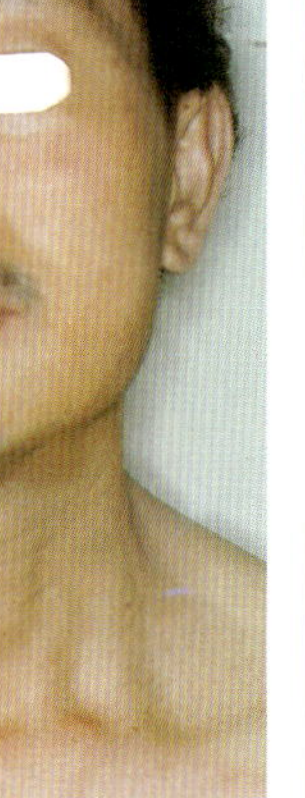

图 268

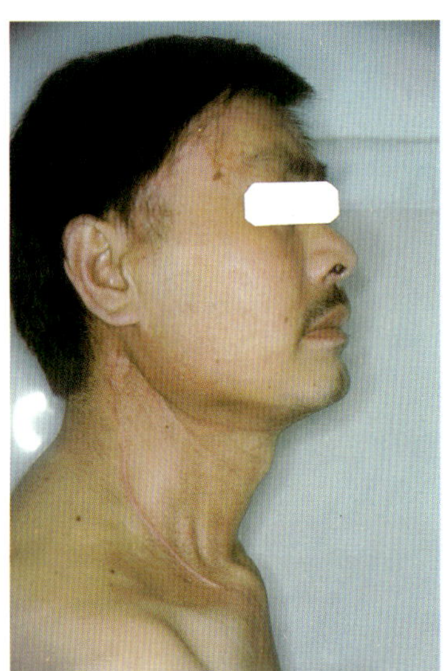

图 269

**图 268, 269** 患者术后 1 年的正、侧面观。

**Fig. 268, 269** Frontal and lateral views of 48-year-old patient 1 year after operation.

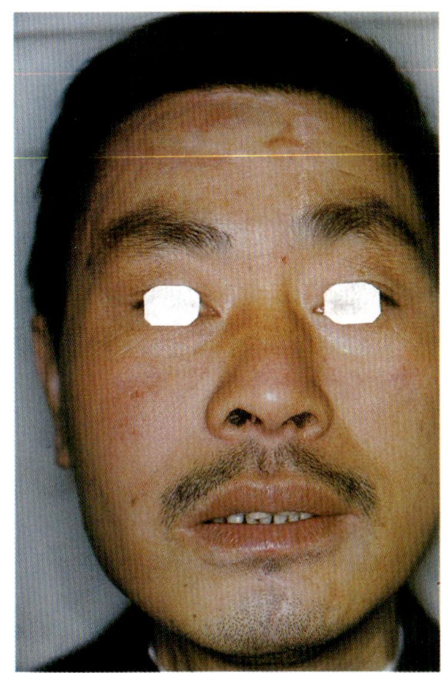
图 270

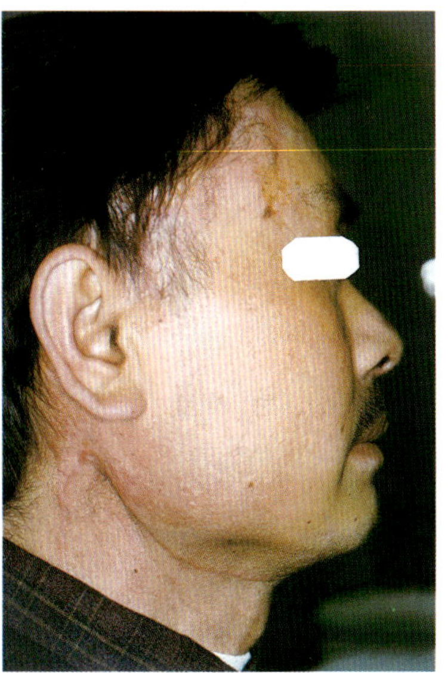
图 271

图 270，271 患者术后 2 年的正侧面观。

Fig. 270，271 Frontal and lateral views of 48-year-old patient 2 years after surgery.

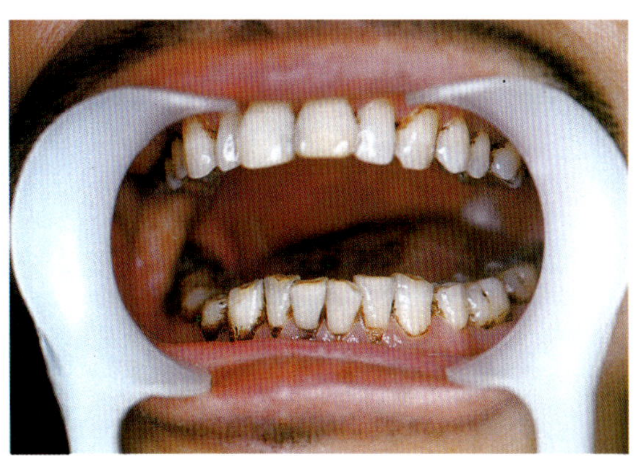

图 272 患者术后 2 年的张口情况。

Fig. 272 The condition of 48-year-old male patient's opening mouth 2 years after operation.

# V. 腭部肿瘤

17. 腭隆凸锉除术
18. 腭部小良性肿瘤切除术
19. 软腭混合瘤切除后颊脂垫修复软腭缺损

# V. Palate tumors

17. Removal of the palatal torus
18. Excision of small benign tumors on the palate
19. Use of the buccal fat pad for reconstruction of the soft palate defect after the removal of pleomorphic adenoma in the soft palate

# 17. 腭隆凸铿除术

# 17. Removal of the palatal torus

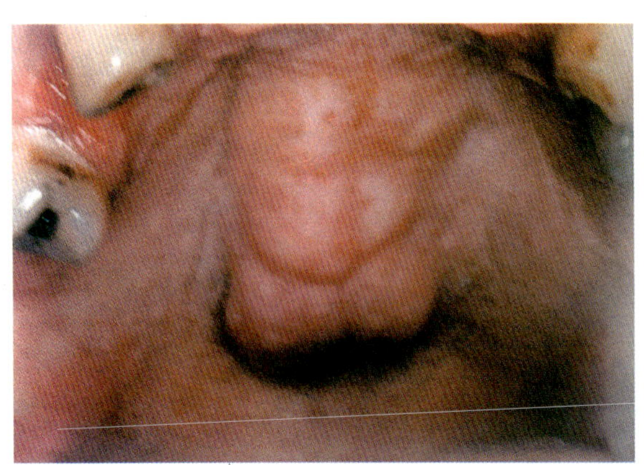

图 273

**图 273** 偶尔，在患者的硬腭部可见一个大而不规则、分叶状的腭隆凸，该隆凸常导致镶牙困难，必须经手术将硬腭隆凸铿除

Fig. 273 Occasionally, large, irregular, lobed tori are seen which are existing or potential prosthetic problems. The palatal torus must be removed.

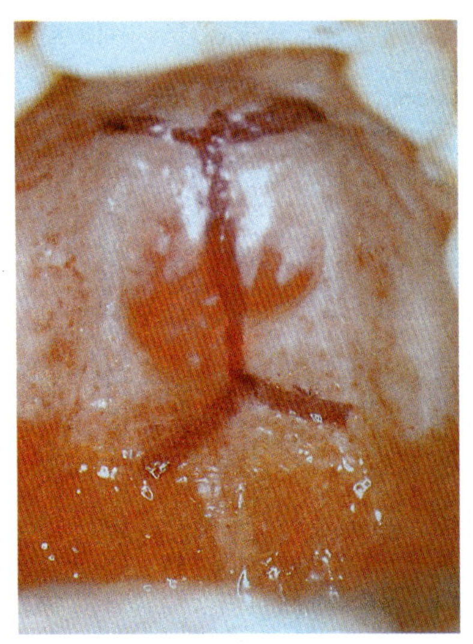

图 274

**图 274** 在硬腭正中作一垂直切口，切口深达骨膜下，切口向前向后分别伸达病变的外缘，前后末端分别呈“Y”切开。病变后端切口的两臂应终止在腭动脉的内侧。可用手指触摸腭大孔以确定动脉的位置是有帮助的。

Fig. 274 A subperiosteal incision is made exactly in the midline and is extended beyond the lesion to end in a " Y" at each end. The limbs of the posterior incision should stop short of the palatine arteries. This will be assisted by palpating the palatal foramen with the finger to localize the line of the artery.

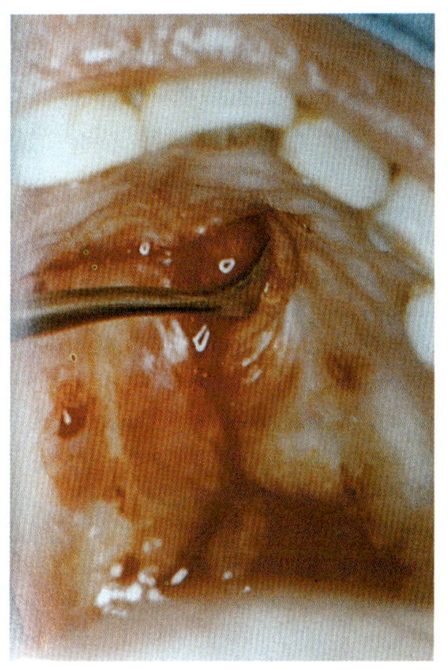

图 275

**图 275** 在腭隆凸的表面细心地将薄的粘骨膜与其下的腭隆凸骨质分开。分离粘骨膜的剥离器必须小到能伸入到腭隆凸各分叶的基部。

**Fig. 275** Careful elevation of the thin mucoperiosteum is required to lift the flap off the bone, the elevator must be sharp and small enough to penetrate into the irregular fissures between each lobe of the torus which commonly have deep undercuts at their base.

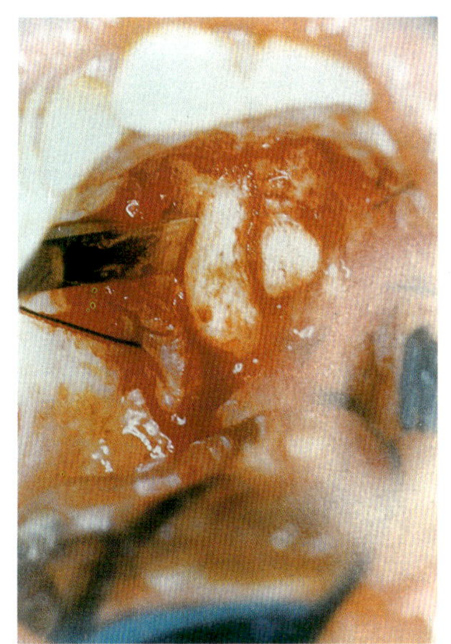

图 276

**图 276** 将骨锉放在腭隆凸的基部，用骨锤敲击 2－3 次，腭隆凸的中央部位将会与其下的骨质分离。

**Fig. 276** Placing the chisel against the large torus, two or three taps with the chisel along its periphery weakened its attachment and a central blow completed its separation.

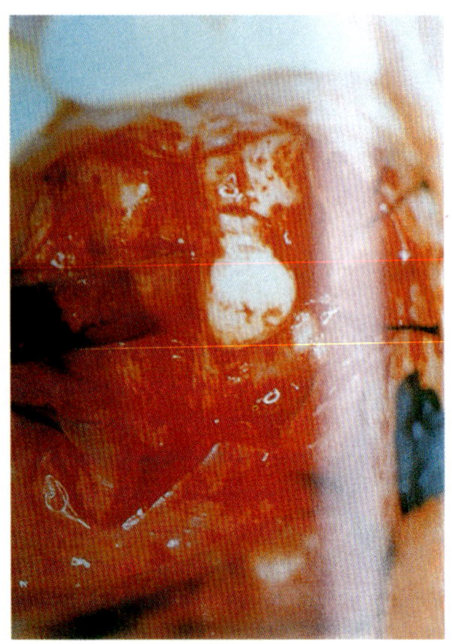

图 277

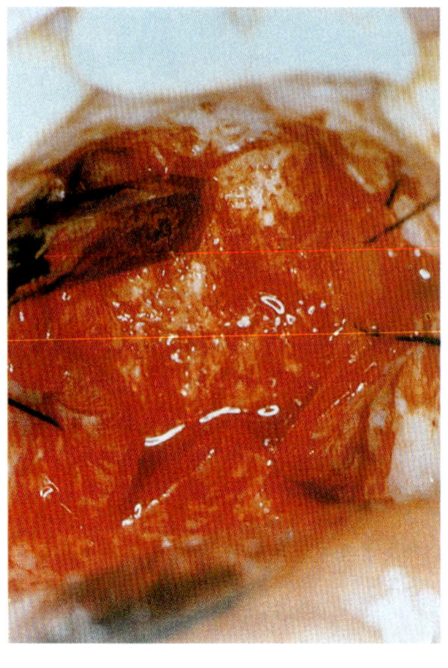

图 278

**图 277** 大的骨隆凸被锉除之后，小及中等大小的骨隆凸可将骨锉放在其基部后，轻击骨锉便可将骨隆凸去除。

**图 278** 小的骨隆凸也被去除之后，可用小球钻或骨锉将其骨隆凸的基部锉平。

**Fig. 277** The large lobe having been removed, the smaller torus is now accessible. Small to moderate shaped tori may be separated by one firm blow with the chisel.

**Fig. 278** Remaining small bone irregularities should be removed by a chisel and the palatal vault smoothed with a bone bur or file.

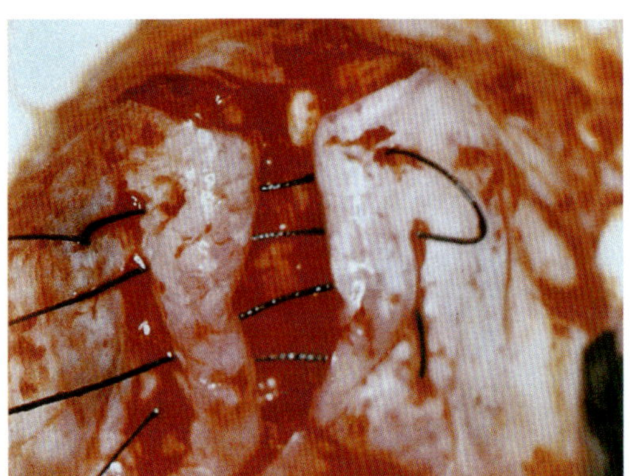

图 279

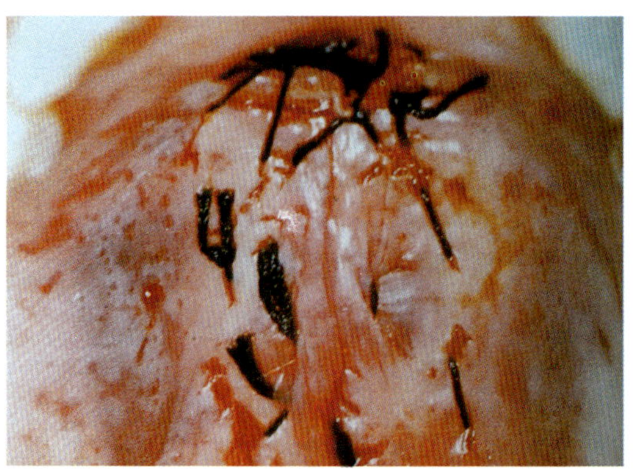

图 280

**图 279** 在腭隆凸的基部，可有多个小的渗出性出血点。软组织的出血点可用电凝止血。沿瓣作水平褥式缝合关闭创面。

**图 280** 采用水平或垂直外翻褥式缝合使粘膜瓣的边缘外翻性对合。假若需要，可修剪多余粘膜瓣的边缘使其创缘更好地对合。

**Fig. 279** The multiple, small bleeding points at the base the tori will ooze rather than bleed briskly. Any soft tissue bleeding points should be coagulated. Horizontal mattress sutures are inserted midway along the flaps to assist in holding them against the palate.

**Fig. 280** The mucosal flap edges are closed by horizontal or vertical mattress sutures which produce eversion of the wound edges. Surplus mucosa may now be trimmed away from the wound edges of necessary. This was not necessary here.

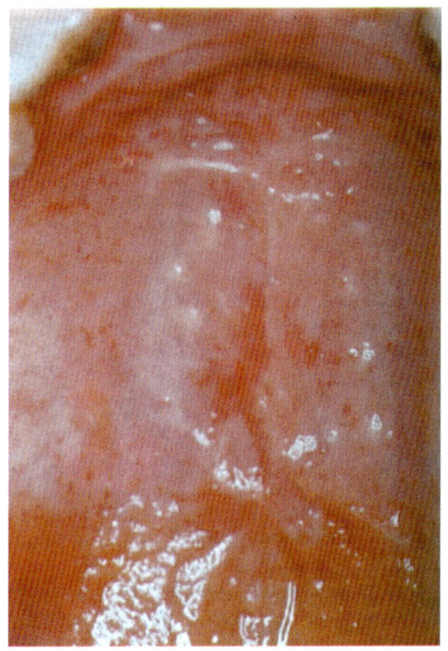

图 281

**图 281** 术后 3 个月腭部恢复的情况。

**Fig. 281** The healing condition of the palate 3 months postoperatively.

# 18. 腭部小良性肿瘤切除术

# 18. Excision of small benign tumors in the palate

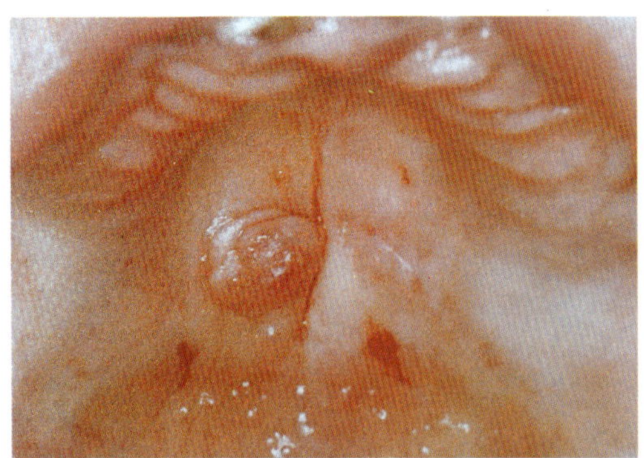
图 282

**图 282** 在硬软腭联合或腭部因假牙创伤所致纤维组织反应性增生，将病变切除后让其创面再上皮化而修复。

用局麻药行腭大孔和门齿管神经阻滞麻醉为首选。

**Fig. 282** Hyperplastic fibrous tissue reaction to denture trauma to the junction of the hard and soft palate and in the palate. The lesions were excised and their bases allowed to re-epithelialise.

The periphery of the lesion was infiltrated with local analgesic solution. The greater palatine and incisive nerve blocks could be used. Peripheral infiltration was used for local haemostasis.

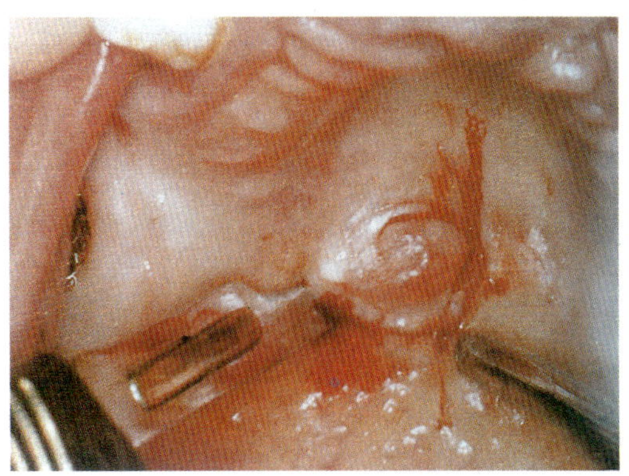
图 283

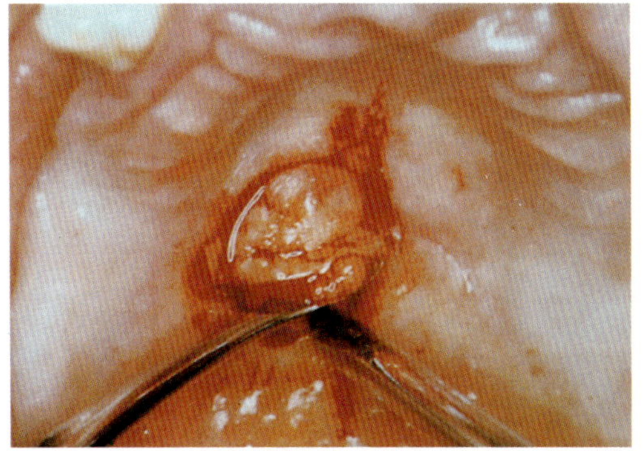
图 284

**图 283, 284** 绕病变周围包括少许正常腭部粘膜组织在内作切口，在切口内将一扁的骨膜剥离器伸入骨与骨膜之间，将骨膜连病变组织完全去除；也可使用一钝性匙状骨膜剥离器将病变组织掀起。

**Fig. 283, 284** A peripheral incision is made around the lesion including a small collar of normal palate. In view of the shallowness of the mucosa the blade was taken down to bone so that the periosteum could be elevated and the lesion removed completely. The lesion is elevated off the palate using a sharp spoon-shaped elevator.

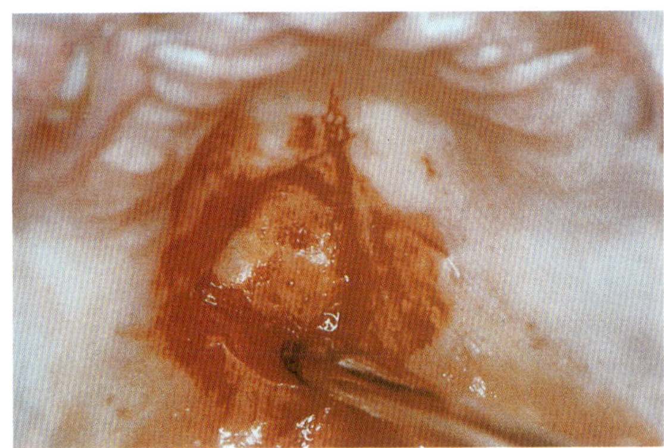

图 285

图 285, 286 行创面止血后，将含碘仿的纱包放在缺损中，在上缝合 1－2 针固定。纱包保留 2 周以使骨质上有肉芽组织形成。

Fig. 285, 286 The palatal bone is exposed and haemostasis achieved. A pack of gauze impregnated with pigmentum iodoform paint is placed in the defect, compressed and then held by one or two overlying sutures. The pack will be retained for 2 weeks by which time the bone should be covered by granulation tissue.

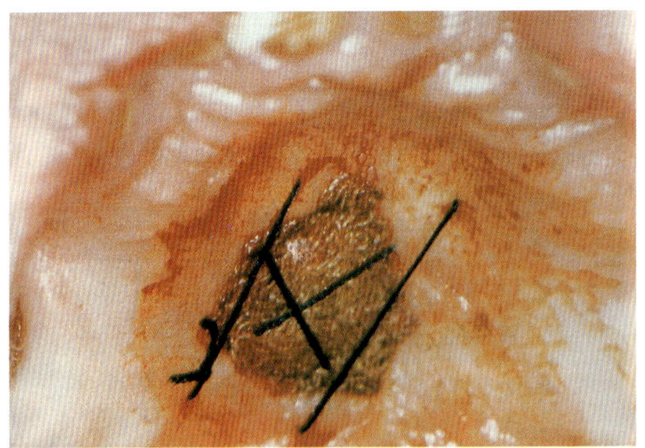

图 286

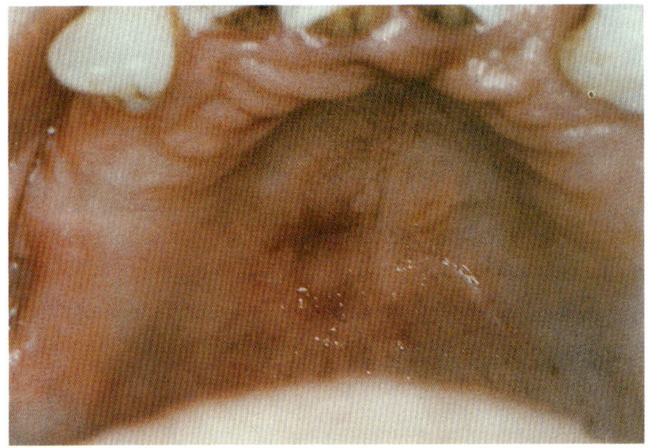

图 287

图 287 3 周之内，腭部缺损已完全愈合。

Fig. 287 The palate defect had healed completely within 3 weeks.

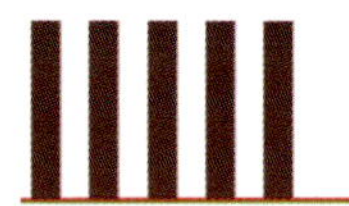



# 19. 软腭混合瘤切除后颊脂垫修复软腭缺损

## 19. The use of the buccal fat pad for reconstruction of the soft palate defect after the removal of pleomorphic adenoma in the soft palate

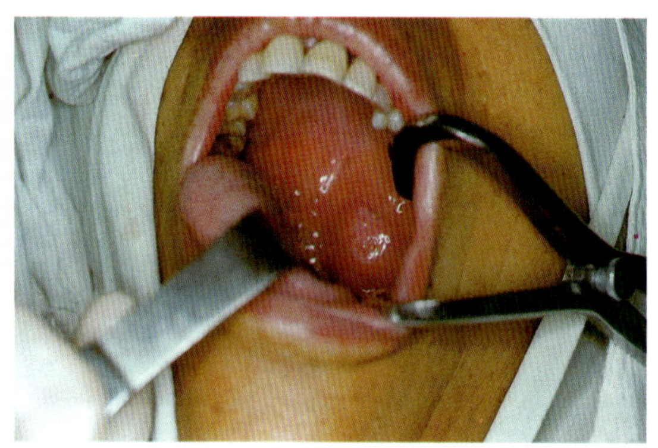

图 288

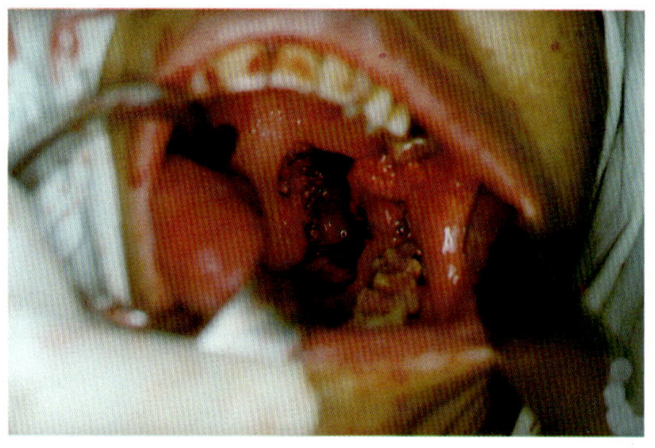

图 289

**图 288** 一患左软腭混合瘤的 46 岁女性患者见软腭部有一约 3×4 cm 大小的肿物，表面粘膜正常。

**图 289** 在肿瘤外约 1cm 将软腭肿瘤完全切除后，在左上颌结节区前庭沟做切口。

**Fig. 288** Intraoral view of a 46-year-old female patient with the pleomorphic adenoma in the soft palate shows a large hard, 3×4 cm mass on the left palate extending from the soft palate to the hard palate. The overlying mucosa is normal.

**Fig. 289** After the tumor is excised, a vestibular incision is made in the left maxillary tuberosity area.

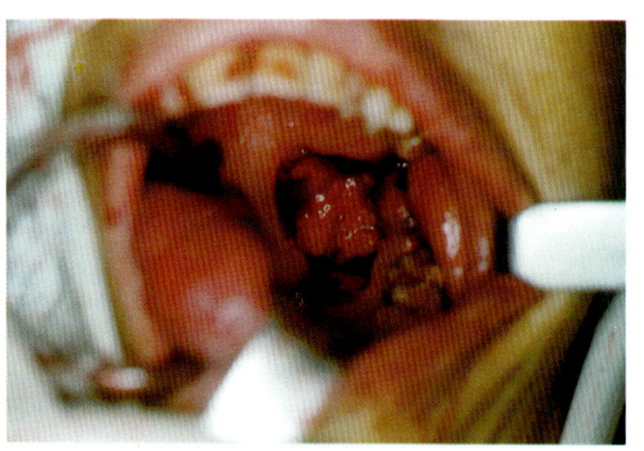

图 290

**图 290** 将颊脂垫从上颌结节区移向缺损区，并与软腭缺损区的各缘相缝合。

**Fig. 290** The buccal fat pad is mobilized from the maxillary tuberosity region and secured to the edges of the soft palate and hard palate wound.

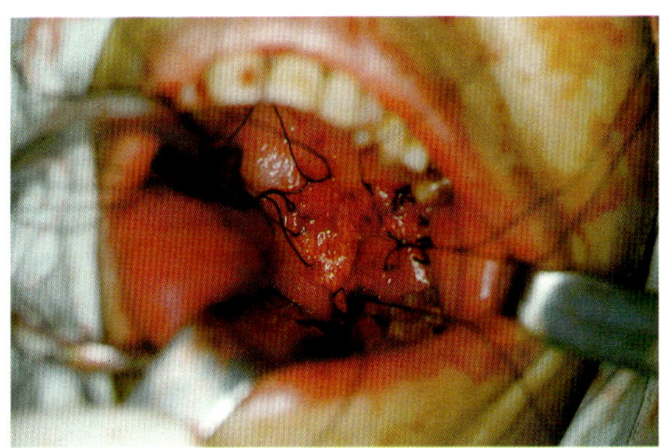

图 291

图 291 颊脂垫被缝合后的情景。

Fig. 291 The condition after the buccal fat pad has been sutured.

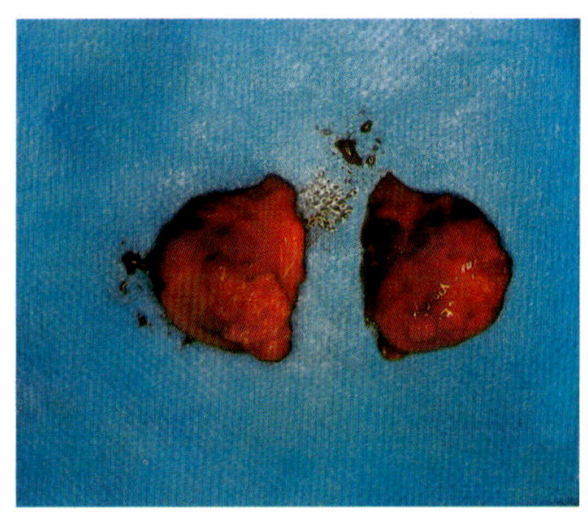

图 292

图 292 被切除肿瘤的外、内侧面观。

Fig. 292 External and internal views of the excised tumor.

# Ⅵ. 舌部肿瘤

20. 淋巴管瘤巨舌症的外科手术治疗
21. 舌前部组织瓣滑行修复半侧舌中部缺损
22. 舌根部癌舌瓣后推修复舌成形术
23. 舌癌切除后侧斜方肌岛状瓣舌重建
24. 舌根部癌切除额岛状瓣转移修复术
25. 口底癌切除后侧斜方肌岛状肌皮瓣转移口底修复术

# Ⅵ. Tongue tumors

20. Surgical excision of lymphangiomatous macroglossia
21. Sliding anterior tongual flap repair in the middle partial defect of the tongue
22. Set-back tongue flap for carcinoma of the tongue base
23. A lateral trapezius-musculocutaneous island flap for partial tongue reconstruction
24. Island forehead flap repair in resection for the cancer of the base of the tongue
25. Immediate trapezius-musculocutaneous island flap repair in resection for the carcinoma of the floor of the mouth

# 20. 淋巴管瘤巨舌症的外科手术治疗

# 20. Surgical excision of lymphangiomatous macroglossia

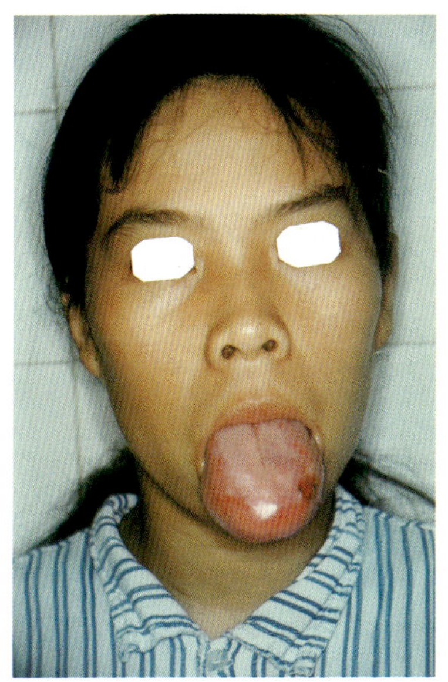

图 293

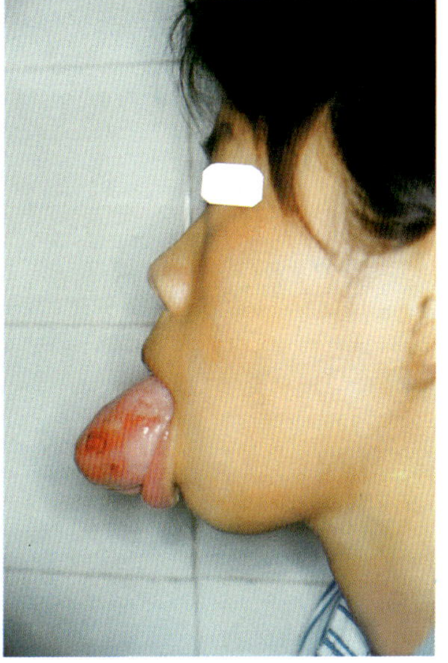

图 294

**图 293，294** 淋巴管畸形形成的淋巴管瘤性巨舌症，舌体增大致舌部分伸出口外。

**Fig. 293，294** Lymphatic malformation producing lymphangiomatous macroglossia. The tongue remains out of the mouth.

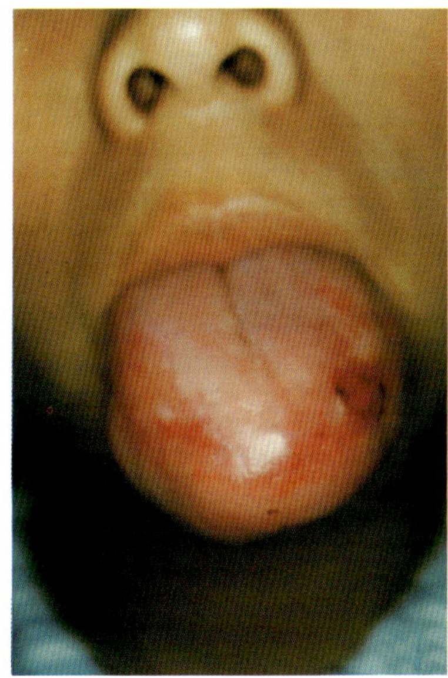

图 295

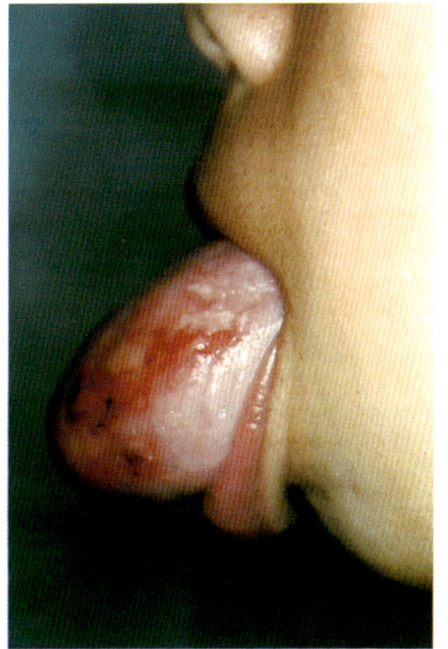

图 296

**图 295，296** 急性上呼吸道感染时淋巴管瘤性巨舌症的表现。突出于口腔外的舌体有出血、干燥、皲裂和坏死。

**Fig. 295，296** Appearance of a lymphatic malformation during an acute upper respiratory infection. The protuberant tongue is hemorrhagic, dried, cracked, and necrotic.

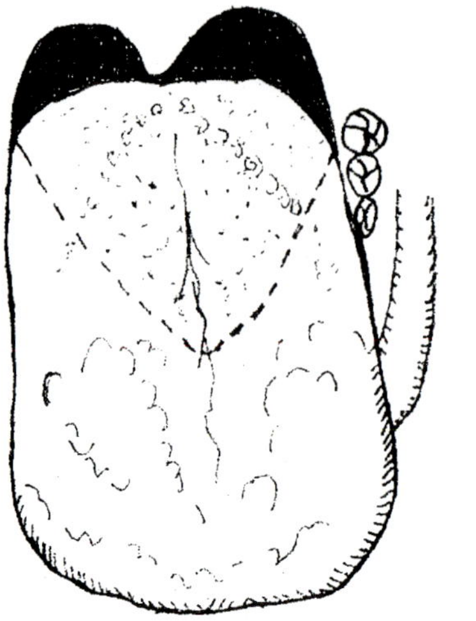

A

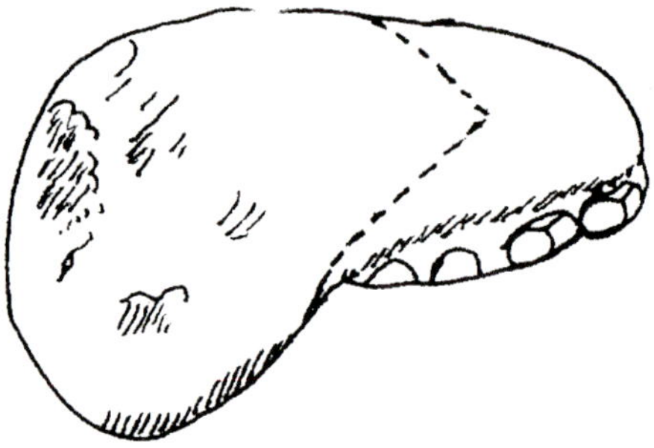

B

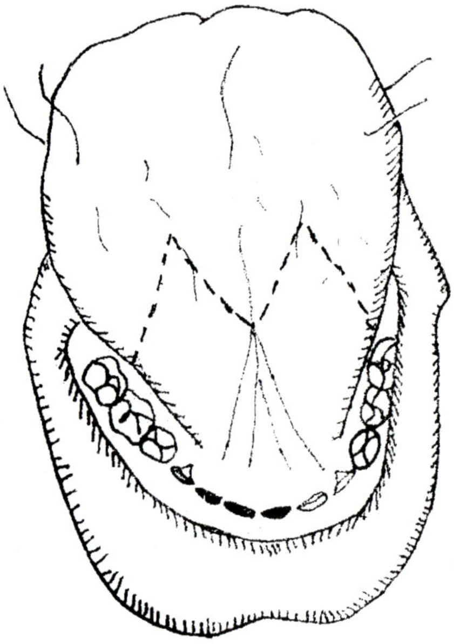

C

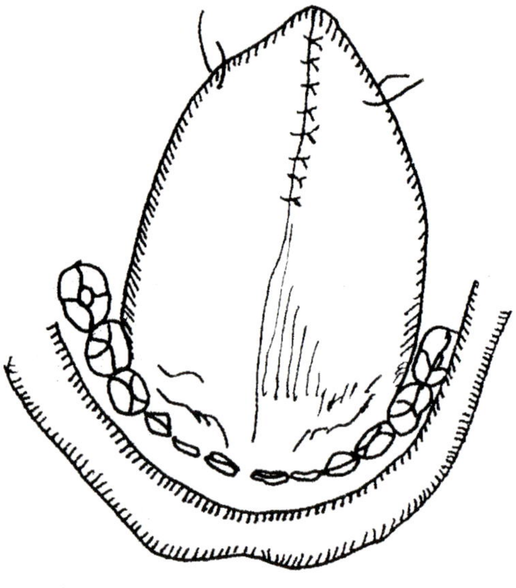

D

图 297

**图 297** 舌切除示意图

A. 舌背面切口设计；B. 舌侧缘切口；C. 舌腹切口设计；D. 缝合后的情景。

**Fig. 297** Diagram of tongue resection.

A. Design of incision on the lingual dorsal surface. B. Incision of lingual lateral margin. C. Design of sublingual incision. D. The condition after suturing.

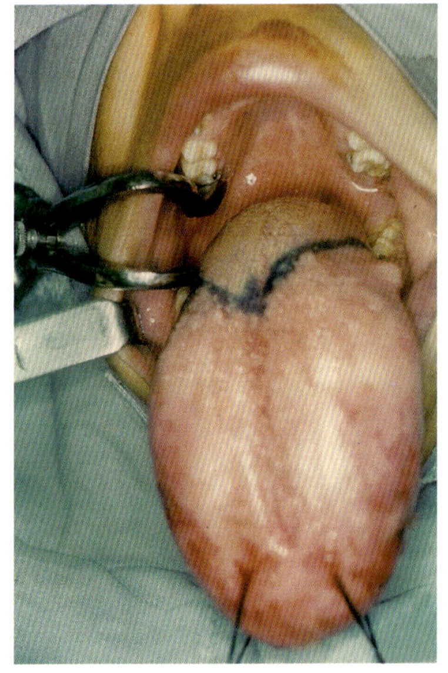

图 298

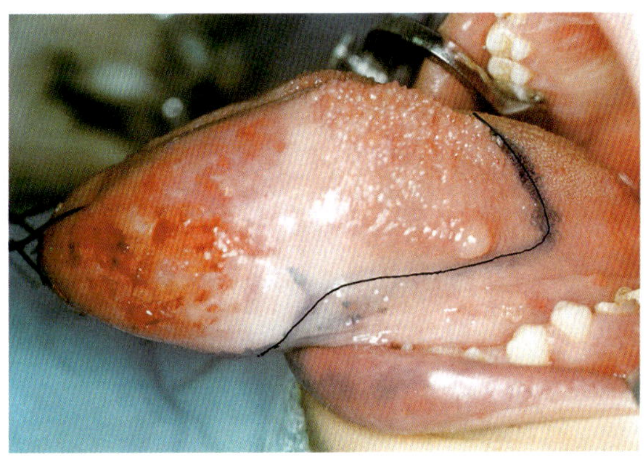

图 299

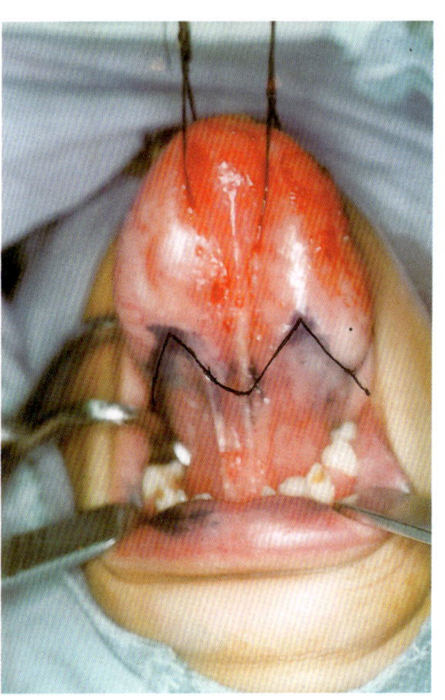

图 300

**图 298－300** 用美蓝画出舌背、舌侧缘及舌腹切口线。在切除舌病变组织之前，在舌后部用 7 号丝线穿过舌后部中线行“8”字结扎以减少出血。

**Fig. 298－300** The patient undergoes surgical resection under general nasotracheal anesthesia. For retraction, two deep sutures are placed in lateral borders of the tongue. A figure-of-eight ligature is placed around the base of the tongue as a temporary method to control bleeding during surgery. Three V-shaped incisions are outlined on the lingual dorsal, lingual lateral, and lingual inferior surfaces of the tongue with methylene blue. The angle of the V on the tongue dorsum is about 1 cm in front of the circumvallate papillae and the inverted V enclosed within it the entire tumor.

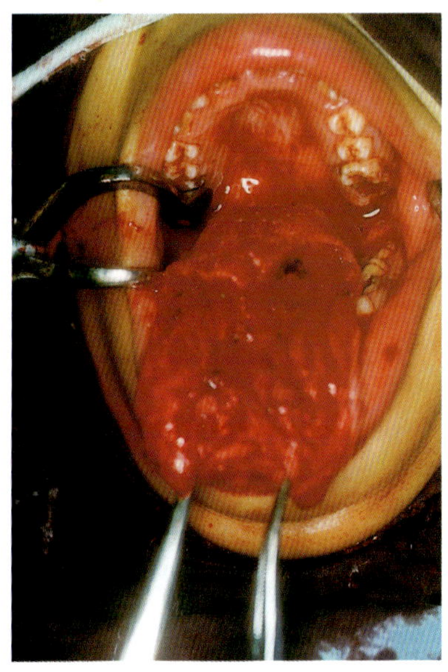

图 301

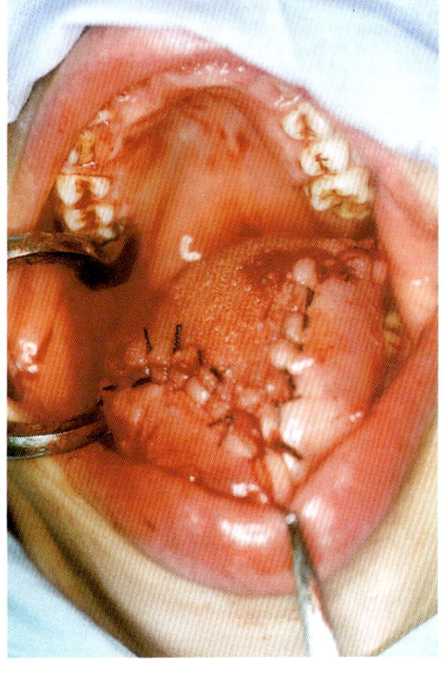

图 302

**图 301，302** 将舌部病变组织切除之后，用电凝彻底止血。将剩余的舌组织用 4 号丝线分三层缝合。缝合后的正常舌前部组织形成了新的舌尖及舌体。

**Fig. 301，302** After completion of the incisions and removal of the lesion, the remaining parts of the tongue is approximated in three layers. The reconstruction provided a new tip of the tongue that consisted of normal tissue.

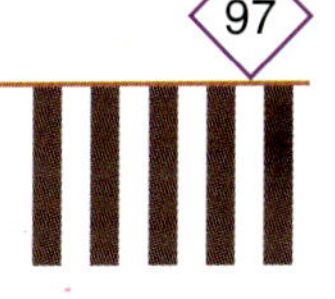

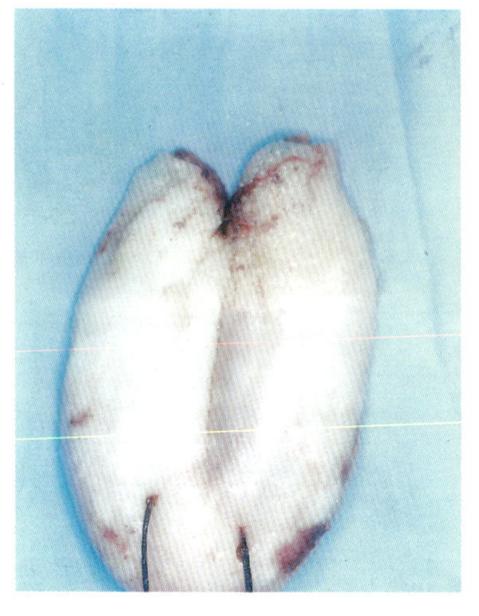

图 303

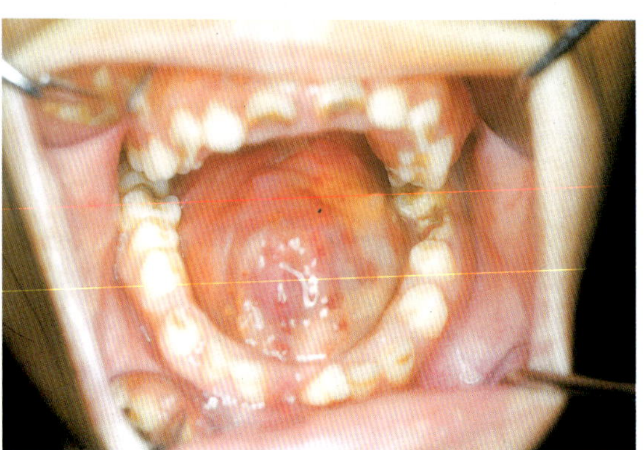

图 304

图 303 切除后的舌病变标本正面观。
图 304 术后 2 周舌愈合情况。

Fig. 303 Frontal view of the operative specimen.
Fig. 304 The condition of the tongue healing 2 weeks after operation.

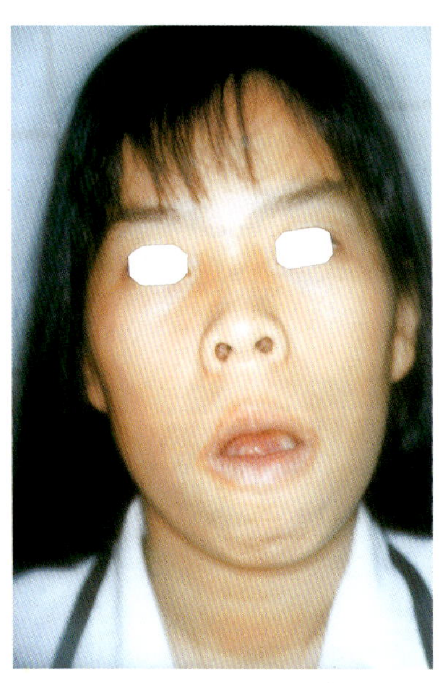

图 305

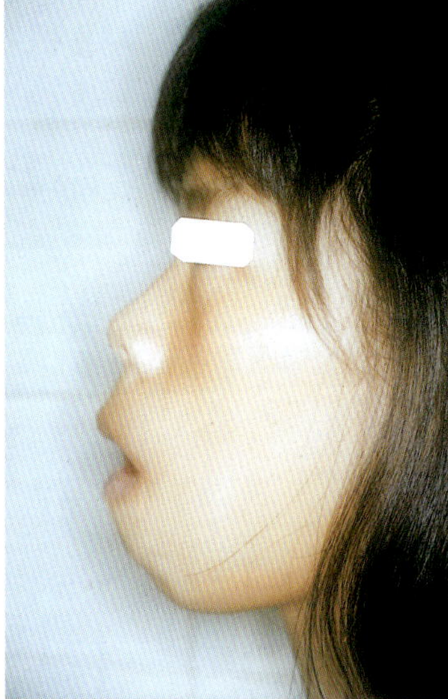

图 306

图 305, 306 手术后 2 周患者的正侧面观见前牙开殆，下颌体部变长，口腔不能完全闭合。下颌体升支角增大，前牙切缘前移位及外倾斜。

Fig. 305, 306 Patient's frontal and lateral views 2 weeks postoperatively. It is found that patient's mouth could not be closed completely and mandibular deformity which was characterized by an anterior open bite, elongation of the mandibular body, increase of the body-ramus angle, anterior displacement and outward tipping of the incisal edges of the anterior teeth.

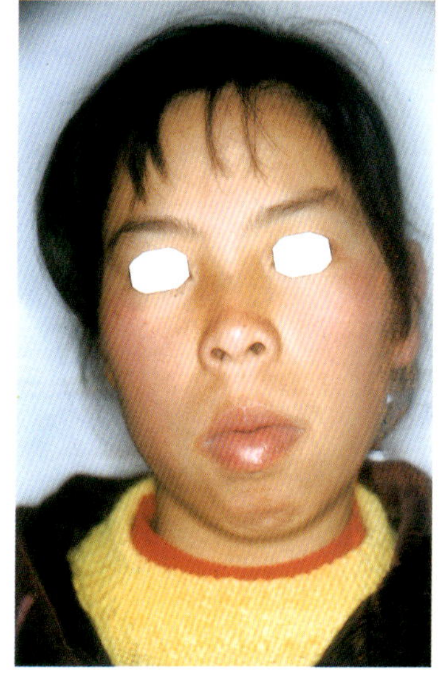
图 307

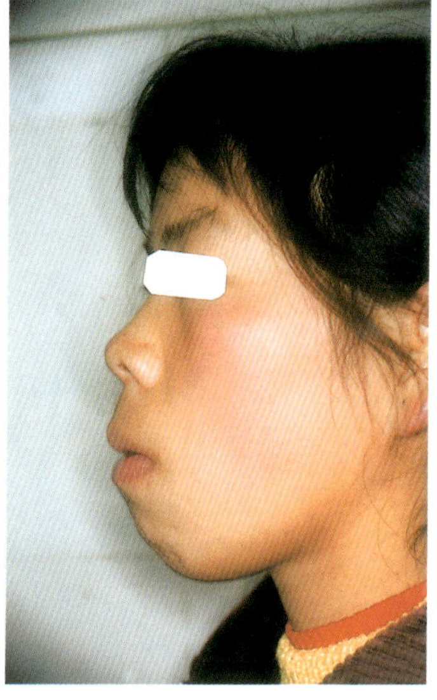
图 308

**图 307, 308** 患者术后 6 个月的正侧面观显示颌骨畸形明显改善,口腔能闭合。

**Fig. 307, 308** Patient's frontal and lateral views 6 months after operation show that mandibular deformity has been improved obviously and her upper and lower lips can close.

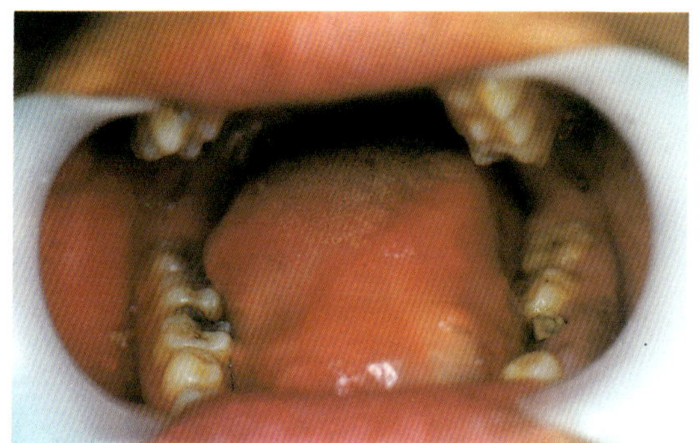
图 309

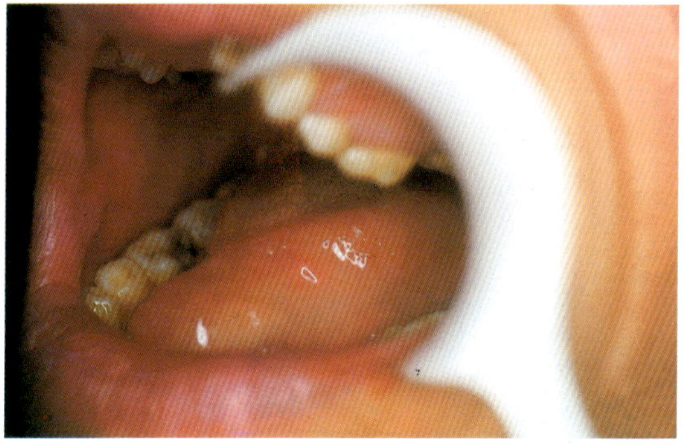
图 310

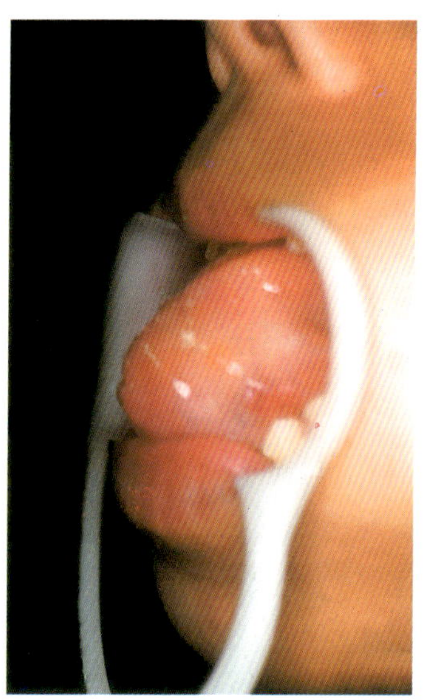
图 311

**图 309 – 311** 术后 6 个月正侧面观舌体形态大小似正常,未见有淋巴管瘤残存;伸舌见舌尖能伸出口外。

**Fig. 309 – 311** Frontal and lateral views of the tongue 6 mouths after operation show a normal-looking tongue in size and shape and the frontal part of the tongue can extend out of the mouth.



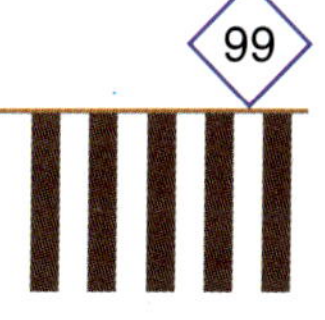

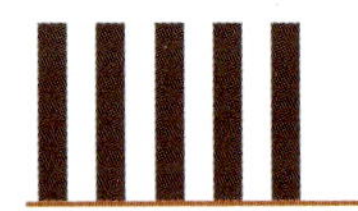



# 21. 舌前部组织瓣滑行修复半侧舌中部缺损

# 21. Sliding anterior tongual flap repair in the middle partial defect of the tongue

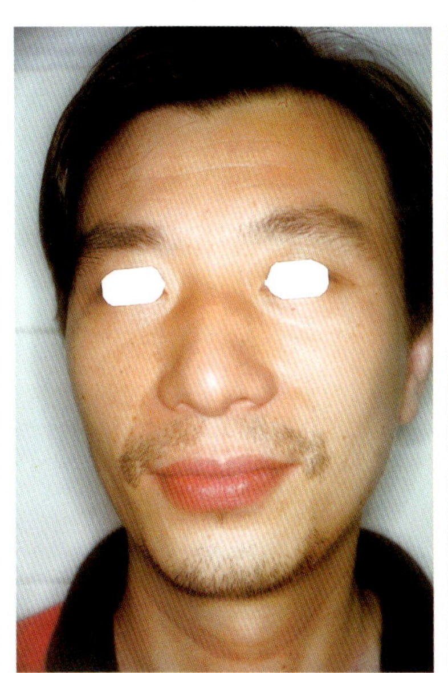

图 312

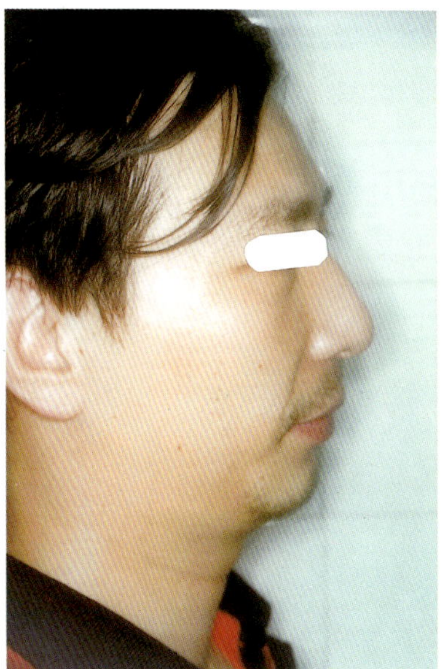

图 313

**图 312, 313** 患有右舌中部鳞状细胞癌的 36 岁的男性患者术前正侧面观。该患者使用舌前部组织瓣滑行修复半侧舌中部缺损。

Fig. 312, 313 Preoperative frontal and lateral views of a 36-year-old man with a squamous cell carcinoma of the right mid-tongue treated by sliding anterior tongual flap.

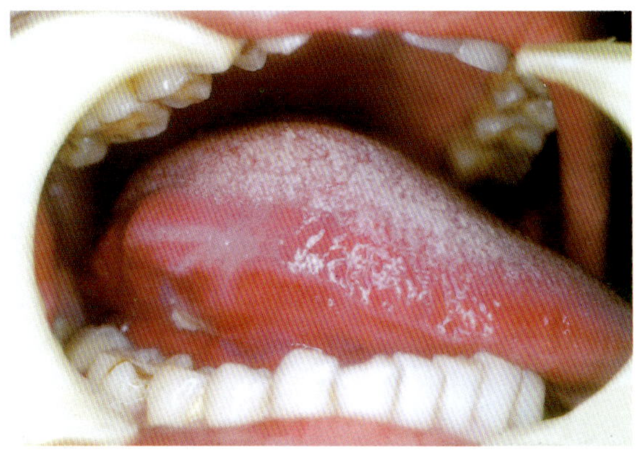

图 314

**图 314** 在舌右侧中部可见一 4cm 的肿瘤。活检显示为中度分化鳞状细胞癌。

Fig. 314 A 4 cm tumor is seen on the right mid-tongue. A biopsy specimen demonstrated a moderately differentiated squamous cell carcinoma.

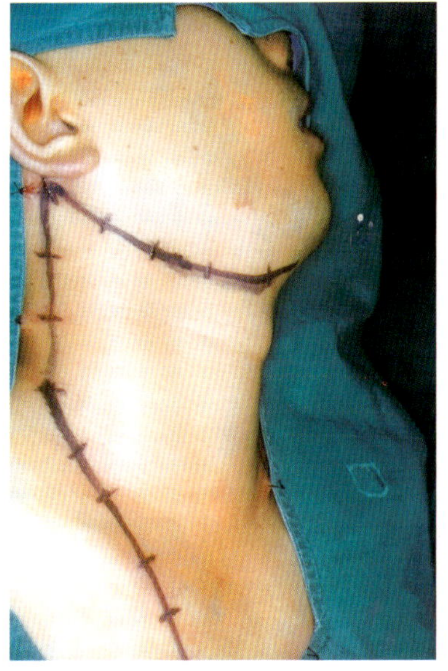

图 315

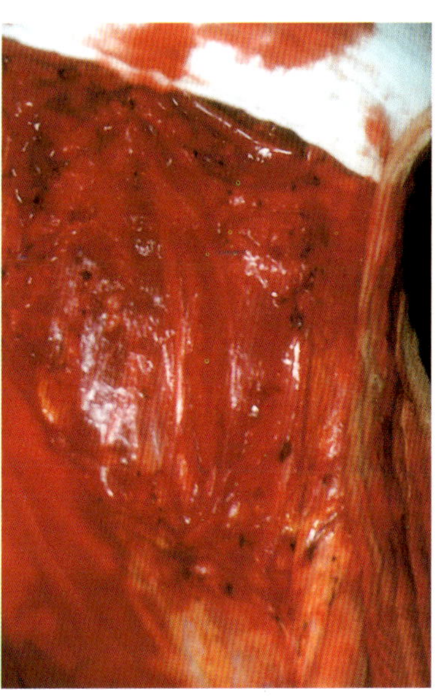

图 316

**图 315，316** 患者采用鼻腔气管内插管全麻。患者仰卧于手术台上，头偏向健侧，颈部中度伸展。颈淋巴清扫术本书作者喜欢采用矩形切口以便于颈部解剖结构有满意的暴露。发生在舌中部的 $T_2$ 病变可常规在口内将肿瘤完全切除而对其缺损进行修复。如果需要行颈淋巴清扫术的话，应先行颈淋巴清扫术。

**Fig. 315, 316** Endotracheal anesthesia is used. The patient is placed on the operative table with his head in moderate extension and rotated away from the operator. The rectangular shaped incision allows satisfactory exposure and is the one we generally prefer. The tumor is resected in usual manner and this can be accomplished transorally in most cases of $T_2$ midtongue lesions. A neck dissection can be done concomitantly if indicated.

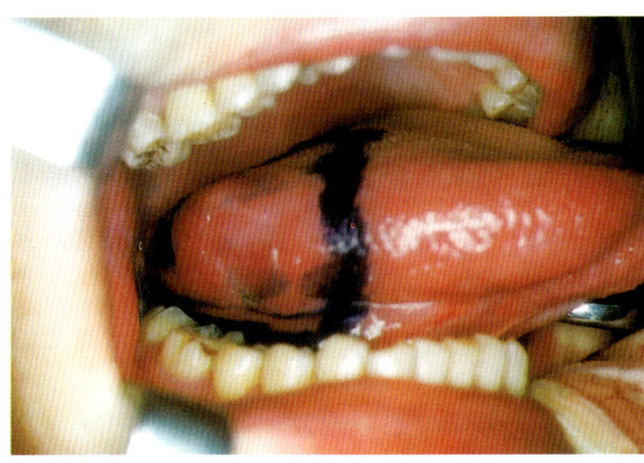

图 317

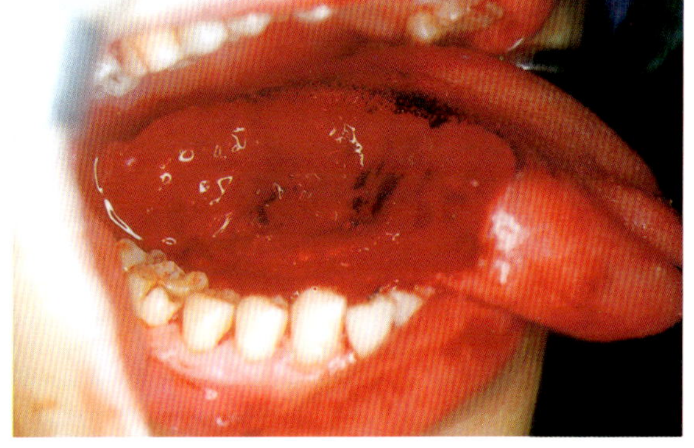

图 318

**图 317** 根据需要切除的病变组织画出切口线。切除局部病变组织时，需在正常组织内 1cm 切除，通常一 4cm 的病变造成的组织缺损是 6cm。

**图 318** 显示切除病变后的舌缺损

**Fig. 317** Incision line is marked out according to resected lesion size. Utilizing a 1 to 2 cm margin for excision, a defect of 5 to 6 cm may result from a 4 cm lesion.

**Fig. 318** View of the lingual defect after the lesion has been resected.

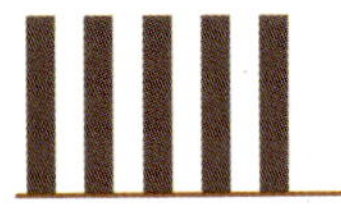



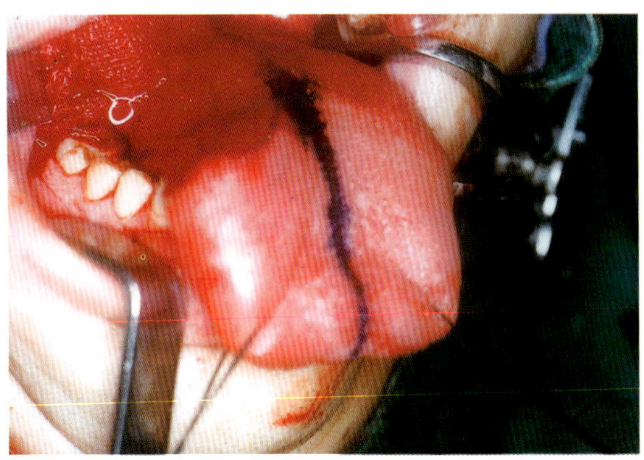

图 319

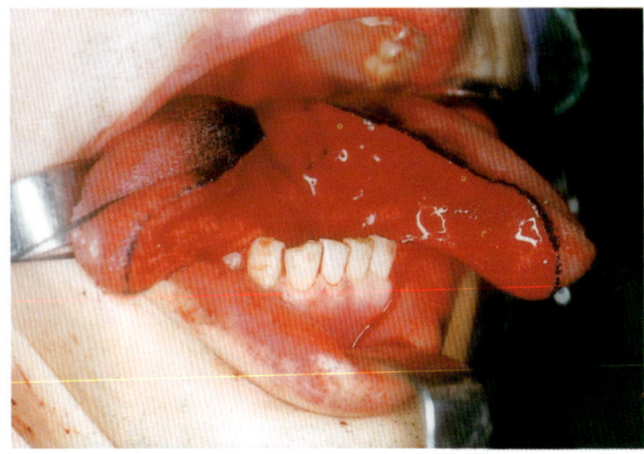

图 320

**图 319** 成人的舌体长约 12－14cm，因此，剩余 8cm 的同侧舌组织可被应用。

**图 320** 由剩余的舌组织正中纤维膈通过颏舌肌向下分开，因为舌神经血管供应来源于舌侧面，舌正中纤维膈不含有大的血管网，可迅速、安全将剩余的舌前部组织分为两瓣几乎无出血。

**Fig. 319** A fully protruding adult tongue has a length of 12 to 14 cm. The remaining ipsilateral tongue would, therefore, have about 6 to 8 cm of usable tissue remaining. The anterior portion of the tongue attaches to the hyoid bone. By releasing a major portion of this origin and maintaining the dorsolingual branch of the lingual artery, this muscle can be slided to back.

**Fig. 320** To complete the slide, the entire ipsilateral tongue flap also be freed from the vertical septum. The dissection continues until adequate release of the tongue flap is obtained.

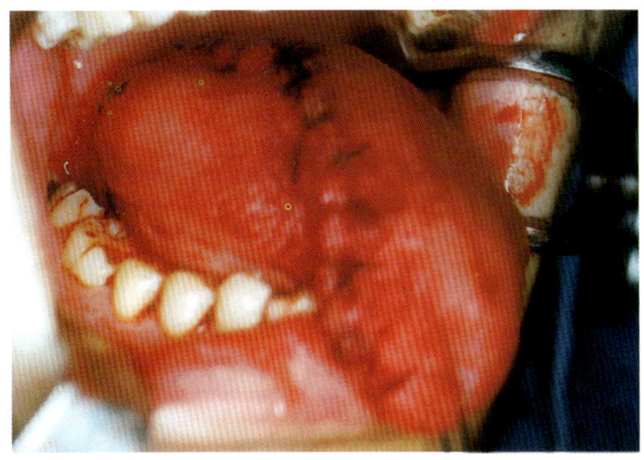

图 321

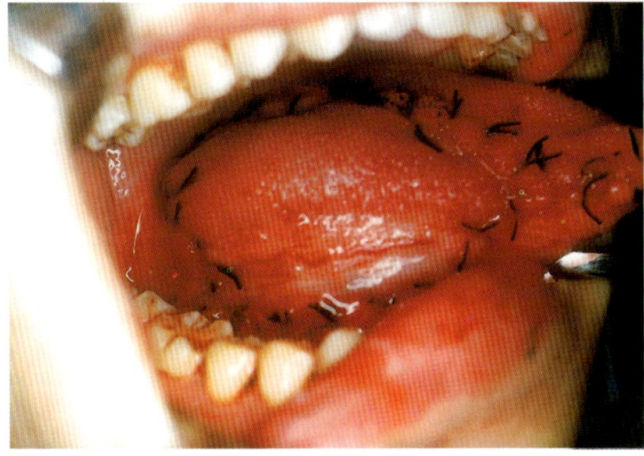

图 322

**图 321，322** 随着舌前部的分开，将前部组织瓣向中部滑行与后部剩余组织及对侧创缘相缝合，前部组织向后滑行后的缺损自身互相对合缝合。

**Fig. 321, 322** The tongue flap is slided to back and the posterior portion of the sliding tongue flap is sutured to the base of the tongue, remaining in a medial portion to the contralateral tongue tissue. The tongue defect on the contralateral anterior side is sutured on itself transorally.

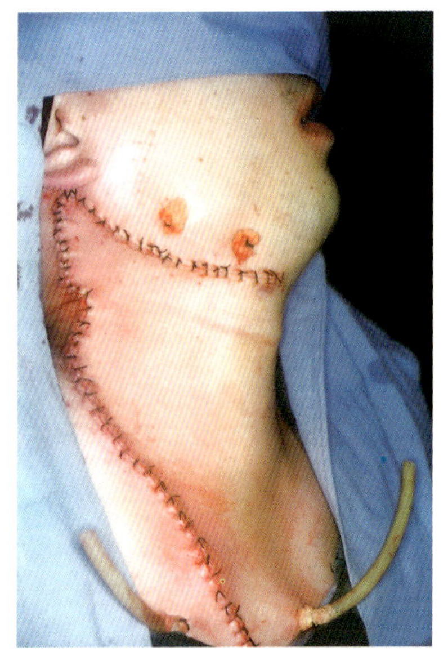

图 323

**图 323** 颈淋巴清扫术颈部创缘缝合后的情景。

**Fig. 323** The condition after suture of the radical neck dissection.

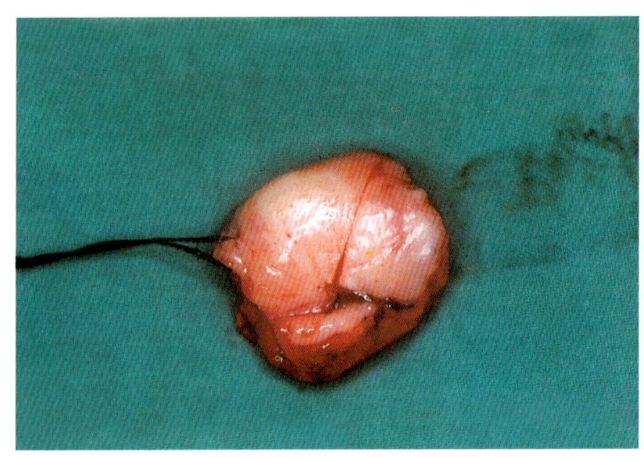

图 324

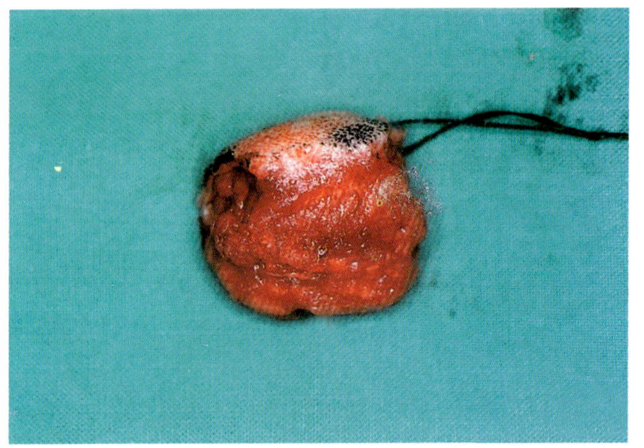

图 325

**图 324, 325** 手术后的舌组织标本。

**Fig. 324, 325** The specimens of the lingual lesion postoperatively.

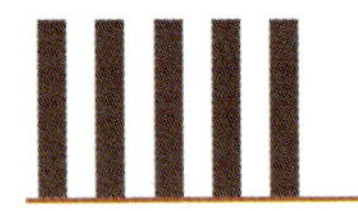



# 22. 舌根部癌舌瓣后推修复舌成形术

# 22. Set-back tongue flap for carcinoma of the tongue base

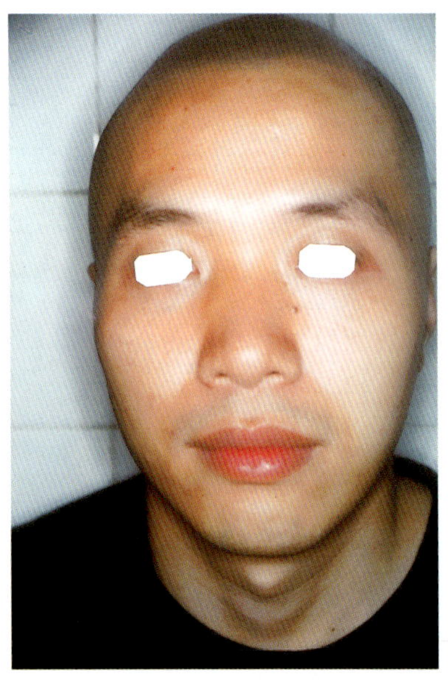

图 326

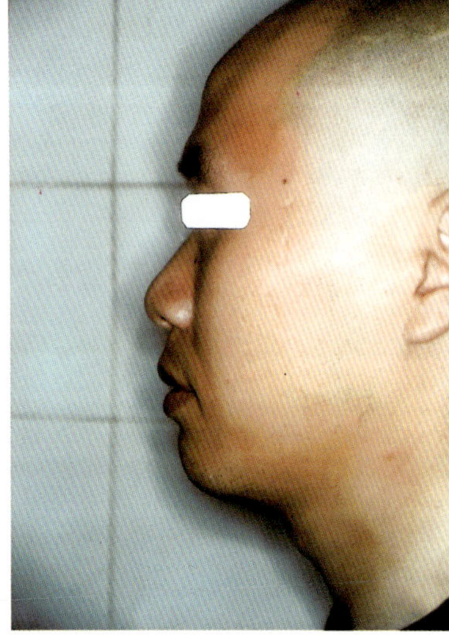

图 327

图 326, 327 一患有左舌根部鳞状细胞癌的患者术前正、侧面观。

Fig. 326, 327 Preoperative frontal and lateral views of patient with a well-differentiated epidermoid carcinoma in the left base of the tongue.

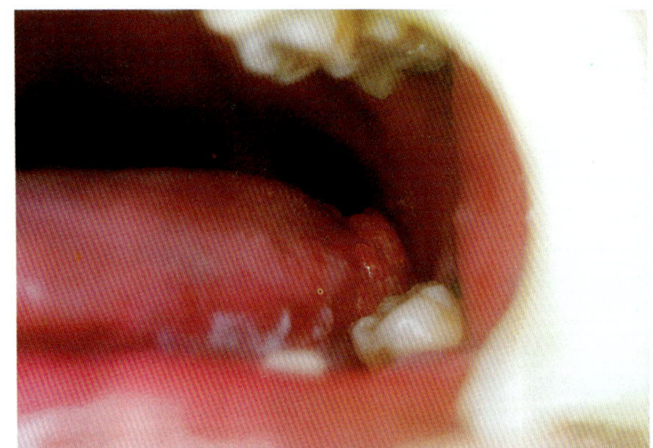

图 328

图 328 左舌根部可见一 4cm 大小的溃疡型病变。活组织切取检查诊断为高分化鳞状细胞癌。

Fig. 328 A 4 cm ulcerated lesion was noted in the left base of the tongue. A biopsy specimen showed a well-differentiated epidermoid carcinoma in the left base of the tongue.

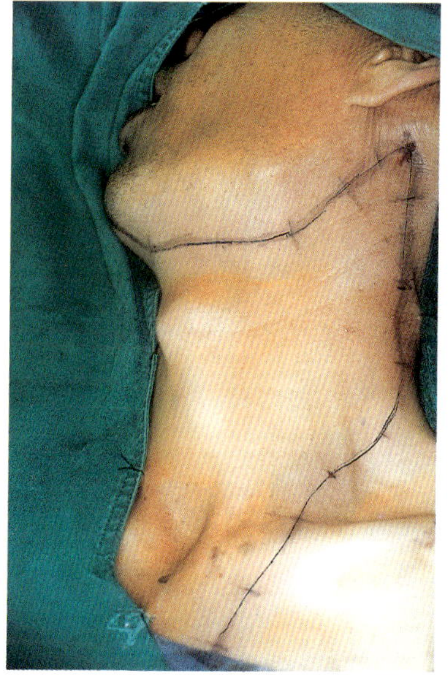

图 329

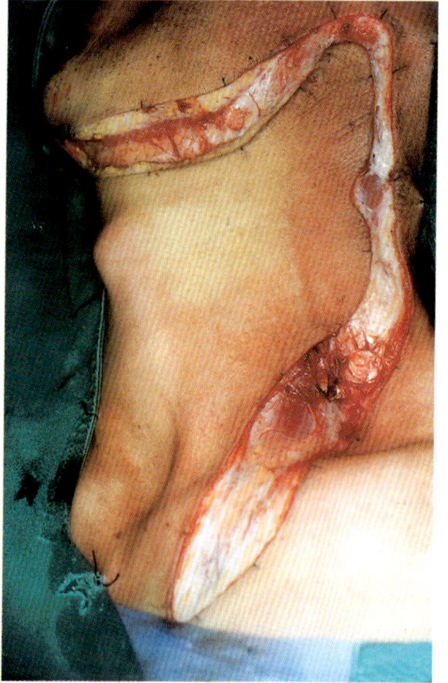

图 330

图 329 颈淋巴清扫术的切口线。
图 330 切开皮肤、皮下组织及颈阔肌。

Fig. 329 Line drawing of the radical neck dissection is outlined.

Fig. 330 The incision of the radical neck dissection is made through the skin and platysma.

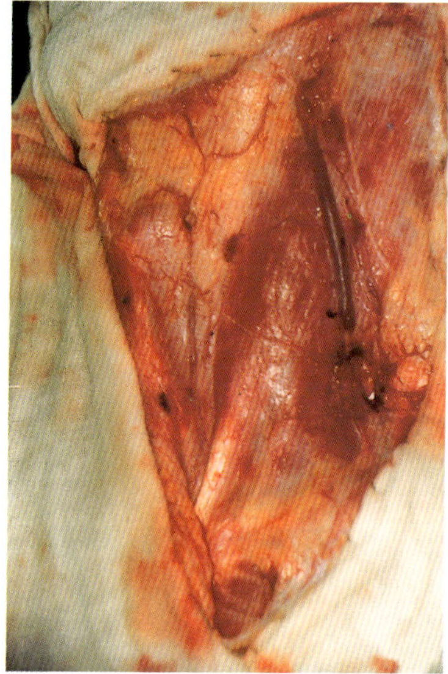

图 331

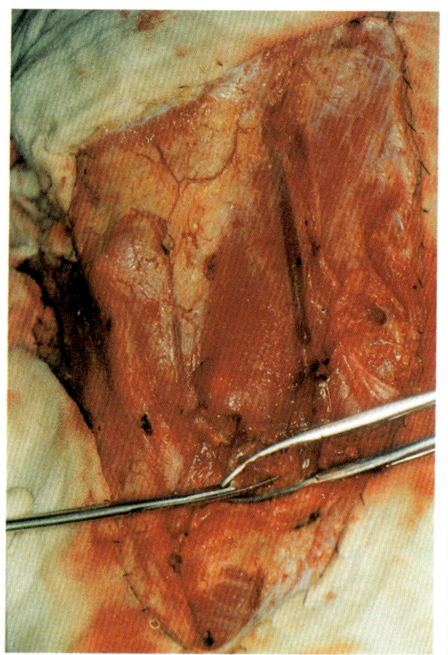

图 332

图 331 由后向前掀起皮肤—颈阔肌瓣，上至下颌下缘，前至颈中线，后至斜方肌前缘，下至锁骨下。

图 332 在锁骨上方约 2cm 处，用弯止血钳将胸锁乳突肌与深层组织分离，于锁骨上约 1cm 分别钳夹，切断胸锁乳突肌胸骨头和锁骨头，且缝扎其残端。

Fig. 331 The flap of skin and platysma is reflected anteriorly and posteriorly to expose the entire lateral region of the neck and the clavicle below. As the upper skin flap is retracted, the ramus marginalis mandibulae of the facial nerve is identified lying on the deep fascia. It is most easily found at the point where it crosses the facial vessels, just below the edge of the mandible. If no gross cancer is present along the course, the nerve is preserved by reflecting it upward with flap of skin and platysma. The flap is dissected a distance of 2 cm, above the inferior border of the mandible. The upper limit of the dissection may be defined by incising the fascia on the lower edge of the mandible dividing the facial vessels, and transecting the tail of the parotid gland. The anterior flap is raised until the anterior midline of the neck is reached. Posteriorly, the platysma is thin and disappears, and fibers of the upper portion of the sternocledomastoid muscle are attached to the skin. Dissection is continued just beneath the skin until the anterior margion of the trapezius muscle is exposed. As the flaps are raised, branches of the anterior and external jugular veins are severed, the veins themselves being left in situ to be removed with the block excision.

Fig. 332 Block dissection of the deep structures of the neck is now commenced. The sternal and clavicular attachments of the sternocleidomastoid muscle are severed at a point 1 cm, above the clavicle, care being taken to protect the underlying carotid sheath. Dissection is then carried posteriorly along the clavicle by incising the superficial layer of the deep fascia.

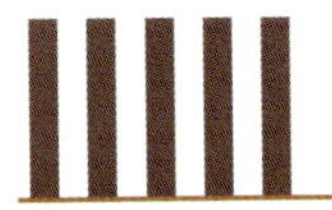



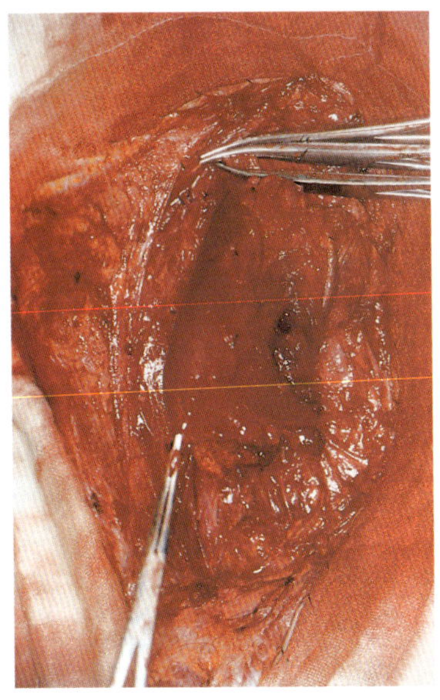

图 333

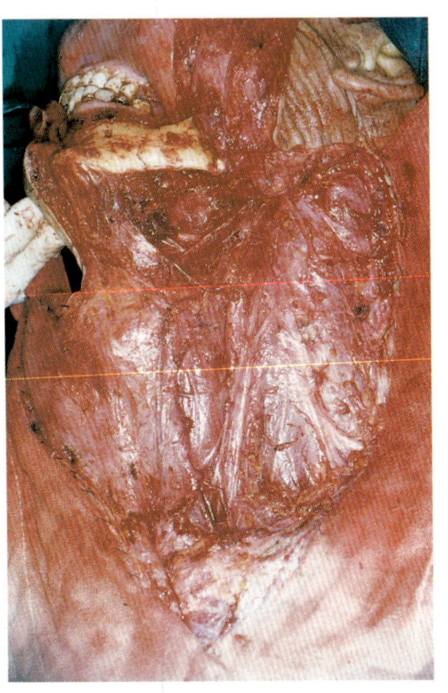

图 334

**图 333** 按颈淋巴清扫术的步骤清扫颈部大块组织后。

**图 334** 于下唇正中曲线切开下唇正中，于下颌龈颊沟处由前向后切开下颌龈颊沟组织达骨膜下，用骨膜分离器分离下颌体部外侧骨膜达嚼肌前缘。分离至颏孔时，游离颏孔穿出的神经血管束，将其切断结扎。

**Fig. 333** View after the block tissue of the neck is removed.

**Fig. 334** The curved lip-splitting incision can be made through the midline of the lower lip, which is the author's technique of choice. The major portion of the body of the mandible may be exposed by blunt dissection. Anteriorly, a few muscular attachments and the mental nerve and artery must be divided with the scalpel. The upper outer surface of body of the mandible is freed by incising the mucosa in the gingivobuccal sulcus.

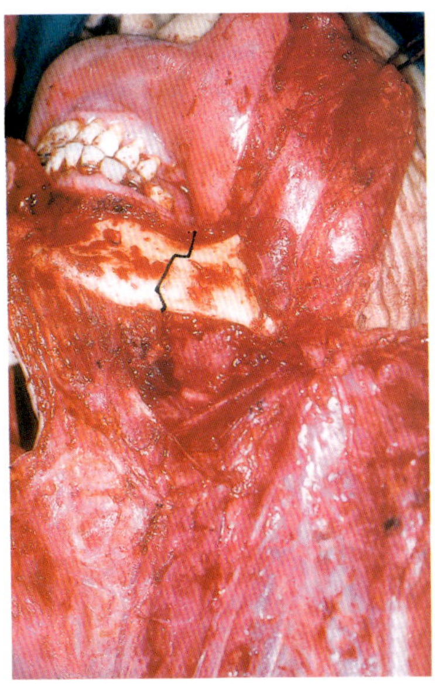

图 335

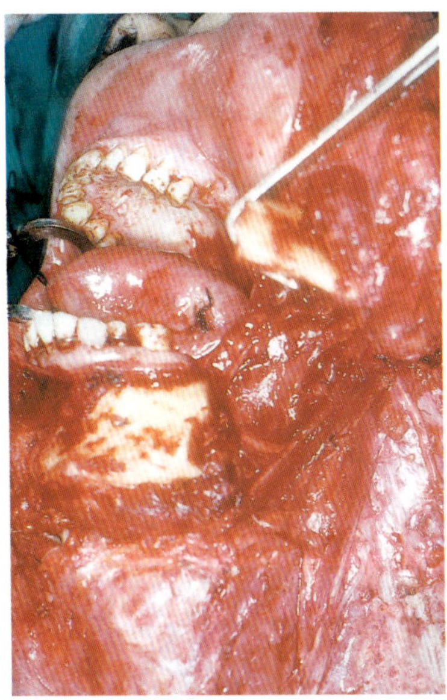

图 336

**图 335, 336** 由下颌体部下缘分离下颌体磨牙后区骨膜，于磨牙后区呈梯形截开下颌体部骨质，将下颌后段向后上牵拉，此时，舌根病变组织便清楚地暴露在手术野。

**Fig. 335, 336** The mandibulotomy may be performed in a stair-step or notched fashion to increase postoperative stability. Howere, with newer plating techniques, a straight vertical osteotomy probably yields comparable stability. The body of the mandible is divided posteriorly with a Gigli saw. The bone is then grasped with a bone-holding forceps and retracted upward. The lesion in the base of the tongue is exposed in the operative field.

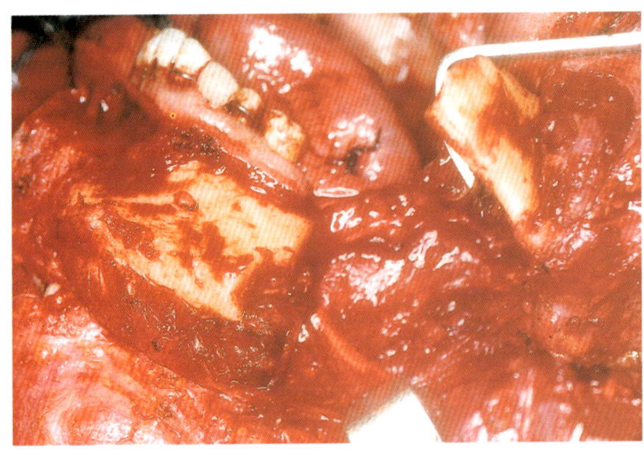

图 337

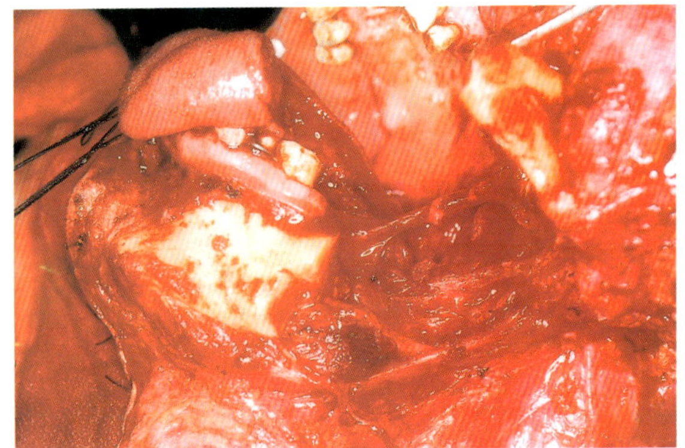

图 338

**图 337** 解剖来自于舌根部的舌下神经和动脉并保护进入舌前 2/3 的舌下神经及动脉。分离舌背动脉分支，将其结扎、切断。切断进入舌根的舌下神经小分支。完成病变部位的暴露。

**图 338** 在切除肿瘤时，牵开舌根部被保护的神经血管结构。

Fig. 337 The hypoglossal nerve and lingual artery are dissected from the base of the tongue and preserved as they enter the anterior half to two thirds of the tongue. The dorsal lingual artery branch is isolated, ligated and cut. Small branches from the hypoglossal nerve that enter the base of the tongue are also severed. Exposure of the lesion is accomplished through mandibulotomy.

Fig. 338 The neurovascular structures that were preserved are retracted from the tongue base as the tumor is resected.

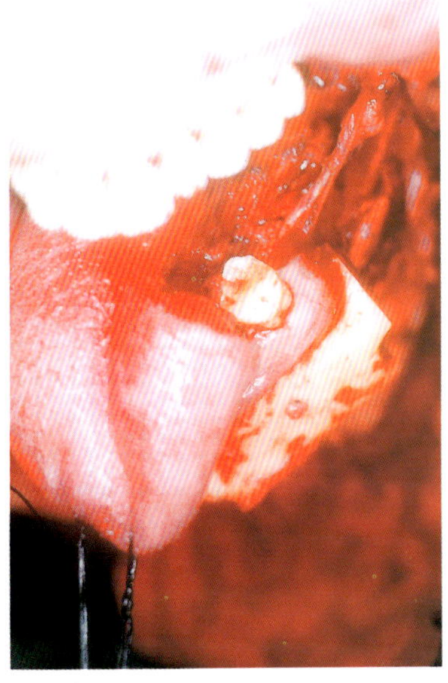

图 339

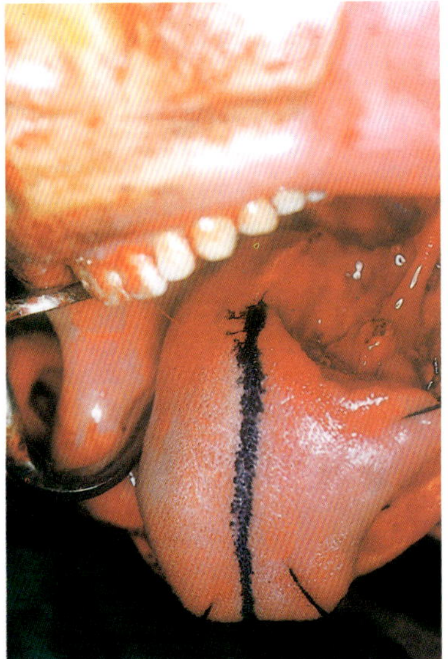

图 340

**图 339, 340** 将舌前部组织向前牵出口腔之外，将剩余的同侧舌前部组织作正中矢状切开达舌骨并使其瓣与对侧分离。

Fig. 339, 340 The anterior tongual tissue is retracted outer the oral cavity forward. The remaining ipsilateral anterior portion of the tongue is isolated from its contralateral side by a sagittal incision down to the hyoid bone.

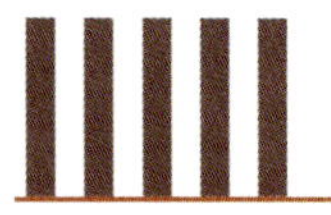



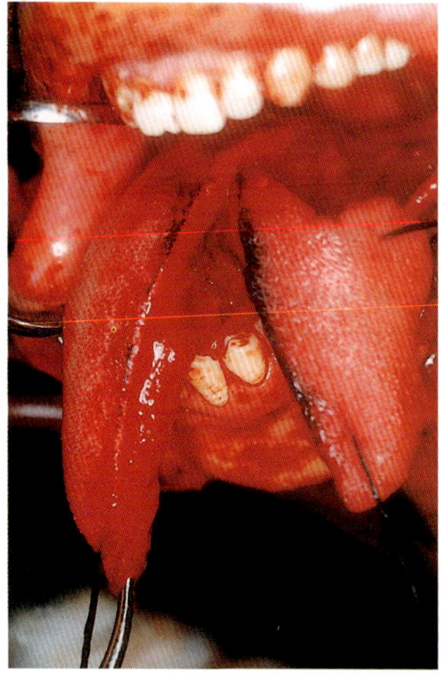

图 341

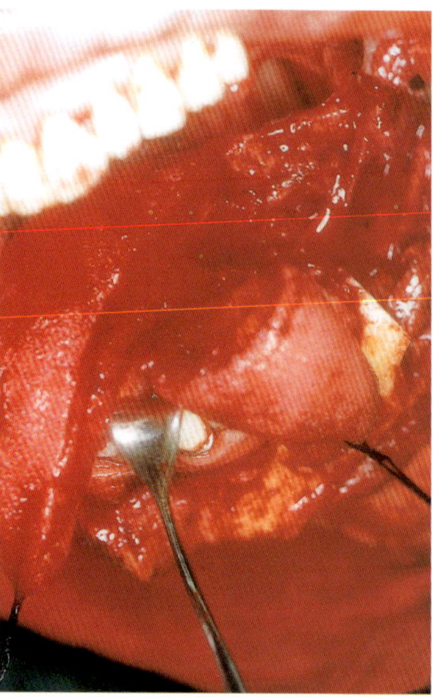

图 342

**图 341，342** 形成的舌前剩余组织瓣通过腱膜经舌下与舌骨相连。将瓣后推于舌根部的缺损。当瓣被用来充填 50% 到 60% 的舌根部缺损时，重点考虑舌下前部粘膜的可用性是必要的。

**Fig. 341，342** The resulting flap pivots on its fascial attachments via the hyoglossus to the hyoid bone. The flap is then set back into the base of the tongue defect. It is necessary to consider the use of the mucosa at the anterior portion of the tongue root when the flap is used to fill in more than a 50% to 60% tongue base defect.

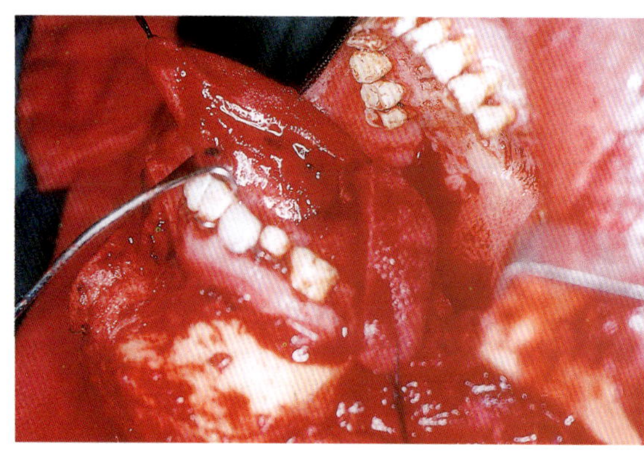

图 343

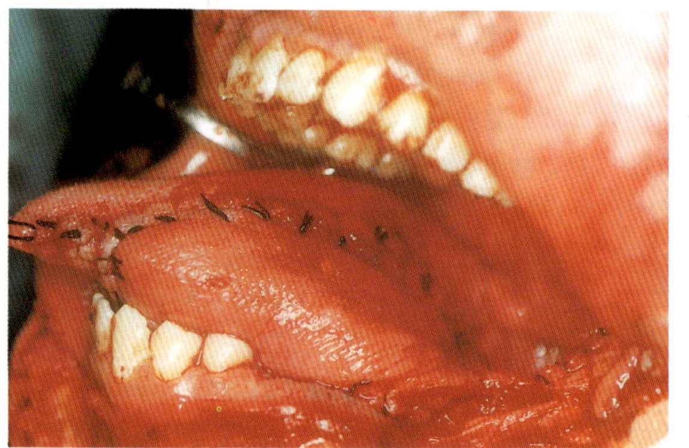

图 344

**图 343, 344** 后推的舌瓣后部与会厌部、内侧与对侧舌组织、外侧与口底组织相缝合。对侧前部的舌缺损自身之间互相缝合。

**Fig. 343, 344** The flap is sutured to the epiglottis posteriorly, the remaining in a medial position to the tongue base and in a lateral position to the tonsilpharyngeal mucosa. The tongue defect on the contralateral anterior side is sutured on itself transorally.

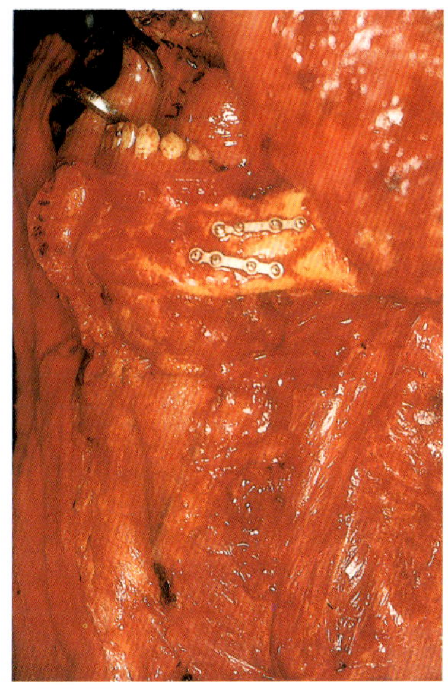

图 345

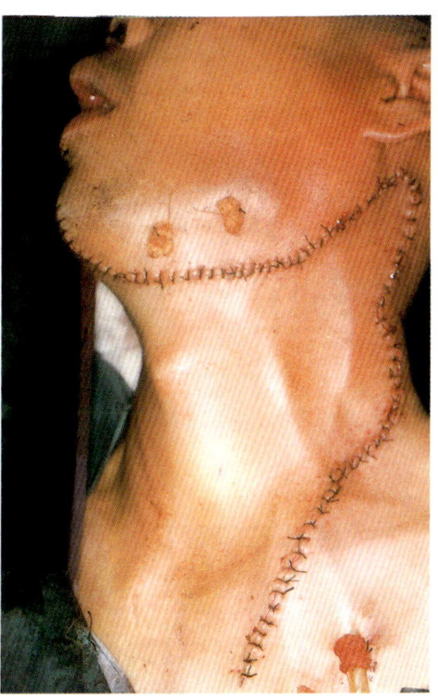

图 346

**图 345** 在被锯开的下颌骨体两端上各上、下钻 4 个孔，然后将微型钛板用螺钉固定。

**图 346** 大量生理盐水反复冲洗手术创面，彻底止血，并用 10% 氮芥湿敷创面；安置双管负压引流管并予以固定，将下唇、颊部及皮肤—颈阔肌瓣复位，分层间断缝合，以消毒纱布覆盖创口。

**Fig. 345** The four-holes in each end of the two ends to be divided the body of the mandible are drilled and the mandible is then reapproximated using the fitted plate. The lower lip is reapproximated by first reattaching the orbicularis oris by means of a permanent suture and then realigning the vermilion border accurately.

**Fig. 346** The entire wound is inspected for hemostasis, after which it is irrigated with saline solusion. Two Penrose drains are placed in the wound, one directed anteriorly and the other posteriorly. The drains may be brought out through the lower angle of the wound or through a stab wound in the lateral skin flap. The flaps are then approximated with buried sutures in the platysma and interrupted sutures of fine silk in the skin. A bulky pressure dressing is applied to the neck.

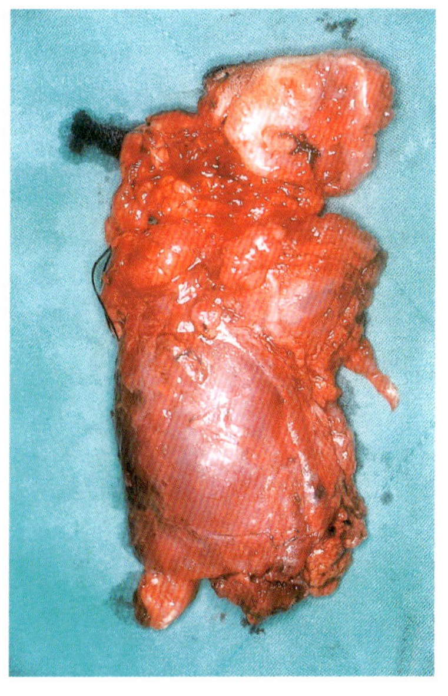

图 347

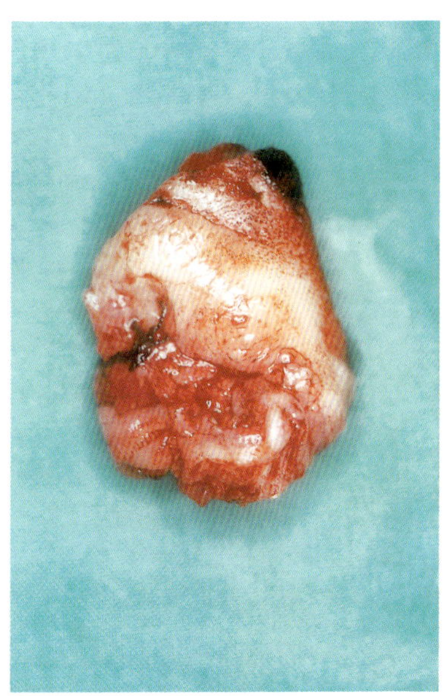

图 348

**图 347, 348** 手术后的组织标本。

**Fig. 347, 348** The specimens postoperatively.

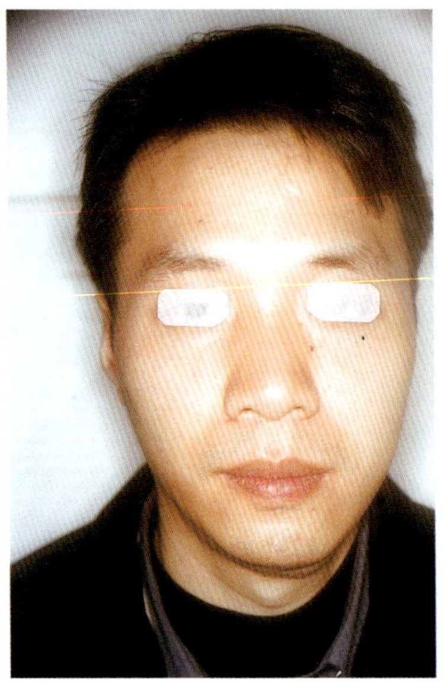

图 349

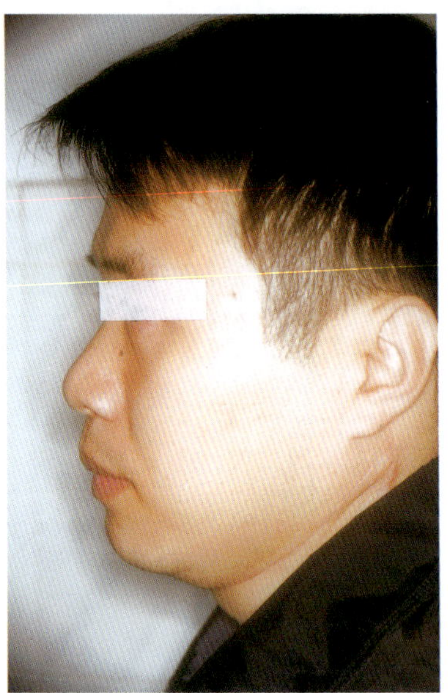

图 350

图 349, 350 手术后 1 年患者的正、侧面观。

Fig. 349, 350 Postoperative frontal and lateral views of patient with a well-differentiated epidermoid carcinoma in the left base of the tongue 1 year after surgery.

# 23. 舌癌切除后侧斜方肌岛状瓣舌重建

# 23. A lateral trapezius-musculocutaneous island flap for partial tongue reconstruction

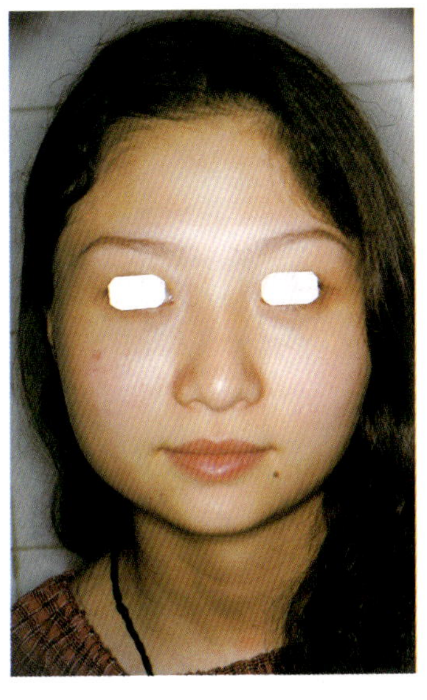

图 351

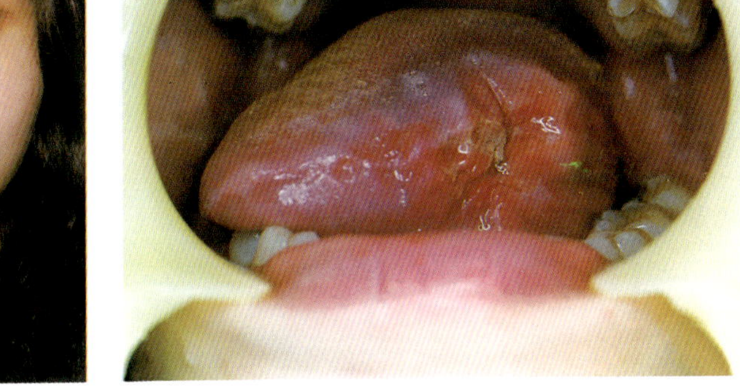

图 352

**图 351** 患舌左半侧鳞状细胞癌的 19 岁女性患者术前正面观。

**图 352** 见舌左侧前 2/3 舌组织溃疡，溃疡前部可见白斑。

**Fig. 351, 352** Frontal view of a 19 girl patient with squamous cell carcinoma at the posterior end of a patch of leukoplakia at the left side of the tongue.

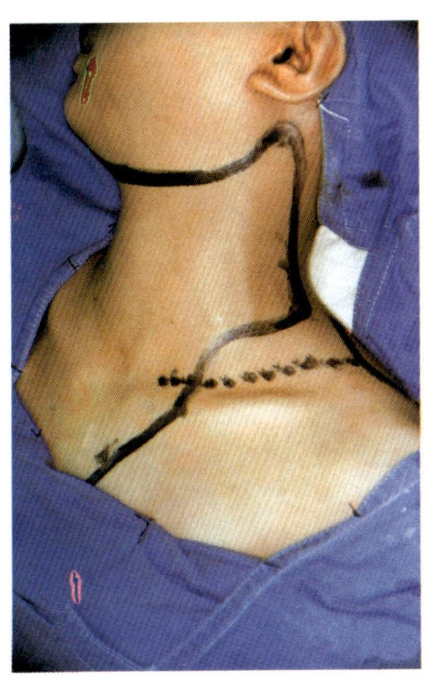

图 353

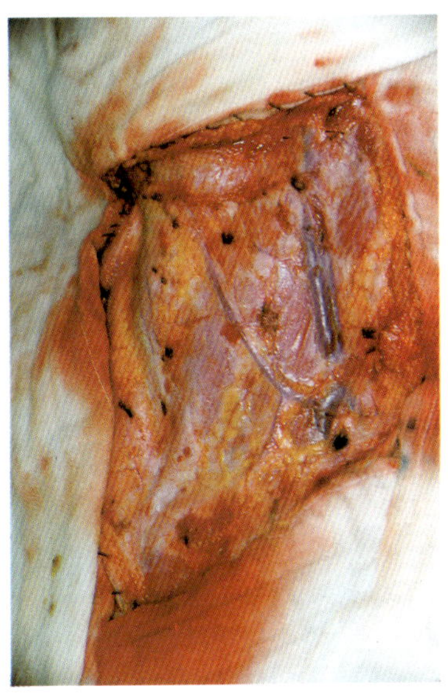

图 354

**图 353, 354** 当决定对舌癌进行治疗时，首先行颈部根治性淋巴清扫术，颈淋巴清扫术按常规方法进行。

**Fig. 353, 354** When decided to treate tongue carcinoma, radical neck dissection will be firstly performed according to the routine way. Neck dissection is completed except for the contents of the digastric triangle. The specimen of the neck dissection remains attached to the submandibular tissues. The inner aspect of the body of the mandible is freed by dissection close to the bone.

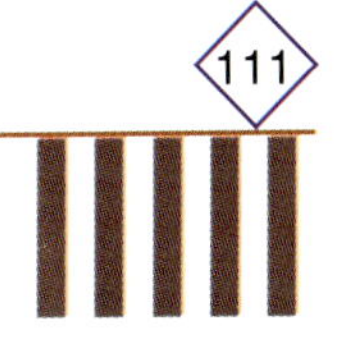

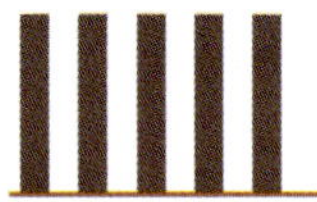



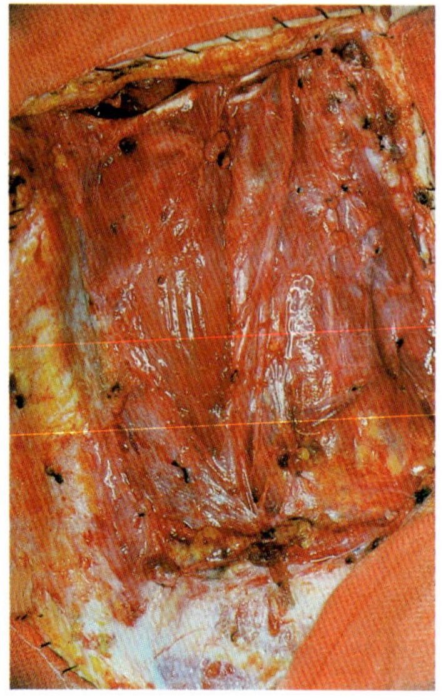

图 355

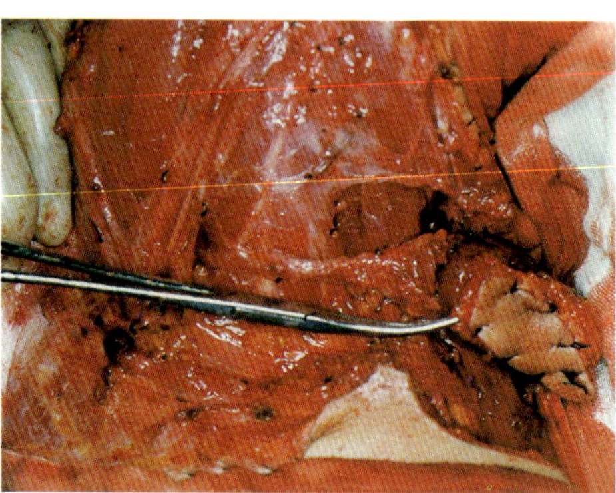

图 356

**图 355** 颈淋巴清扫术被完成之后，进行侧斜方肌岛状肌皮瓣的制取，当行根治性颈淋巴清扫术时，外科医师在清除颈后三角和切除胸锁乳突肌的过程中，可清楚地看到颈横动脉；另外，下后三角临床上很少有淋巴结转移。

**图 356** 本肌皮瓣是以颈横动－静脉系为基础的外侧斜方肌皮瓣。皮瓣的前缘与斜方肌的前缘相一致，从此处向后下沿肩胛棘的方向扩展。为了确定肌皮瓣中所含的血管，应该记住的是颈横动脉在锁骨上大约 5cm 处进入斜方肌的深面。

在手术过程中，为了确定蒂血管的存在和长度，手术的第一步是在其近端先解剖蒂，然而，解剖不必扩大到颈后三角达血管的全长，一旦血管的全程已经被确定，留着由软组织包围的静脉可能是最好的。知道了血管到达肌肉是在锁骨上 5cm，就能精确地计算出三角蒂的长度。蒂的长度必须足够以保证肌皮瓣到达受植区而无张力。从提肩胛肌上掀起与肌肉相连的皮岛，继续向前掀起蒂的肌肉，其宽度应与皮岛的宽度一致。

**Fig. 355** After radical neck dissection has been completed, the island flap of the lateral trapezius is performed. When a radical neck dissection is being carried out it is in the process of clearing the posterior triangle and resecting sternocleidomastoid that the area in which the transverse cervical vessels run becomes visible to the surgeon. The lower posterior triangle is virtually never the site of metastasis in the clinical situation potentially suitable for the flap so that its use is unlikely to compromise resection.

**Fig. 356** This flap is based on the transverse cervical arteriovenous system and is raised from more or less the same skin area as the upper trapezius island myocutaneous flap. Its anterior border corresponds approximately to the anterior margin of trapezius and from there it extends backwards and downwards in the general direction of the spine of the scapula. In order to be certain of including the vessels in the flap both the muscle element and the skin should extend above the point at which the transverse cervical vessels disappear deep to trapezius, i. e. approximately 5 cm above the clavicle.

During the procedure, the course of the artery is reliable generally. Because of the uncertainties it is probably wise as a first step to dissect the pedicle at its medial end in order to establish both its presence and length. The dissection however need not extend over the entire length of the vessels in the posterior triangle. Once the course of the vessels has been established medially it may be best to leave the vein surrounded by some of the soft fat present in the area. Knowing that the vessels reach the muscle approximately 5 cm above the clavicle the length of the pedicle in the posterior triangle can be measured accurately and the pivot point pin-pointed. This allows the skin island to be positioned on trapezius at a suitable distance from its anterior border so that the overall pedicle length, part muscle and part purely vascular are sufficient to allow the flap to reach its destination without tension.

The island of skin with the underlying muscle is raised from levator scapulae and elevation of the muscle segment of the pedicle is continued forward at a width similar to that of the island to the anterior border of trapezius. There it becomes continuous with the purely vascular element of the pedicle.

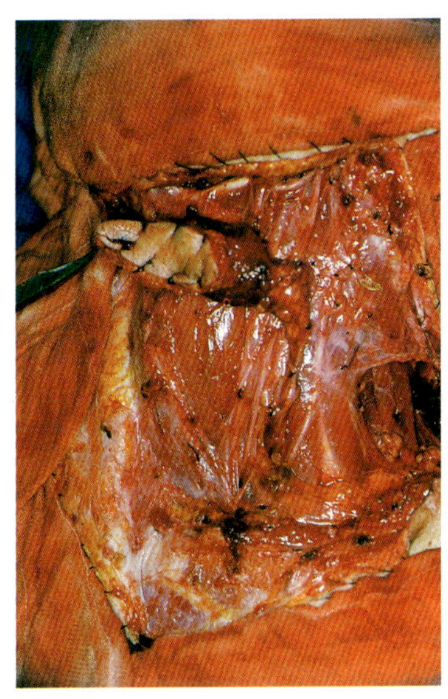

图 357

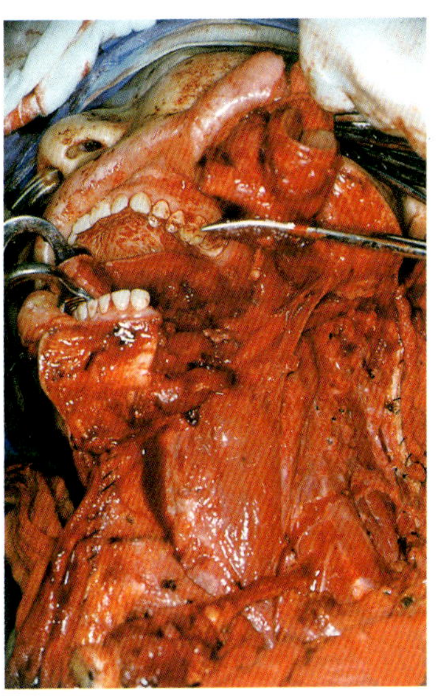

图 358

**图 357, 358** 在下唇正中弧形全层切开达颏下并与颈淋巴清扫术的颌下切口相连。于下颌正中患侧唇颊沟偏颊侧粘膜由前向后切开达下颌第二前磨牙处，于下颌下缘向上分离颊侧骨膜，暴露患侧颏神经。在下颌第一、二前磨牙之间分离舌侧骨膜。拔除第一双尖牙，穿入线锯，锯断患侧下颌骨，止血后用剪刀剪开口底粘膜及下颌舌骨肌达舌腭弓前缘。将下颌骨短骨段向上牵开，暴露患侧舌体部。在正常范围内将舌病变组织完全切除，止血。将制备好的侧斜方肌岛状瓣旋转 180°后达舌缺损区。由后向前缝合肌层，然后把岛状皮瓣的内侧边缘与舌缺损边缘缝合，外侧与复位后的口底粘膜肌层断端缝合。在患侧两断端下颌骨上分别钻孔后钢丝结扎。

**Fig. 357, 358** The lower lip is split in the midline and a cheek flap is elevated by an incision in the gingivobuccal gutter and dissection along the body of the mandible as far as the mental foramen and the mandibular periosteum is incised anterior to the mental foramen. The periosteum is elevated, ensuring that the mental nerve is not compromised. A pharyngeal pack is inserted to prevent aspiration of blood. The mandible is divided well anterior to the mental foremen with a Gigli saw. A teeth must be extracted before the mandible is divided.

At this stage, a mucosal incision is made in the lateral floor of the mouth extending posteriorly toward the anterior tonsillar pillar. It is important to preserve a cuff of mucosa on the alveolar ridge to permit a watertight closure when the incision is closed. The mandible is now swung laterally by dividing the mylohyoid muscle. Once the segment of mandible has been freed posteriorly, an incision is outlined around the tumor, leaving at least 1.0 cm of normal tissue on all its edges. The incision is carried through the deep musculature of the tongue and the floor of the mouth. The lingual nerve is sacrificed and the lingual artery is divided and ligated. The lingual tumor has been freed from all attachments and is removed. Hemostasis is obtained by ligating all bleeding vessels.

The lateral trapezius-musculocutaneous island flap is preferable to correct the initial rotation in order to reach comfortably the site to be repaired. A few sutures are placed between the muscular island and the neck muscles thus ensuring a good protection for the carotid artery all along its course. Then the skin island will be sutured to the defect of the tongue and the floor of the mouth. The mandibular split is repaired with lowprofile titanium plates and screws.



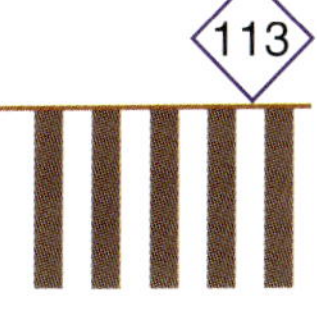

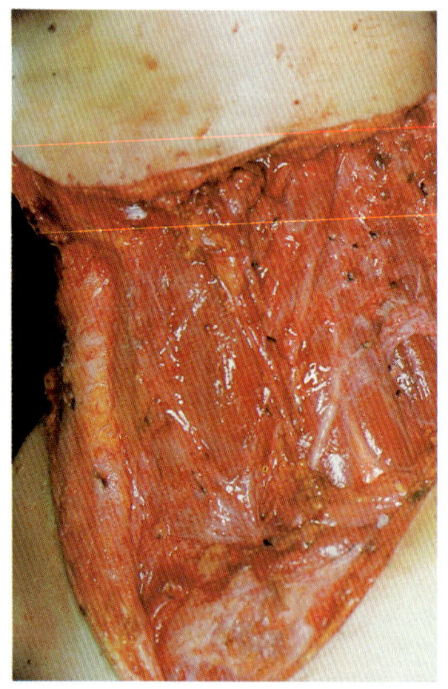
图 359

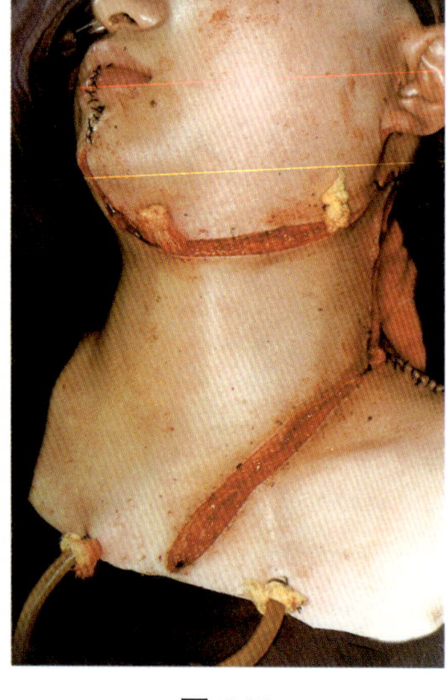
图 360

**图 359，360** 将颊瓣复位后由后向前缝合龈颊及唇颊沟粘膜。缝合下唇内侧粘膜，然后缝合肌层，最后缝合皮肤。将颈部肌皮瓣复位，在其下放入两根负压引流管后缝合颈阔肌、皮下组织及皮肤。局部稍加压包扎。手术结束。

**Fig. 359, 360** Closure of the gingivobuccal gutter is accomplished with interrupted mucosal sutures of fine silk. The lip is reconstructed with buried chromic sutures in the orbicularis muscle and fine silk sutures in the skin and mucosa. Care is taken to align accurately the vermilion-skin junction. The pharyngeal pack is removed. The neck wound is drained and closed in the usual manner.

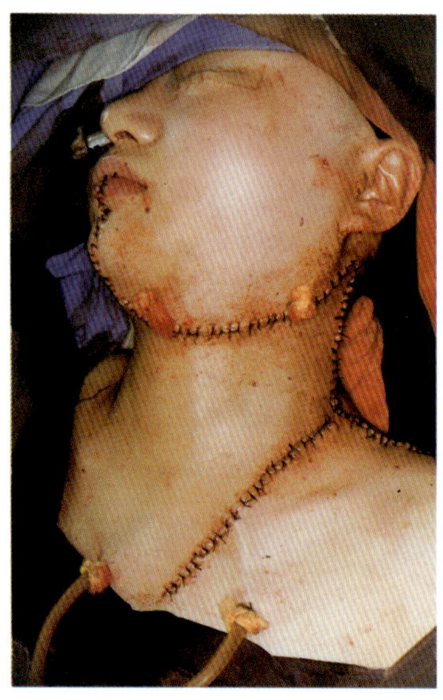
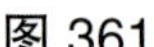
图 361

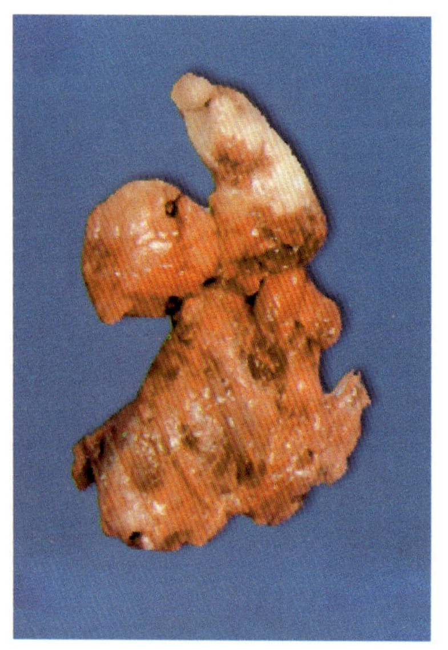
图 362

**图 361，362** 缝合后情景及术后组织标本。

**Fig. 361, 362** Condition after sutures and postoperative specimen.

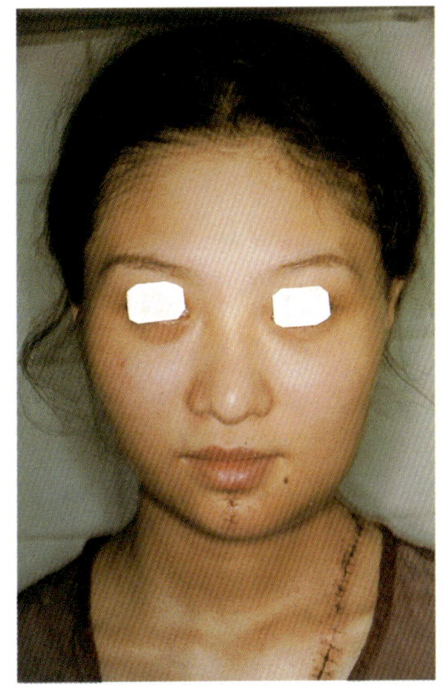

图 363

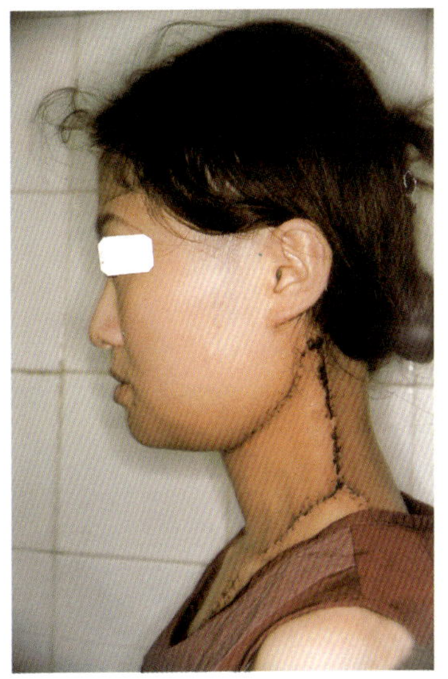

图 364

**图 363, 364** 患者手术拆线后正面及侧面观。

Fig. 363, 364 Patient's frontal and lateral views after sutures have been removed.

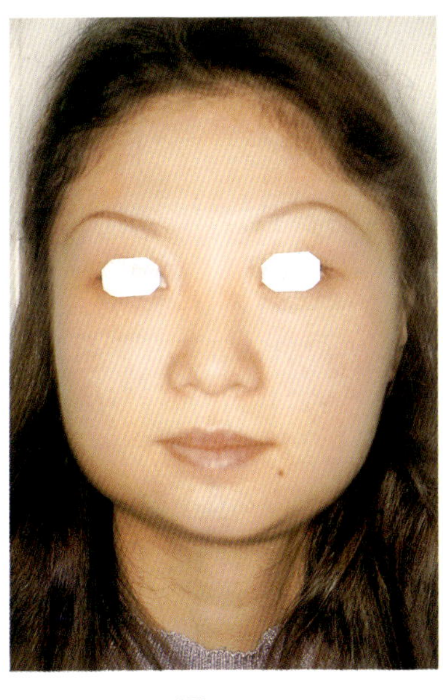

图 365

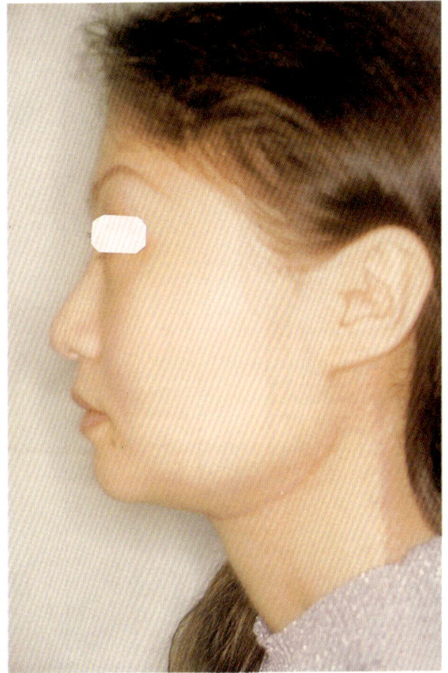

图 366

**图 365, 366** 患者术后一年正面及侧面观。

Fig. 365, 366 Patient's frontal and lateral views 1 year postoperatively.

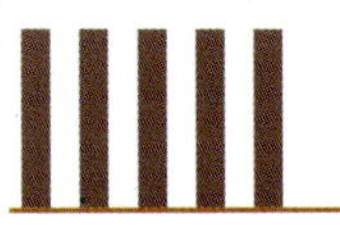



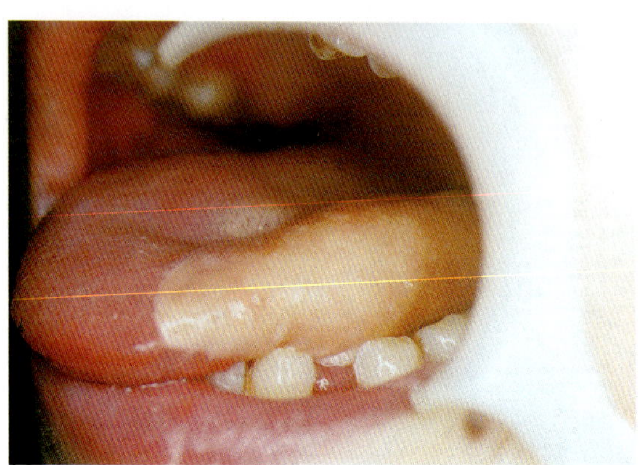

图 367

**图 367** 患者术后一年舌修复后的情景。舌体形态良好，肿瘤无复发。语言、吞咽功能正常。

**Fig. 367** Lingual healing of the repaired lingual defect 1 year postoperatively.

# 24. 舌根部癌切除额岛状瓣转移修复术

# 24. Island forehead flap repair in resection for the cancer of the base of the tongue

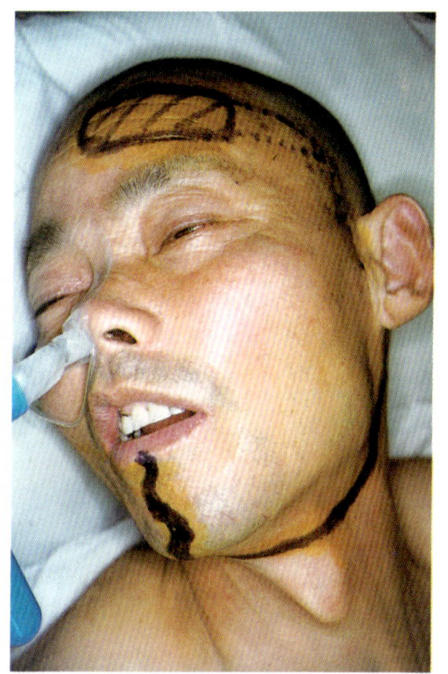

图 368

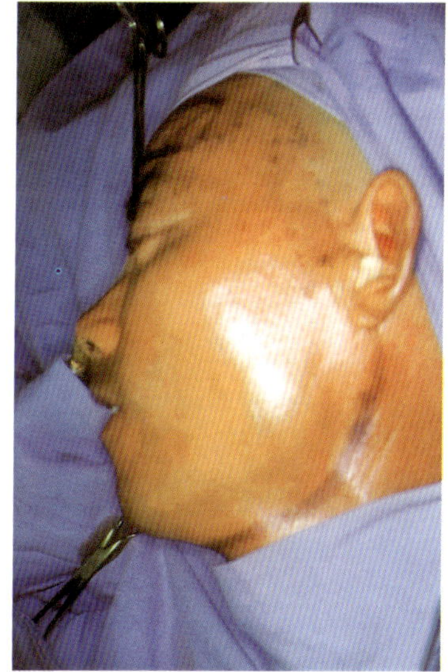

图 369

图 368，369 用美蓝画出额岛状瓣及手术切口线的正、侧面观。

Fig. 368, 369 Island forehead flap and incision lines are designed with methylene blue.

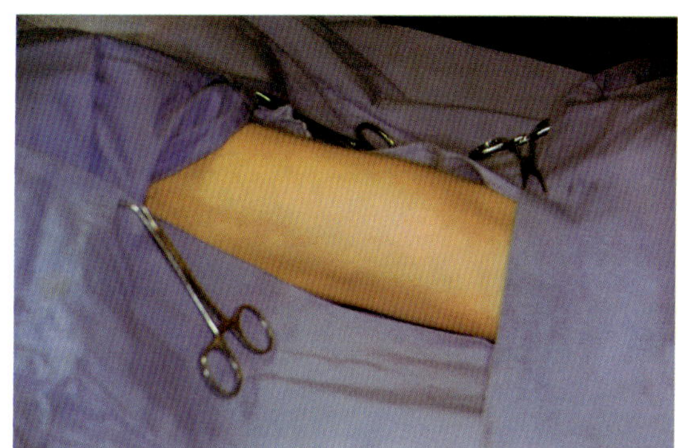

图 370

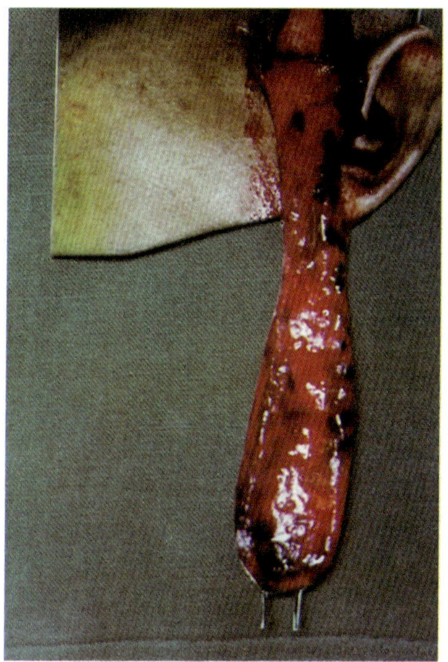

图 371

图370, 371 额岛状皮瓣的制备被完成之后，将额瓣蒂部的上皮组织还回原处后对位缝合，缺损区植前臂全厚皮片以覆盖额部缺损区。

Fig. 370, 371 After the preparation of the island forehead flap has been completed, the dermal layer of the forehead portion of the island is returned in place and is sutured each other. A thick split thickness skin graft is tightly applied to the donor area and secured with flutted gauzes.

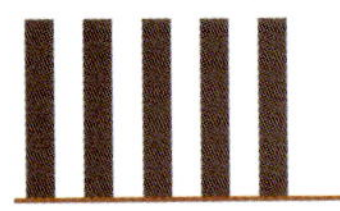



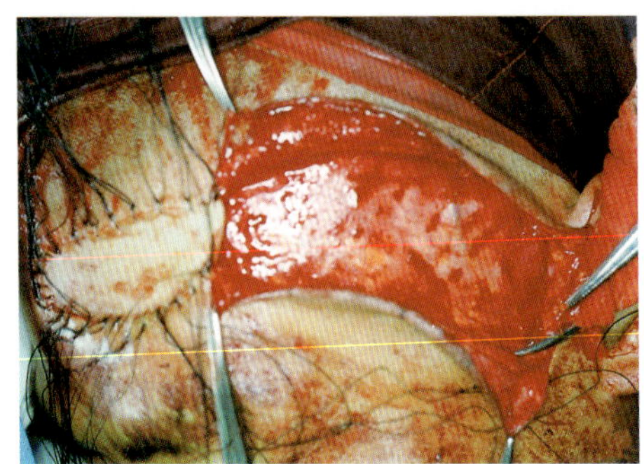

图 372

**图 372** 全厚前臂皮片被缝合于额供瓣缺损区后的情景。

**Fig. 372** The condition after a thick split thickness skin graft is sutured to the donor area.

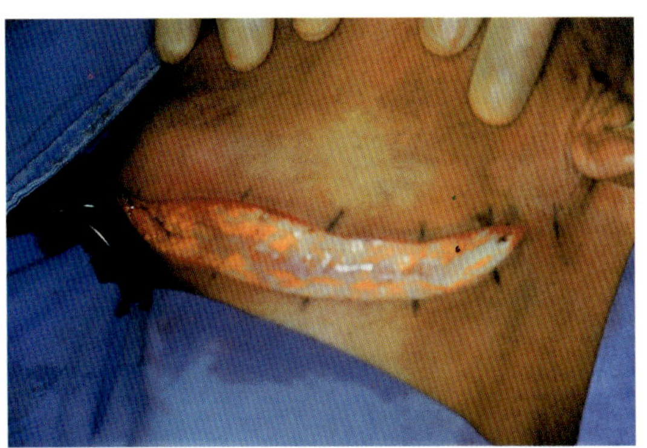

图 373

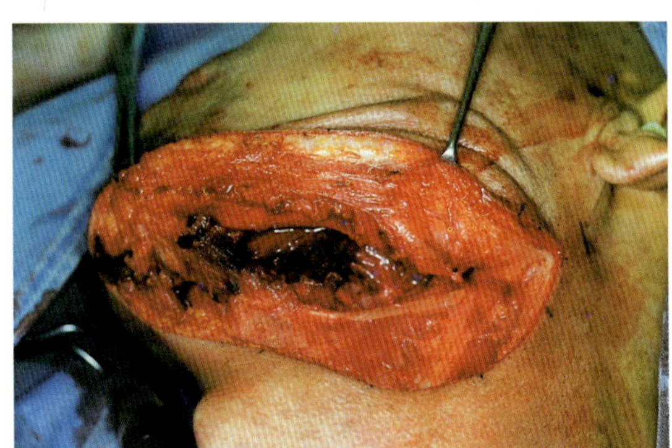

图 374

**图 373, 374** 在下颌体下缘约 2cm 平下颌骨体从下颌升支下缘开始向前延伸达颏下做切口，切口深达颈阔肌之下。在颈阔肌深面与覆盖颌下腺的颈筋膜之间的平面解剖皮瓣，注意保护面神经的下颌缘支。在嚼肌前缘处分离颌外动脉并切断结扎。

**Fig. 373, 374** The incision is made below and parallel to the body of the mandible, extending from the lower segment of the ramus of the mandible forward to beneath the chin. It is deepened through the skin and platysma. The skin flaps are dissected on a plane between the undersurface of the platysma and the cervical fascia covering the submandibular gland. The mandibular branch of the facial nerve must be identified and protected. The external maxillary artery and vein are dissected at the anterior border of the masseter, divided and ligated.

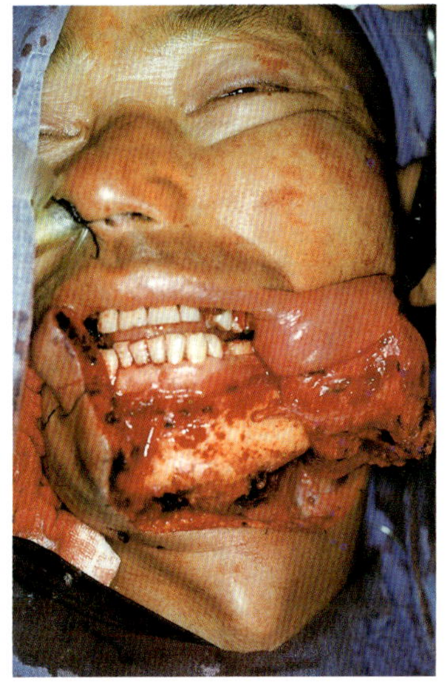

图 375

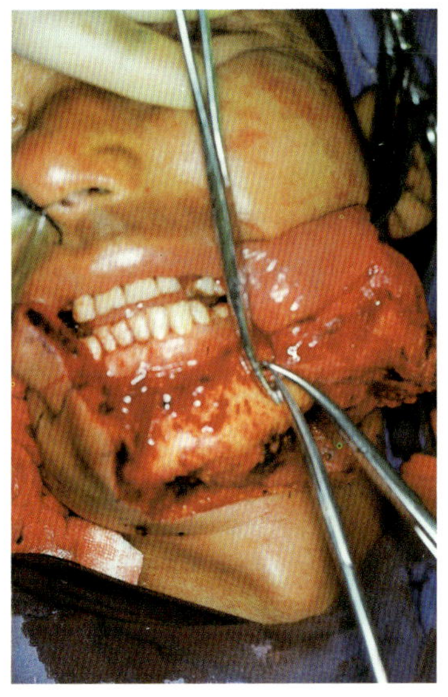

图 376

**图 375, 376** 在下唇正中弧形全层切开达颏下并与颌下切口相连。于下颌正中患侧唇颊沟偏颊侧由前向后切开达下颌第二磨牙处，于下颌下缘向上分离颊侧骨膜，暴露患侧颏神经，并将其切断、结扎。

**Fig. 375, 376** The lower lip is split in the midline to under the chin and associated with the submandibular incision. A cheek flap is elevated by an incision in the gingivobuccal gutter and dissection along the body of the mandible as far as the mental foramen and the mandibular periosteum is incised anterior to the mental foramen. After the mental nerve is divided, the periosteum is elevated.

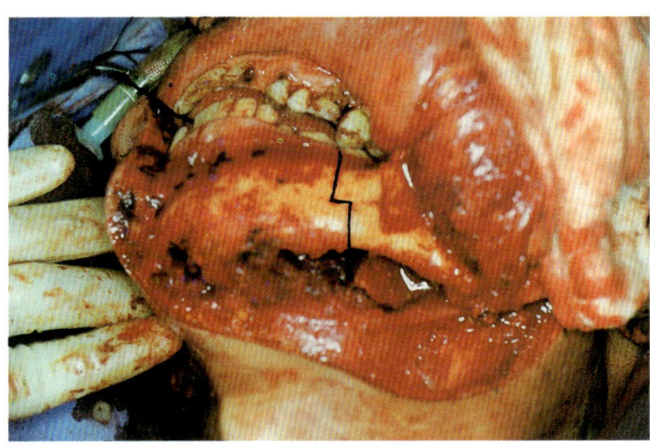

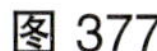

图 377

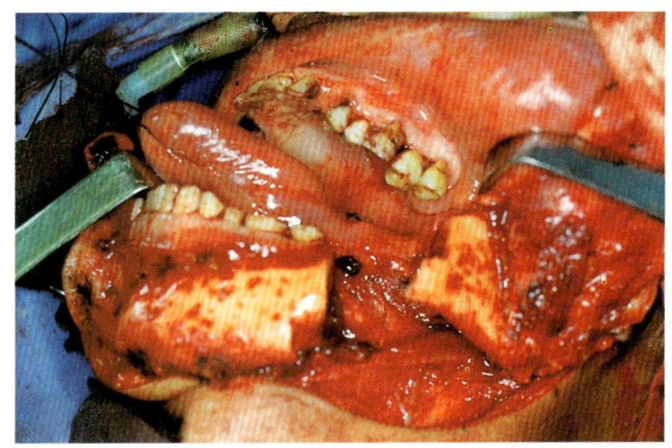

图 378

**图 377** 在下颌第二磨牙的远中分离舌侧骨膜，穿入线锯，锯断患侧下颌骨，止血后用剪刀剪开口底粘膜及下颌舌骨肌达舌腭弓前缘。

**图 378** 将下颌骨短骨段向上牵开，暴露患侧舌根部。

**Fig. 377** The mandible is divided well anterior to the angle of the mandible with a Gigli saw. At this stage, a mucosal incision is made in the lateral floor of the mouth extending posteriorly toward the anterior tonsillar pillar. It is important to preserve a cuff of mucosa on the alveolar ridge to permit a watertight closure when the incision is closed.

**Fig. 378** The mandible is now swung laterally by dividing the mylohyoid muscle.

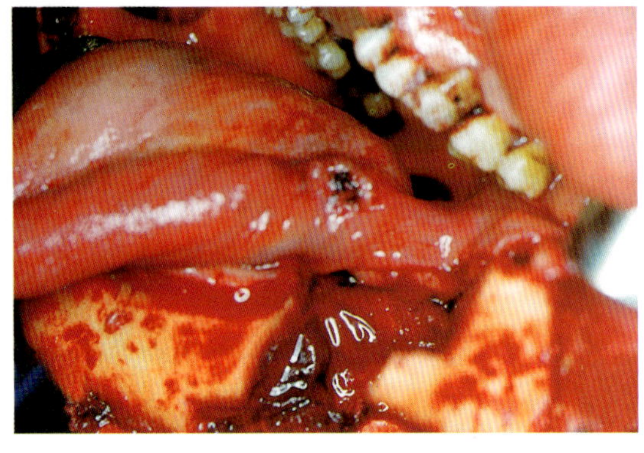

图 379

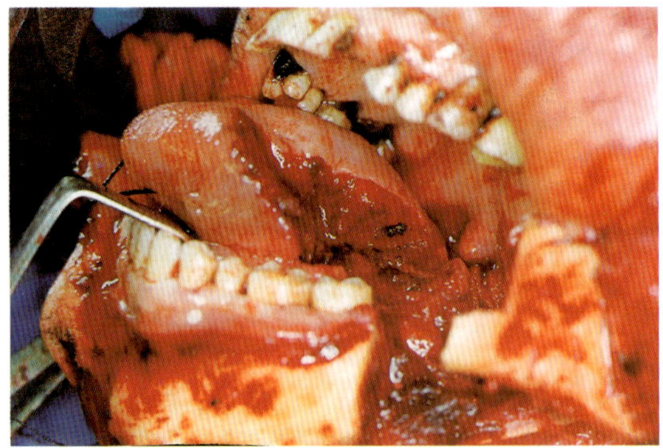

图 380

**图 379** 将舌体向前拉，整个舌根部病变组织完全暴露在手术野中。

**图 380** 在正常范围内将舌病变组织完全切除，止血。

**Fig. 379** After the body of the tongue was pulled forward, the lesion in the base of the tongue is completely exposed in the field of operation.

**Fig. 380** Once the segment of mandible has been freed posteriorly, an incision is outlined around the tumor and leaving at least 1.0 cm of normal tissue on all its edges. The incision is carried through the deep musculature of the tongue and the floor of the mouth. The lingual tumor has been freed from all attachments and is removed. Hemostasis is obtained by ligating all bleeding vessels.

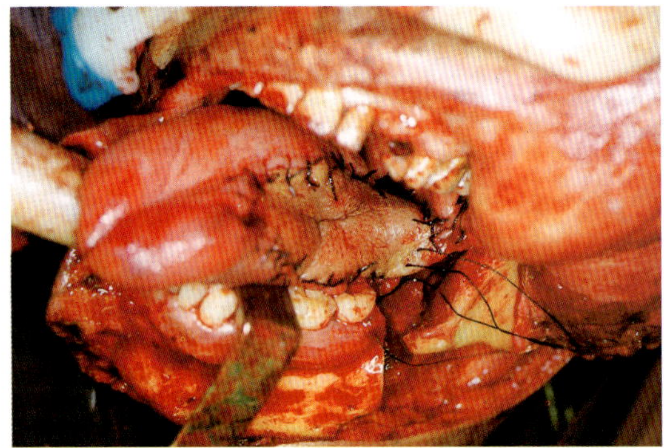

图 381

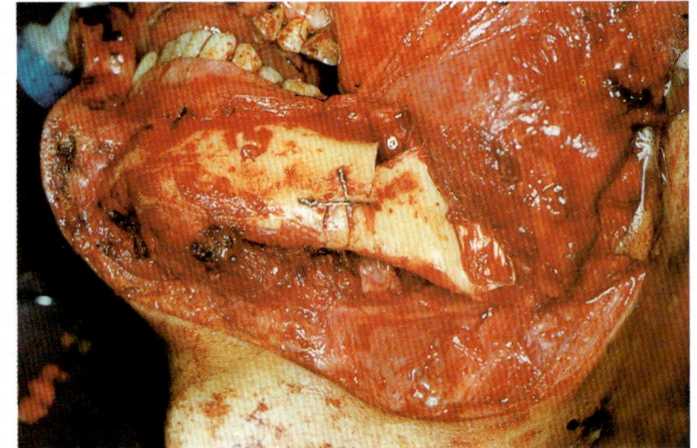

图 382

**图 381** 将岛状额瓣导入口腔后放置于舌根缺损区，额瓣的周缘与舌切除边缘创面相缝合。

**图 382** 将下颌骨断端复位后用钢丝将下颌骨断端固定。将颊瓣还回后缝合龈颊沟粘膜。生理盐水冲洗创面，分层缝合颈部创口。放置橡皮引流管一根引流 48 小时。

**Fig. 381** After the island forehead flap has reached the oral cavity through a tunnel, the island forehead flap will be sutured to the defect of the base of the tongue and the floor of the mouth.

**Fig. 382** The mandibular split is fixed with wires placed through holes drilled in the bone. Closure of the gingivobuccal gutter is accomplished with interrupted mucosal sutures of fine silk. The lip is reconstructed with buried chromic sutures in the orbicularis muscle and fine silk sutures in the skin and mucosa. The wound is drained with a rubber tube for 48 hours.

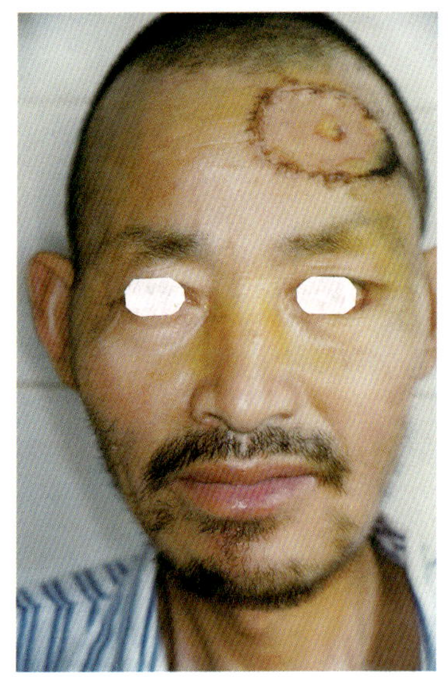

图 383

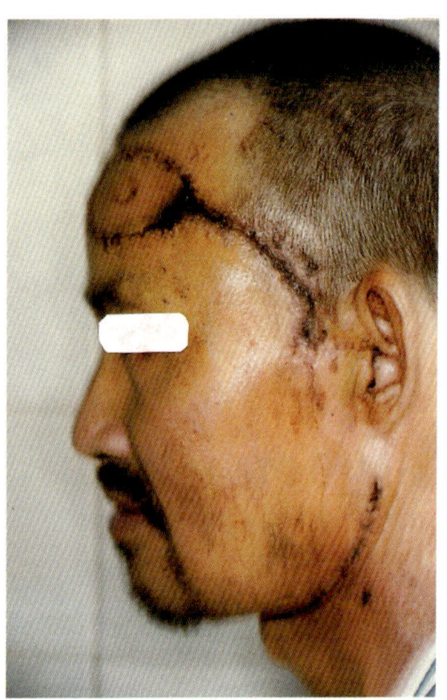

图 384

图 383, 384 术后 10 天患者的正、侧面观。

Fig. 383, 384 Frontal and lateral views of the patient 10 days after operation.

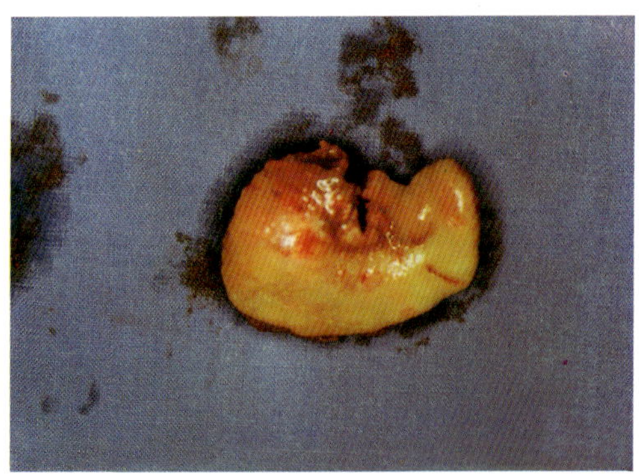

图 385

图 385 术后标本的正面观。

Fig. 385 Frontal view of the specimen postoperatively.

# 25. 口底癌切除后侧斜方肌岛状肌皮瓣转移口底修复术

# 25. Immediate trapezius-musculocutaneous island flap repair in resection for the carcinoma of the floor of the mouth

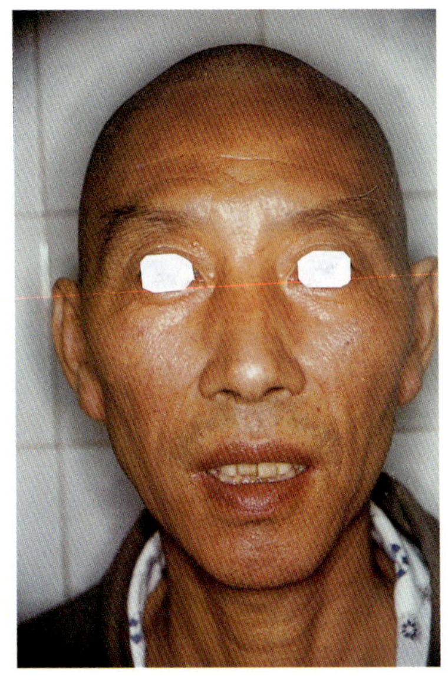

图 386

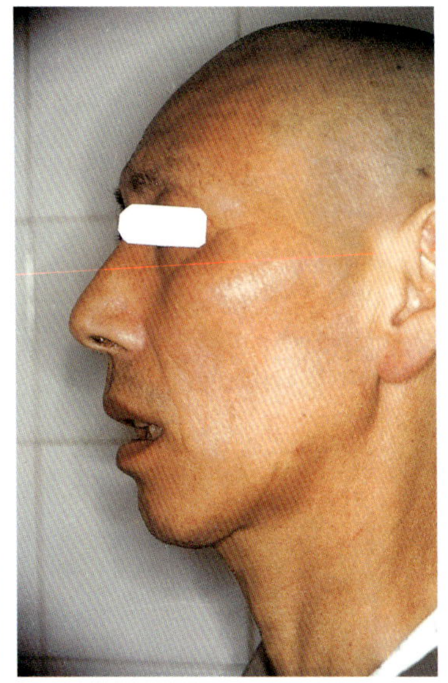

图 387

**图 386，387** 一患口底鳞状细胞癌的 62 岁男性患者的正、侧面观。

**Fig. 386, 387** Frontal and lateral views of a 62-year-old male patient with squamous cell carcinoma of the anterior floor of the mouth.

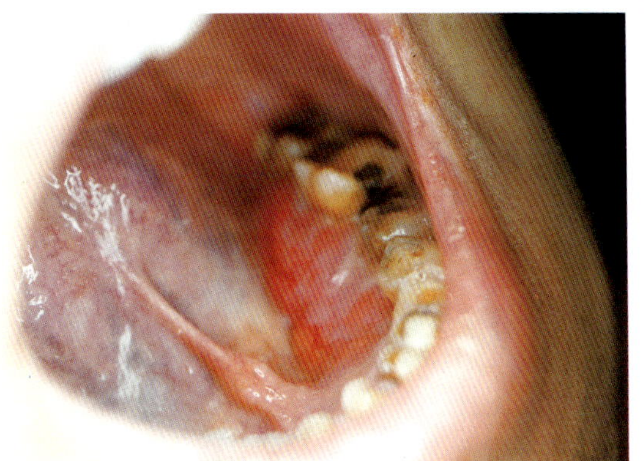

图 388

**图 388** 发生于口底前部的鳞状细胞癌。

鳞状细胞癌位于口底前部的正中线及左侧，病变呈溃疡状并向口底深层及舌体腹面扩展。

**Fig. 388** The squamous cell carcinoma occurs in the anterior portion of the floor of the mouth.

The squamous cell carcinoma is located in the anterior portion of the floor of the mouth in the region of the junction with the tongue. As the tumor spreads on to the side of the tongue and deep spreads into hyoglossus and genioglossus.

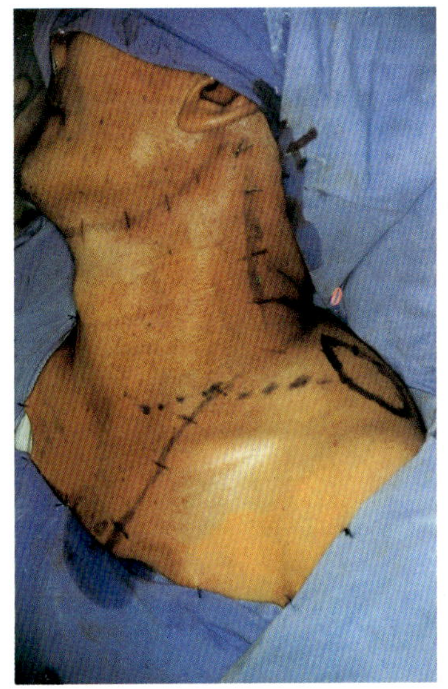

图 389

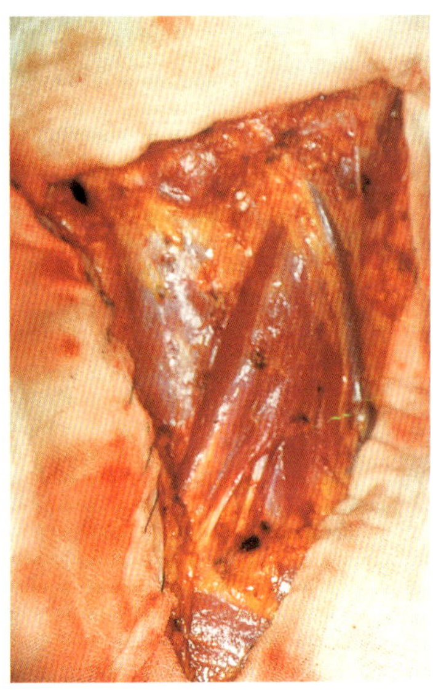

图 390

**图389** 设计出颈清扫术和侧斜方肌岛状瓣制备的切口线。

**图390** 按设计的颈淋巴清扫术的切口线切开颈部皮肤、皮下组织及颈阔肌，在颈阔肌深面由后向前掀起皮肤 - 颈阔肌瓣。暴露颈侧区域。

**Fig. 389** Incision line of the radical neck dissection and the trapezius-musculocutaneous island flap is marked out with the methylene blue.

**Fig. 390** After incision line has been marked out, the upper curved incision of the radical neck dissection is made through the skin and platysma. The vertical portion of the incision is made and flaps of skin and platysma are reflected anteriorly to expose the entire lateral region of the neck and the clavicle below.

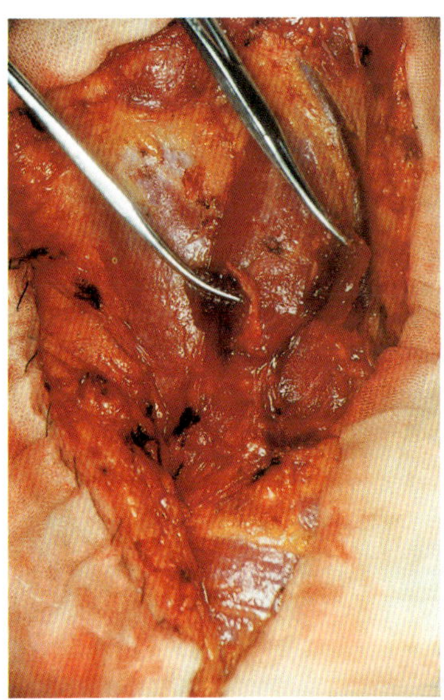

图 391

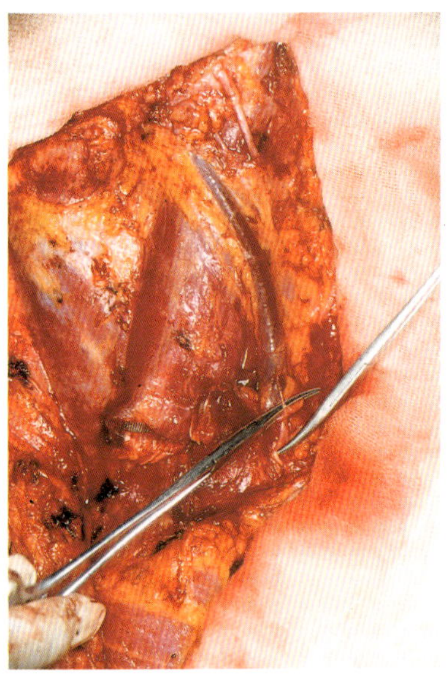

图 392

**图391** 在锁骨上方约2cm处，用弯止血钳将胸锁乳突肌与深层组织分离，于锁骨上约1cm分别钳夹、切断胸锁乳突肌胸骨头和锁骨头，且缝扎其残端。

向上翻起切断的胸锁乳突肌下端，即可见到斜行于血管鞘浅层的肩胛舌骨肌，切断其肩胛端并顺其方向游离。细心分层切开颈血管鞘，显露颈内静脉、颈总动脉和迷走神经。小心分离颈内静脉，分别用7号、4号丝线结扎颈内静脉，然后切断，再用1号丝线结扎其近心断端并将其固定在胸锁乳突肌的残端深面以保护。

**图392** 从颈内静脉近心端平面向斜方肌前缘作横形切口，切开颈深筋膜和脂肪，切断锁骨上皮神经分支。结扎、切断颈外静脉近心端。在脂肪组织内显露出颈横动脉、静脉，切断其分支后予以保留。继续向下解剖分离至斜角肌浅面，显露在斜角肌表面、椎前筋膜下的由外上方向内下方越过的膈神经和该肌外侧的臂丛神经，均予以保护。此平面即为手术区的底界。最后再横断斜方肌前缘处的脂肪和蜂窝组织。至此，整个手术区的下界已全部被解剖游离。

**Fig. 391** Block dissection of the deep structures of the neck is now commenced. The sternal and clavicular attachments of the stenocleidomastoid muscle are severed at a point 1 cm above the clavicle. Care being taken to protect the underlying carotid sheath. Dissection is then carried posteriorly along the clavicle by incising the superficial layer of the deep fascia.

The external jugular vein is exposed and divided near the midpoint of this incision. Laterally, the omohyoid muscle is encountered and is severed just above its scapular attachment where it meets the anterior edge of the

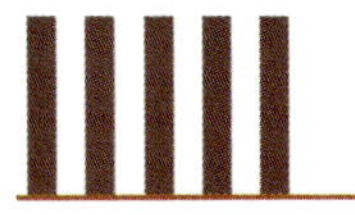



trapezius muscle. This point is the posterior corner of the block dissection. The carotid sheath is entered about 1 cm above the clavicle. The internal jugular vein is isolated at this point by careful blunt dissection. The vein is divided between ligatures. After division of the vein, its lower end is additionally secured with a transfixion suture.

Fig. 392 The common carotid artery and vagus nerve are identified within the carotid sheath. The anterior portion of the sheath is elevated a short distance. Dissection is once again carried laterally through the fatty areolar tissue of this deep plane to outline the lower limits of the block excision. As dissection proceeds from the carotid artery outward, three important structures are encountered. The thyrocervical artery trunk or its transverse cervical branch must be divided and ligated just lateral to the carotid sheath. The phrenic nerve is noted coursing downward in an oblique direction from the posterior toward the anterior edge of the scalenus anterior muscle and is preserved. Near the outer third of the clavicle, the brachial plexus is seen in the same plane as the scalene muscles. The fatty and areolar tissue overlying the brachial plexus is continuous with the contents of the axilla. This tissue is transected at the lower outer corner of the operative field and the branches of the transverse servical vessels encountered being clamped and ligated.

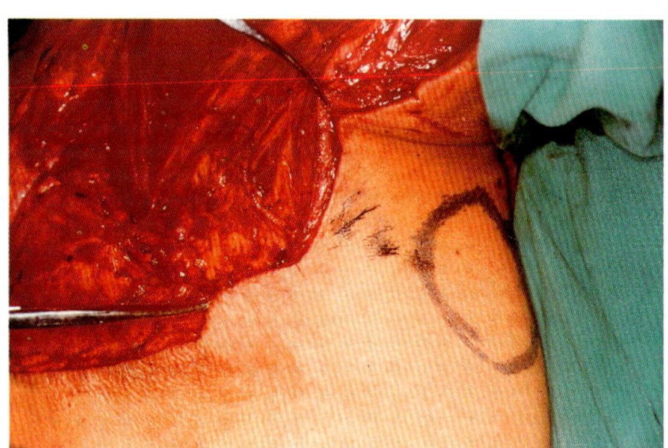

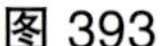

图 393

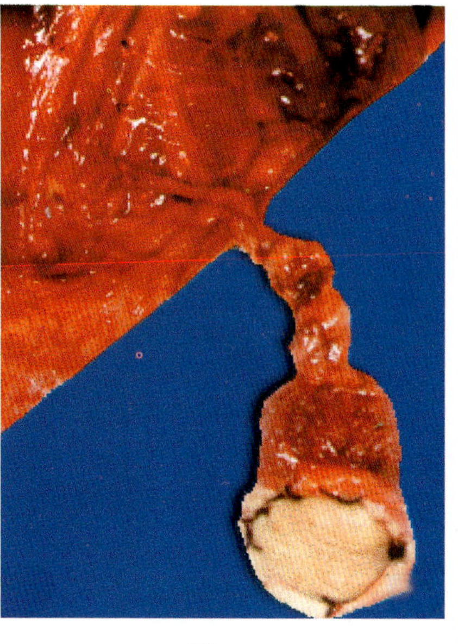

图 394

图 393, 394 按常规方法完成颈淋巴清扫术。颈淋巴清扫术被完成之后，进行侧斜方肌岛状肌皮瓣的制取。在手术过程中，为了确定蒂血管的存在和长度，手术的第一步是在其近端先解剖蒂，然而，解剖不必扩大到颈后三角达血管的全长，一旦血管的全程已被确定，留着由软组织包围的静脉可能是最好的。蒂的长度必须足够以保证肌皮瓣达受植区而无张力。在切开皮岛的皮肤之前，把皮岛的皮肤与其下的肌肉缝合固定几针以防其下的供血与其上的皮肤分离是有帮助的。在肩锁关节上做切口，肌皮瓣大小的确定需由被修复的组织量来决定。从提肩胛肌上掀起与肌肉相连的皮岛，继续向前掀起蒂的肌肉，其宽度应与皮岛的宽度一致。

Fig. 393, 394 A radical neck dissection is completed in the usual manner. After radical neck dissection has been completed, the island flap of the lateral trapezius is performed. During the procedure, it is probably wise as a first step to dissect the pedicle at its medial end in order to establish both its presence and length. The dissection however need not extend over the entire length of the vessels in the posterior triangle. Once the course of the vessels has been established medially, it may be best to leave the vein surrounded by some of the soft fat present in the area. This allows the skin island to be positioned on trapezius at a suitable distance from its anterior border so that the overall pedicle length, part muscle and part purely vascular are sufficient to allow the flap to reach its destination without tension. A few sutures are placed between the muscular island and the neck muscles thus ensuring a good protection for the carotid artery all along its course. The incision is placed in·the acromioclavicular joint and its borders are defined by the amount of tissue required. The island of skin with the underlying muscle is raised from levator scapulae and elevation of the muscle segment of the pedicle is continued forward at a width similar to that of the island to the anterior border of trapezius.

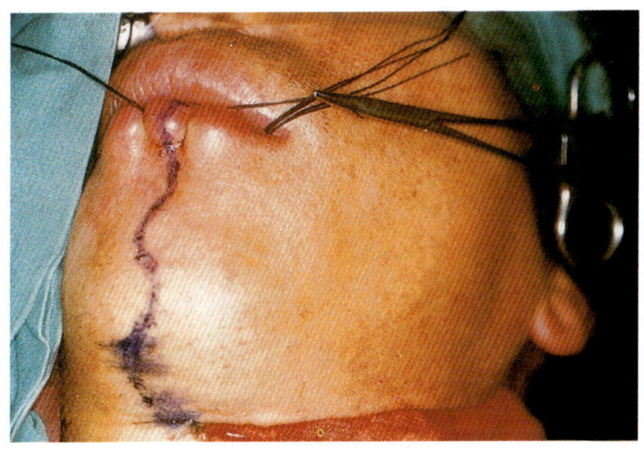

图 395

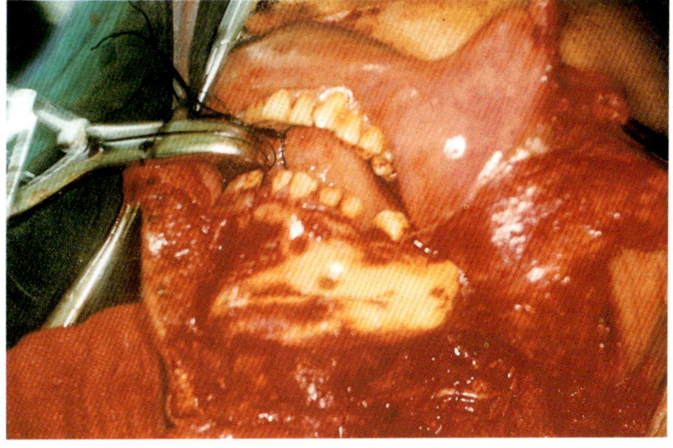

图 396

**图 395, 396** 在下唇正中弧形全层切开达颏下并与颈淋巴清扫术的颌下切口相连。于下颌正中患侧唇颊沟偏颊侧粘膜由前向后切开达下颌第二磨牙处，用骨膜分离器分离颊侧骨膜，暴露患侧颏神经并将其剪断结扎。从下颌正中分离舌侧骨膜达第二磨牙，拔除第一磨牙，用线锯去除病变侧上半部分下颌骨，骨蜡止血。

**Fig. 395, 396** The lower lip is split in the midline and a cheek flap is elevated by an incision in the gingivobuccal gutter and the mucoperiosteum on the lingual side of the mandible is incised and dissection along the body of the mandible. Rim resection of the mandible is made.

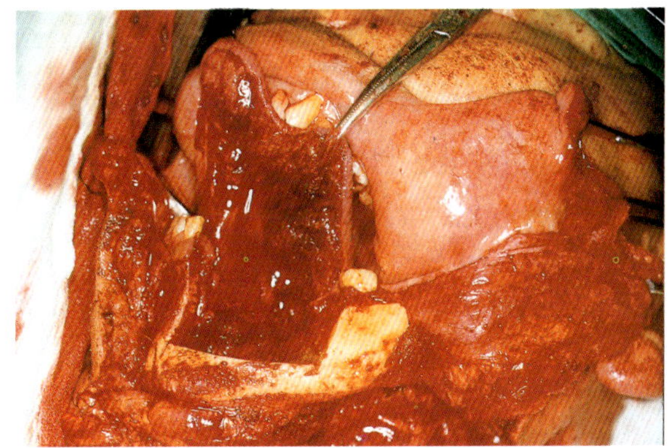

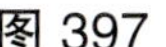

图 397

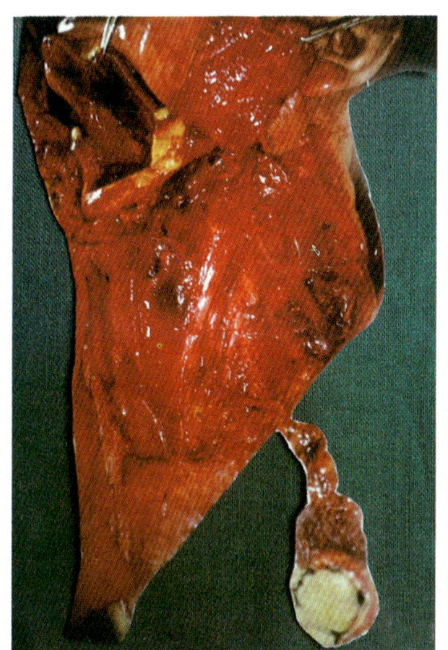

图 398

**图 397, 398** 在肿瘤外 1cm 切除口底病变组织，彻底止血后，将颈侧斜方肌岛状瓣经下颌内侧入口底缺损区。

**Fig. 397, 398** An incision is outlined around the tumor, leaving at least 1.0 cm of normal tissue on all its edges. The incision is carried through the deep musculature of the floor of the mouth. The intra-oral tumor and resected mandibular segment have now been freed from all attachments and are removed. Hemostasis is obtained by ligating all bleeding vessels with ties of fine chromic catgut. The wound is thoroughly irrigated with saline solution. Trapezius-musculocutaneous island flap is then maneuvered into the defective area of the floor of the mouth through the mandibular internal surface.

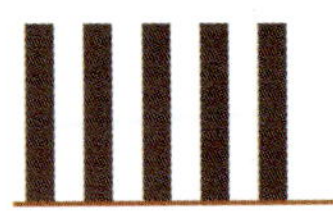



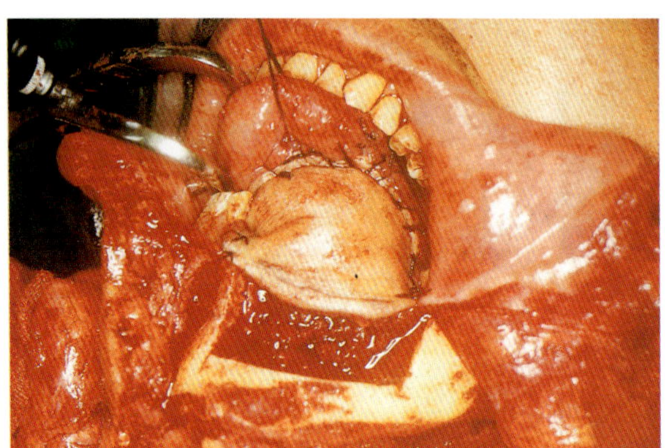

图 399

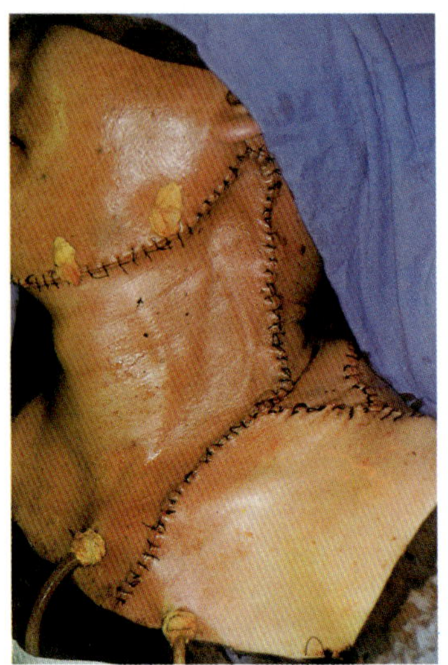

图 400

**图 399** 将侧斜方肌岛状瓣的皮岛边缘与舌及口底粘膜缝合，还回颊瓣，将侧斜方肌岛状瓣的皮肤外侧缘与颊粘膜缝合。

**图 400** 按常规方法缝合下唇颊部及颈淋巴清扫术后的创缘。局部轻压。

**Fig. 399** After trapezius-musculocutaneous island flap has reached the defective area of the oral cavity, the flap is then sutured to the surrounding mucosa with interrupted suture.

**Fig. 400** Closure of the gingivobuccal gutter is accomplished with interrupted mucosal sutures of fine silk. The lip is reconstructed with buried chromic sutures in the orbicularis muscle and fine silk sutures in the skin and mucosa. Care is taken to align accurately the vermilion skin junction. The radical neck dissection wound is drained and closed in the usual manner.

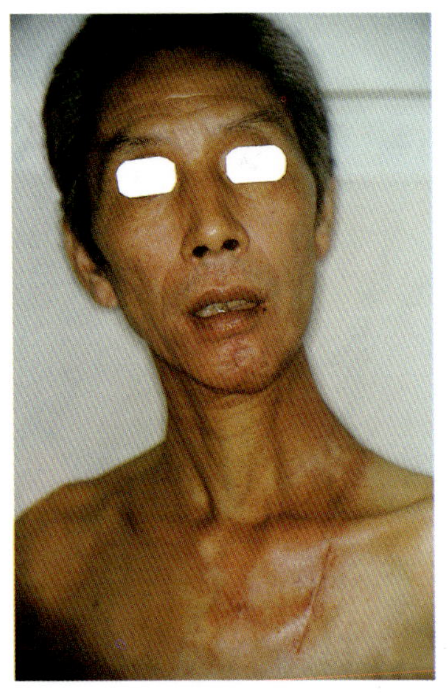

图 401

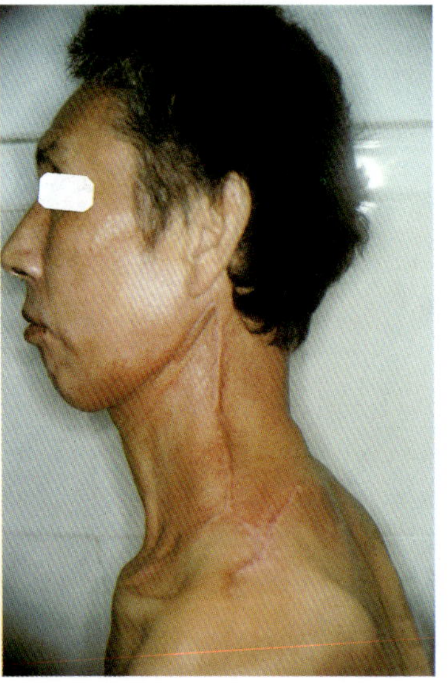

图 402

**图 401, 402** 术后 3 个月患者的正、侧面观，面部外形正常。

**Fig. 401, 402** Frontal and lateral views of the patient 3 mouths after surgery show normal facial configuration.

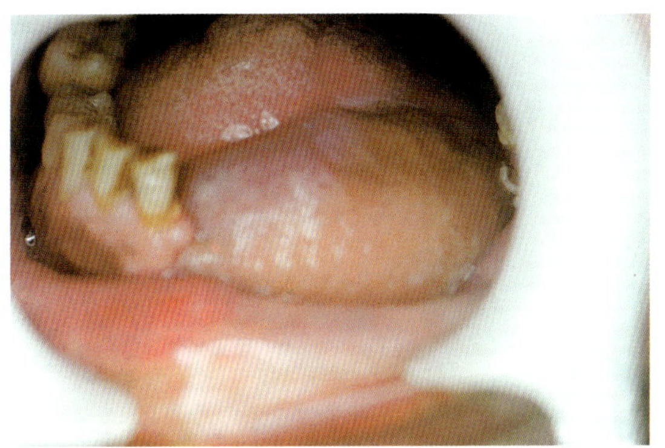

图 403

**图 403** 术后 3 个月患者口腔内口底愈合情况。

**Fig. 403** Healing conditions of the floor of the mouth in the oral cavity 3 mouths after operation.

# Ⅶ. 下颌骨肿瘤

26. 下颌骨隆凸的外科治疗
27. 左下颌骨体部含牙囊肿摘除术
28. 下颌骨造釉细胞瘤下颌骨部分切除后髂骨植入下颌骨重建术
29. 改良 Barbosa 进路手术治疗下颌骨升支造釉细胞瘤
30. 半侧下颌骨切除肋骨移植下颌骨重建术
31. 下颌磨牙后区鳞状细胞癌的颌颈联合根治术
32. 下颌牙龈癌切除后下颌口底缺损岛状额瓣修复
33. 下颌牙龈癌颌颈联合根治术后下颌骨缺损金属植入体即刻下颌骨重建

# Ⅶ. Mandible tumors

26. Surgical treatment of mandibular torus
27. Excision of dentigerous cyst in the body of the mandible
28. Ilium implantation for the mandibular reconstruction after resection of the partial mandible with ameloblastoma
29. Surgical treatment of the recurrent ameloblastoma in the mandibular ramus by the modifying Barbosa approach
30. Rib graft for the reconstruction after hemimandibulectomy
31. Combined operation of radical neck dissection with resection of mandible for the carcinoma arising in the mandibular retromolar trigone
32. The island forehead flap reconstructing the mandibular and the floor of the mouth after resection of the mandibular gingival carcinoma
33. Immediate metal implant for mandibular reconstruction following segmental resection of the mandible for the carcinoma of the lower gingiva

# 26. 下颌骨隆凸的外科治疗

# 26. Surgical treatment of mandibular torus

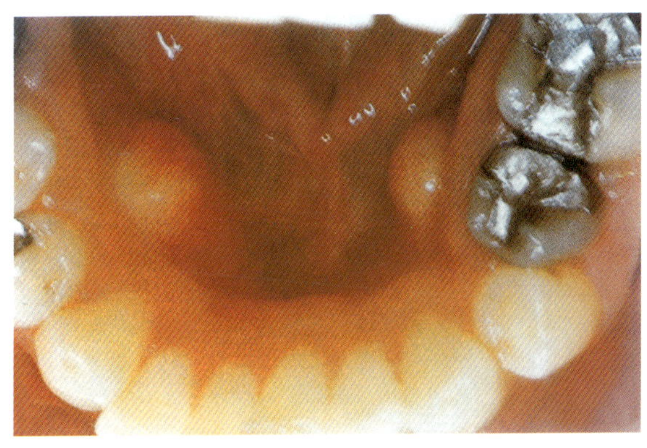

图 404

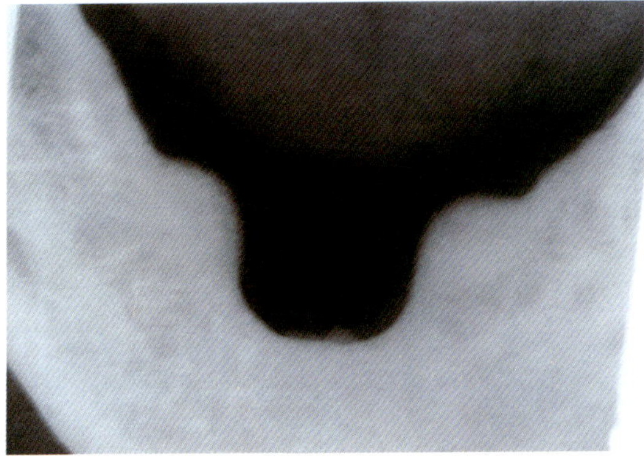

图 405

图 404 该患者因双侧下颌骨隆凸致部分下颌假牙设计困难而行手术治疗。
图 405 X 线片示双侧下颌骨隆凸。

Fig. 404 The patient was referred for surgery because of the design difficulties with the partial lower denture caused by the bilateral tori.
Fig. 405 The compact nature of the bone forming the tori is demonstrated by the radiograph.

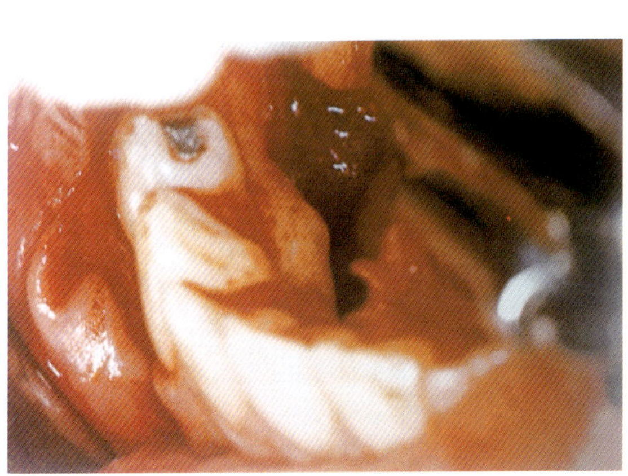

图 406

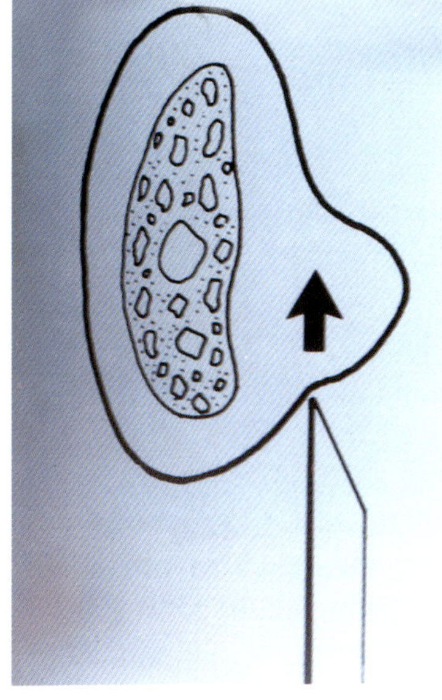

图 407

图 406 由龈缘切口暴露舌隆凸。
图 407 由助手支撑着下颌骨，将 5mm 的锉缘放在舌面隆凸的基部，锉除舌侧隆凸，用骨锉锉平基部。

Fig. 406 The lingual exostosis has been exposed through a gingival margin incision.
Fig. 407 The mandible must be supported by an assistant at the 5mm chisel edges is placed against the base of the torus with the bevel facing the tongue and then the mandibular torus is removed.

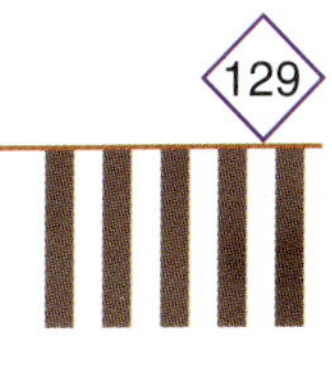

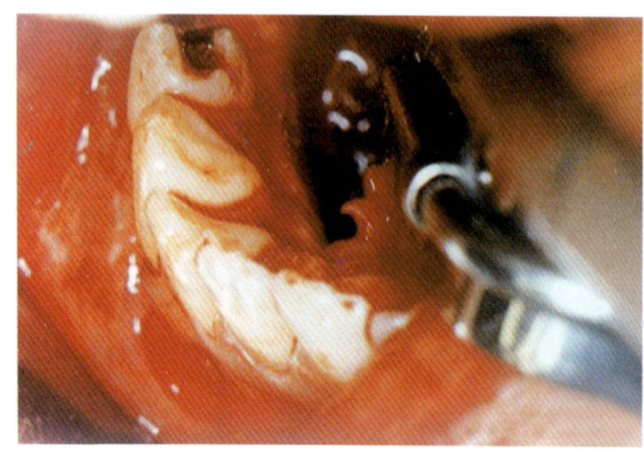

图 408

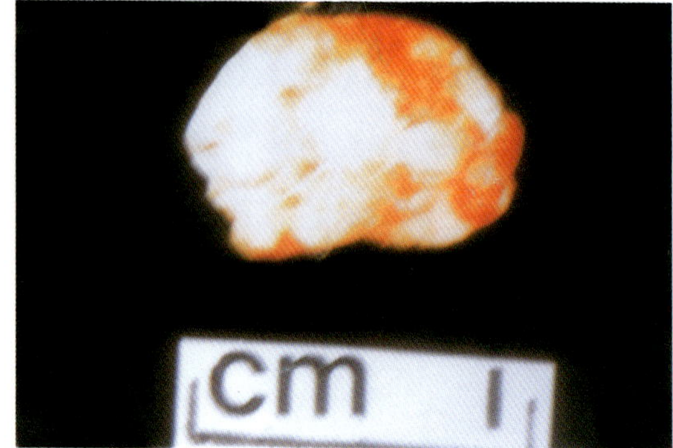


图 409

**图 408** 舌侧骨隆凸被去除之后，将颊、舌侧粘骨膜还回后间断缝合。
**图 409** 被铿除的下颌骨隆凸。

Fig. 408 This exostosis has also been removed by one blow with a chisel. The mucosa should be replaced before suture and sutured with interrupted sutures.

Fig. 409 The lingual exostosis which was separated with one 'pulled' blow from a mallet and chisel.

# 27. 左下颌骨体部含牙囊肿摘除术

# 27. Excision of dentigerous cyst in the body of the mandible

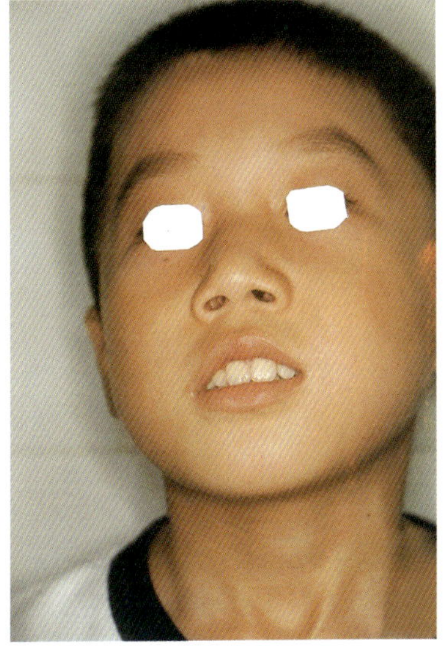

图 410

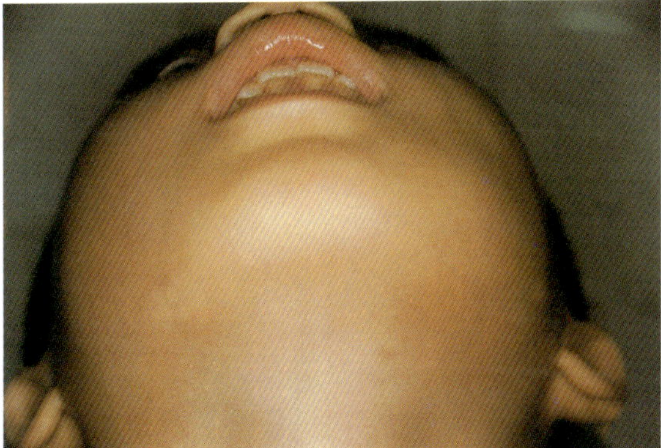

图 411

图 410, 411 一患左下颌骨含牙囊肿 9 岁患者正面及仰面观。双侧面部不对称，左侧下颌骨明显膨隆。患者的左下颌骨缓慢的无痛性膨胀性增大。

Fig. 410, 411 Frontal and submental views of a 9-year-old male patient with dentigerous cyst in the mandibular third molar region.

Both sides of the face are asymmetry and there is the extensive growth of the left mandible.

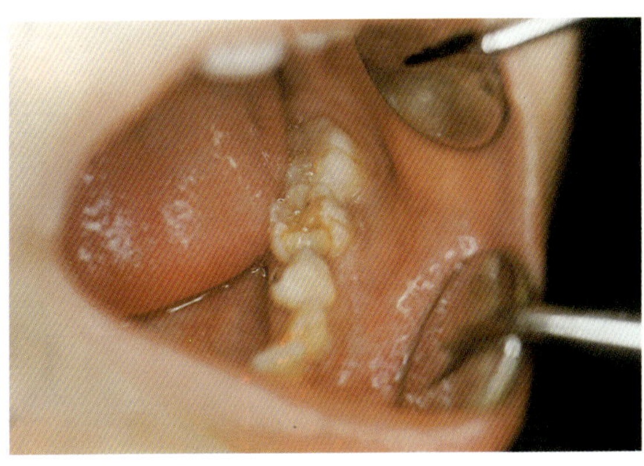

图 412

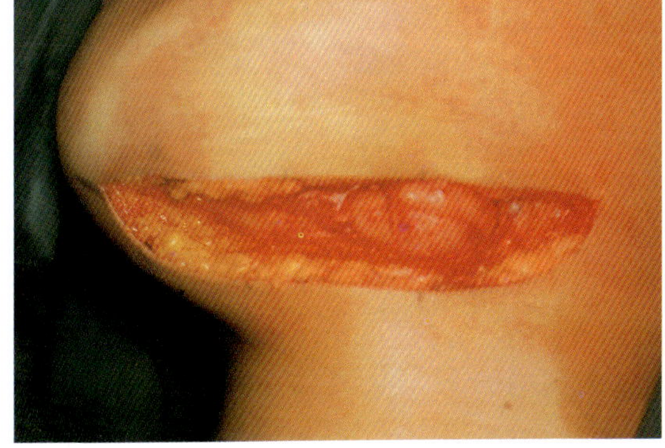

图 413

图412 口内见左下颌磨牙区的前庭沟变浅，下颌牙槽嵴明显增宽。

图413 在下颌骨下缘下1.5cm 处切开皮肤、皮下组织及颈阔肌。在颈阔肌深面向上翻起组织瓣达下颌骨下缘，在此处切开骨膜并加以分离。

Fig. 412 The gingivobuccal sulcus of the left mandibular molar region becomes supperficial and the left mandibular alveolus is widen obviously.

Fig. 413 A incision is made parallel to and 1. 5 cm below the horizontal ramus of the mandible. The mandibular branch of the facial nerve is identified where it crosses the facial vessels and is preserved. The soft parts are elevated away from the bone.

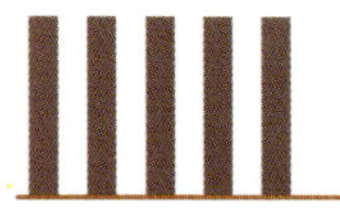



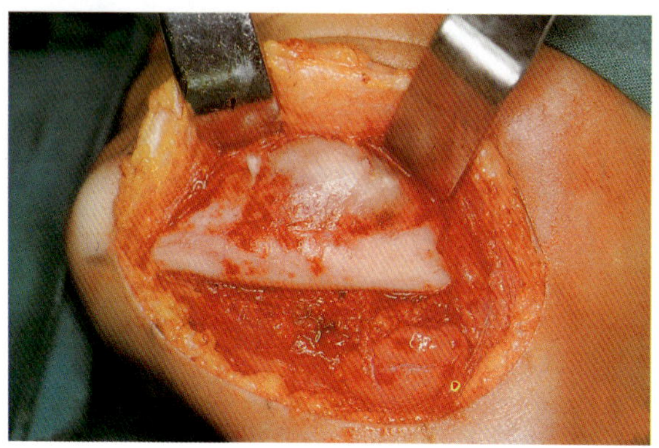

图 414

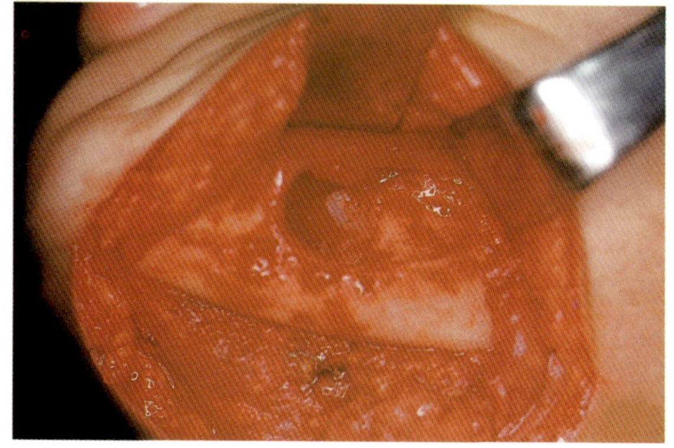

图 415

**图 414** 显露病变的骨壁，用骨凿凿开骨壁，显露囊肿的囊壁。

**图 415** 从凿开骨壁与囊壁组织边缘开始，用骨膜剥离器将囊肿完整摘除。用生理盐水冲洗骨腔，骨蜡止血。

**Fig. 414, 415** After the bony wall of the lesion is exposed, small chisels and rongeurs are used to remove a window of bone over the cyst. Small curved elevators and curettes are then used to enucleate the intact cyst. The bony cavity is irrigated with the saline solusion.

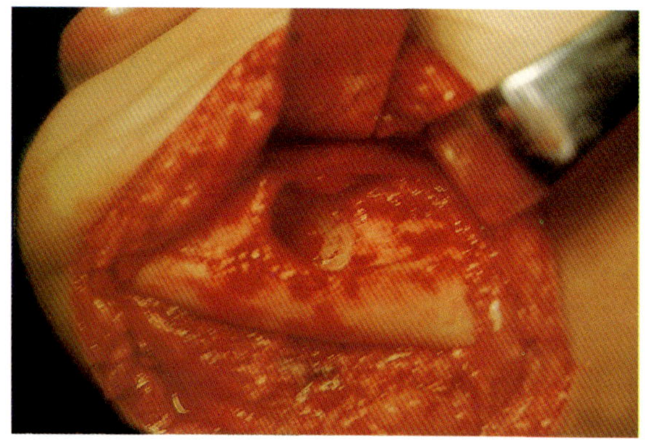

图 416

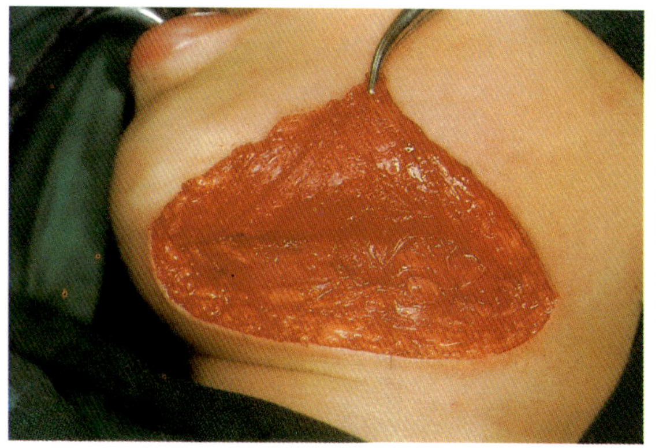

图 417

**图 416** 骨腔内填入明胶海绵后，将组织瓣还回原位，缝合骨膜。

**图 417** 骨膜缝合完成后，放入橡皮引流管一根，缝合颈阔肌、皮下组织及皮肤。

**Fig. 416** After a pack of absorbable gelatin sponge is placed in the cavity, the soft flap is returned in place and the periosteum is sutured with fine chromic catgut.

**Fig. 417** After the suture of the periosteum has been completed, sutures in layers are made with fine silk. A drain is left in the wound for 48 hours.

图 418 创口缝合后情景。

Fig. 418 The condition after the wound suture.

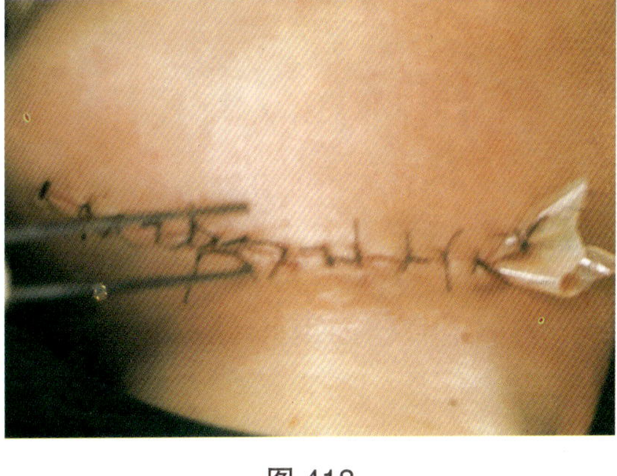

图 418

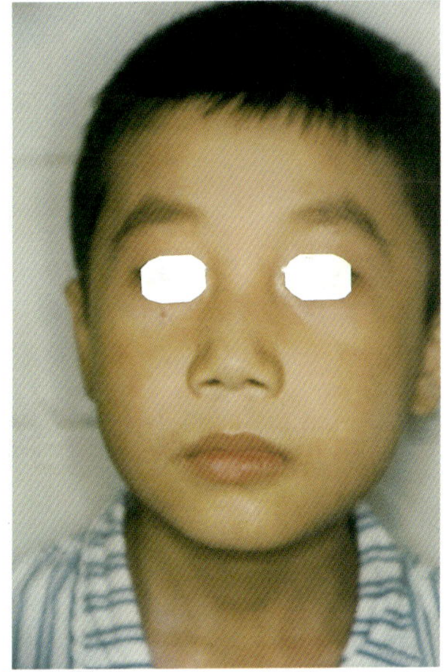

图 419

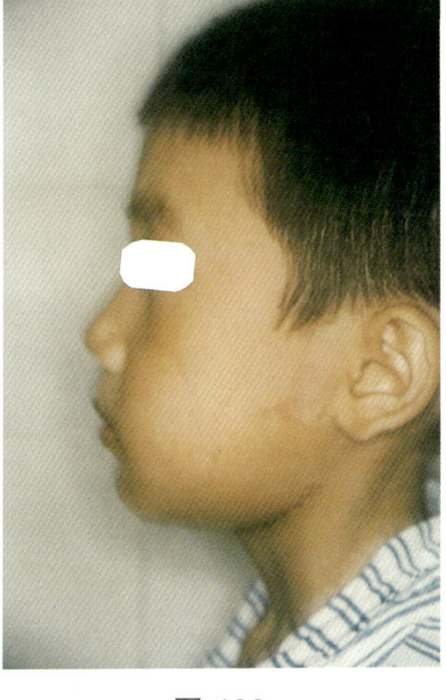

图 420

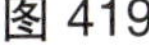

图 419, 420 患者术后第 10 天正面及侧面观显示创口愈合正常。

Fig. 419, 420 Frontal and lateral views of the patient 10 days after surgery show that wound healing is normal.

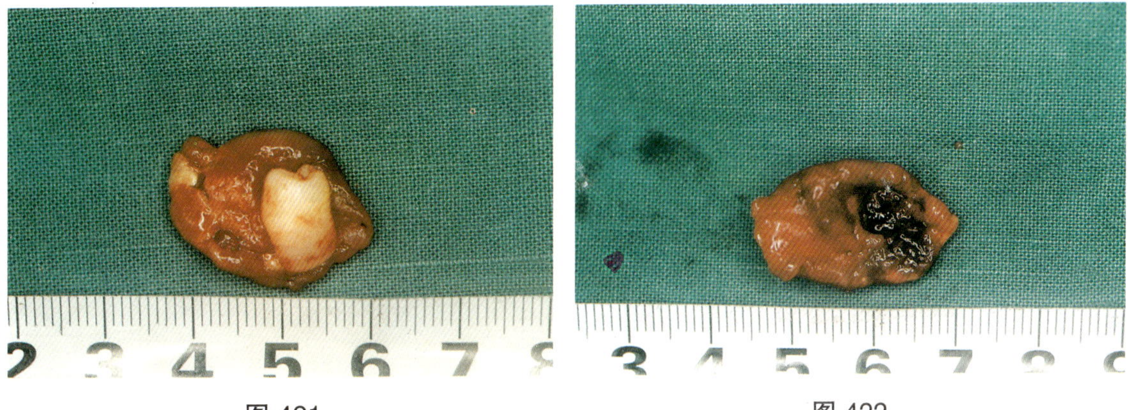

图 421　　图 422

图 421 囊肿位于牙冠的侧面。
图 422 含牙囊肿的内侧面观。

Fig. 421 Lateral dentigerous cyst situated at the side of the crown of the tooth.
Fig. 422 Internal surface view of gross specimen of dentigerous cyst.

# 28. 下颌骨造釉细胞瘤下颌骨部分切除后髂骨植入下颌骨重建术

# 28. Ilium implantation for the mandibular reconstruction after resection of the partial mandible with ameloblastoma

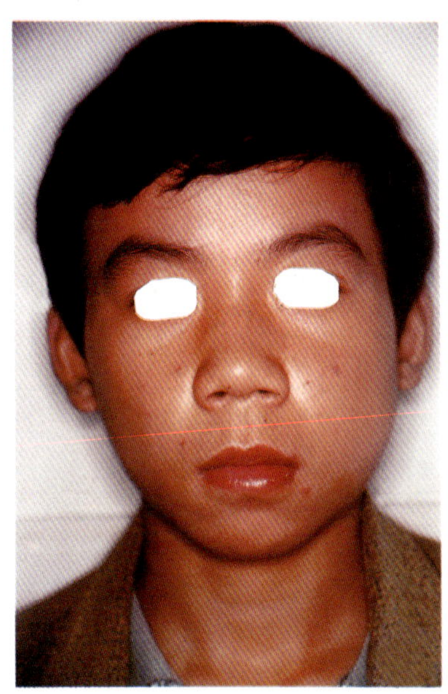

图 423

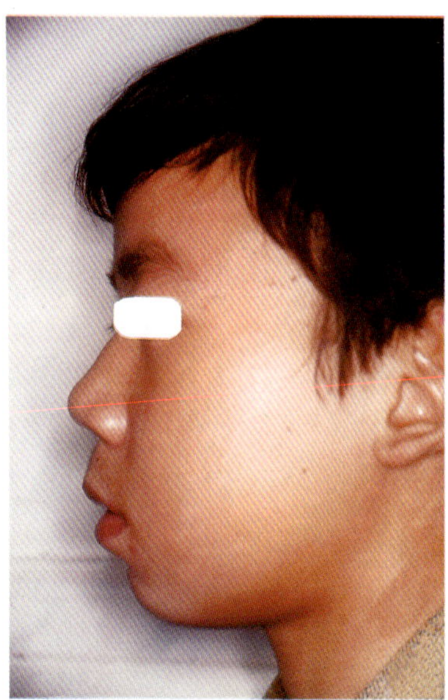

图 424

**图 423, 424** 一患左下颌骨造釉细胞瘤的 17 岁患者的正面及侧面观。

患者本人发现左面部逐渐增大畸形，病变区域的牙齿松动但疼痛不明显。由于造釉细胞瘤的缓慢生长，当肿瘤在发现之前肿瘤就已经存在。因为未进行及时的治疗，肿瘤继续增大使周围骨质变薄而出现蛋壳样感。

**Fig. 423, 424** Frontal and lateral views of a 17-year-old male patient with the left mandibular ameloblastoma.

There is a gradually increasing facial deformity noted by the patient himself and the teeth in the area of the tumor became loosened. Pain is seldom a complaint. Because of the slow growth of the tumor, it is probable that even in apparently early cases it has already been present for an appreciable period before detection. In the absence of treatment the tumor continues to enlarge and the surrounding bone becomes so thin that fluctuation or egg-shell cracking may be elicited.

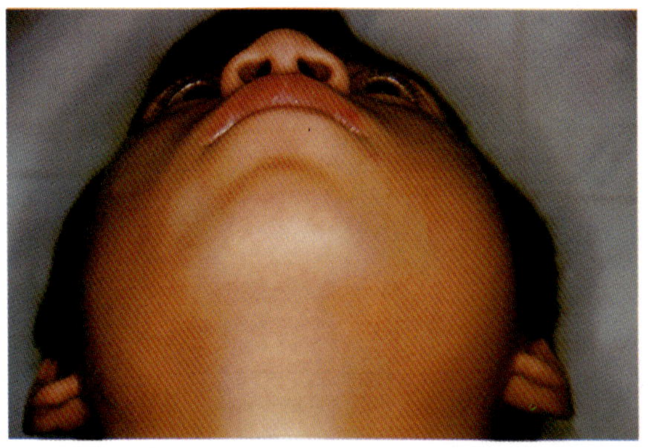

图 425

**图 425** 患者的仰面观显示左面颊部明显膨隆。

**Fig. 425** The Patient's submental view shows obvious expansion of the left facial and buccal region.

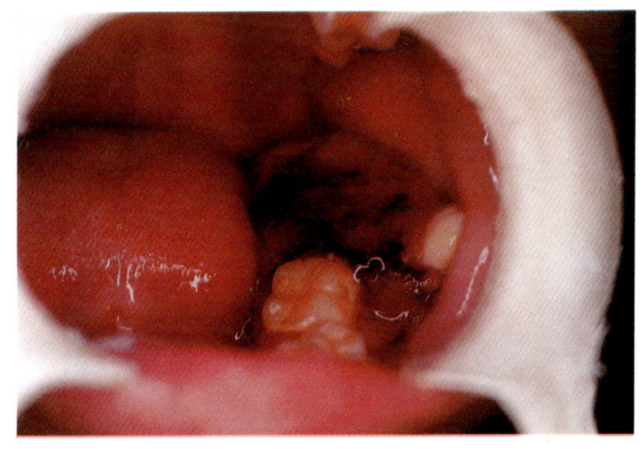

图 426

**图 426** 口内面观显示左下颌骨明显膨隆，下颌骨磨牙后区粘膜破溃，第二磨牙颊侧移位、松动。

Fig. 426 View of the intra-oral cavity shows obvious expansion of the left mandible. The mucosa of the retromolar trigone of the left mandible is ulcerous. The left secondary molar tooth is displaced to the buccal side and loosened.

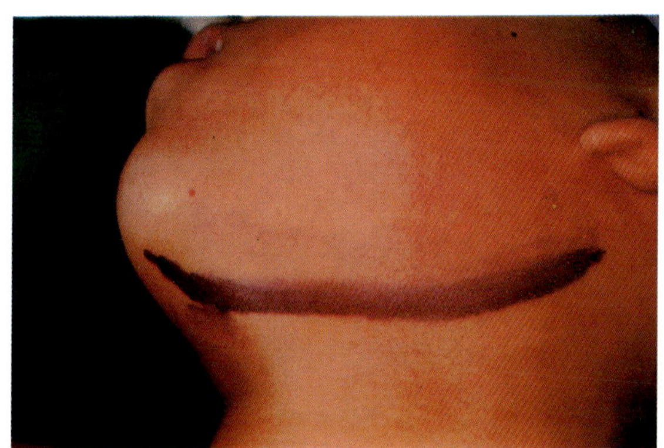

图 427

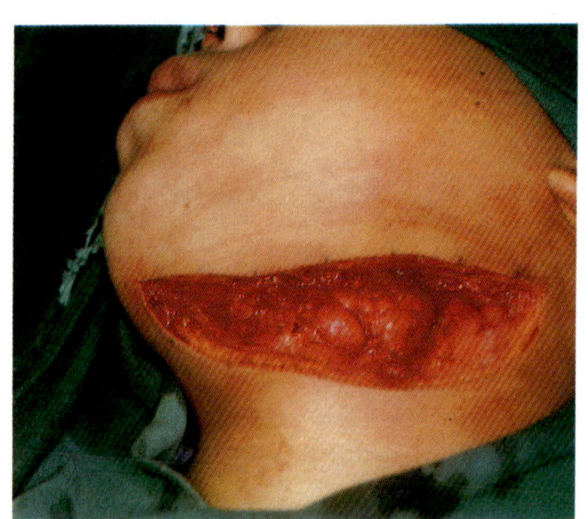

图 428

**图 427** 采用鼻腔插管全麻。取仰卧位，肩下垫枕，头偏向健侧。自耳垂向下，沿下颌升支后缘往下，至下颌角下 2cm 转向前直达颏下做切口。

**图 428** 切开皮肤、皮下组织及颈阔肌；如口腔手术野需有更广泛而良好的暴露时，可作下唇正中的附加切口。

Fig. 427 Endetracheal anesthesia is administered and a pharyngeal pack inserted. An incision is made from the midpoint of the chin to the angle of the mandible, being carried parallel to and 2 cm below the lower border of the bone. The mandibular branch of the facial nerve is identified and preserved.

Fig. 428 The lip-splitting incision can be made through the midline if needed. The incision should extend through the platysma and the superior flap elevated in this plane to protect the marginal mandibular nerve.

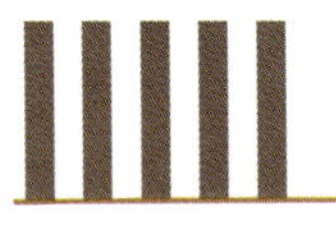



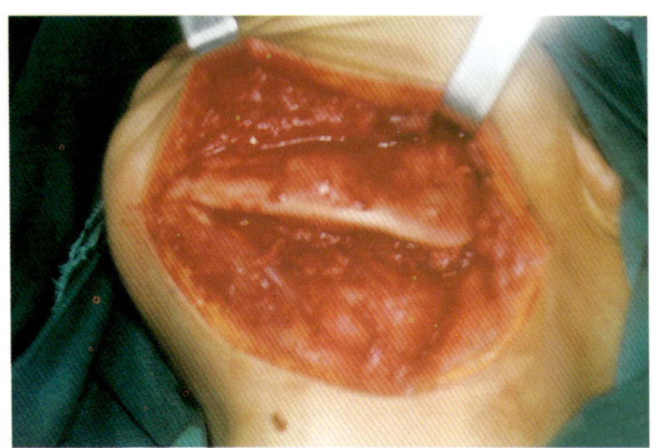

图 429

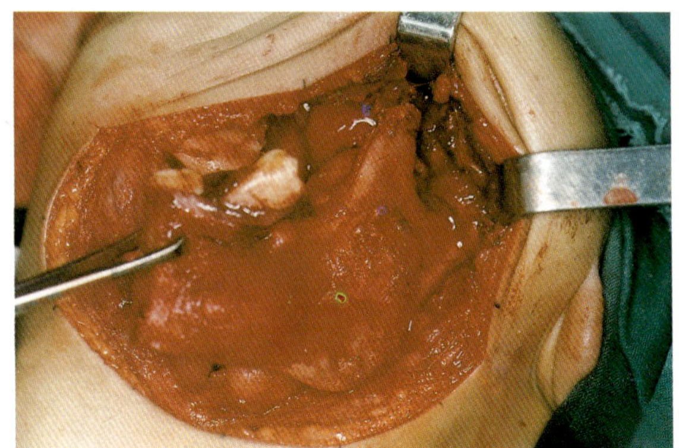

图 430

**图 429** 在嚼肌前下角之下颌切迹处用钝分离显露，游离颌外动脉及面前静脉，在下颌骨下缘下方各用二血管钳夹住动、静脉，切断后分别结扎之。分离下颌骨两侧的软组织，显露并在下颌骨下缘切开骨膜，用骨膜分离器将包括骨膜在内的下颌外侧面软组织向上掀起；然后在病灶外缘切开粘膜使口内外创口相通，途中将颏神经血管束切断结扎。在下颌角及升支部嚼肌附着紧密，需配合锐分离将嚼肌自骨面剥离。继续用同法分离下颌骨内侧的骨膜及翼内肌。

拔除同侧下颌第二双尖牙，用大弯血管钳将线锯从下颌骨下缘经内侧引入口腔，再从已拔牙后的牙槽窝上缘将线锯由下颌骨外侧面引向颌下切口处，拉动线锯，自⌈5之间截断下颌骨，断端用骨蜡止血。

**图 430** 将下颌骨断端向外下方牵引，在病灶外缘切开舌侧粘膜附着，并绕过磨牙后区，使与颊侧粘膜相连。用组织剪切断下颌升支前缘及喙突部的颞肌附着。于下颌升支内侧中部分离下牙槽神经血管束，用血管钳夹住切断、结扎。

**Fig. 429** The major portion of the body of the mandible may be exposed by blunt dissection. Anteriorly, a few muscular attachments and the mental nerve and artery must be divided with the scalpel. Posteriorly, the masseter muscle is severed at its insertion along the angle and ascending ramus. The upper outer surface of the body of the mandible is freed by incising the mucosa in the gingivobuccal sulcus. The mucosa of the floor of the mouth is incised close to the gingiva. After the left mandibular secondary bicanine was extracted, the mandible is divided in the area of the left mandibular secondary bicanine with a Gigli saw.

**Fig. 430** The bone is then grasped with a bone-holding forceps and retracted downward and rotated outward to facilitate disarticulation. The temporalis muscle is located by palpation at its insertion on the coronoid process and is severed with strong curved scissors. The condyle is then freed by incision of its attachments at the temporomandibular joint.

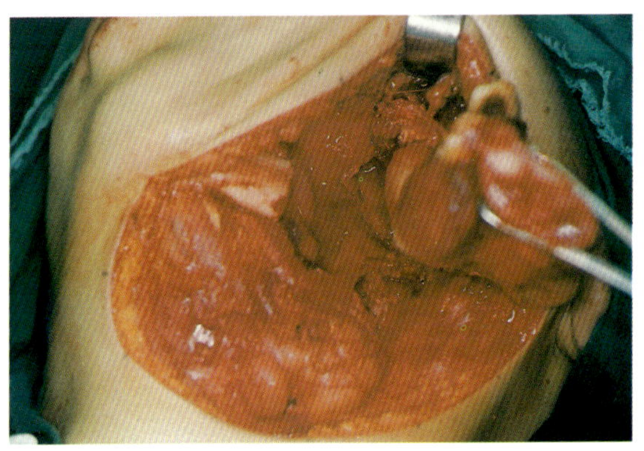

图 431

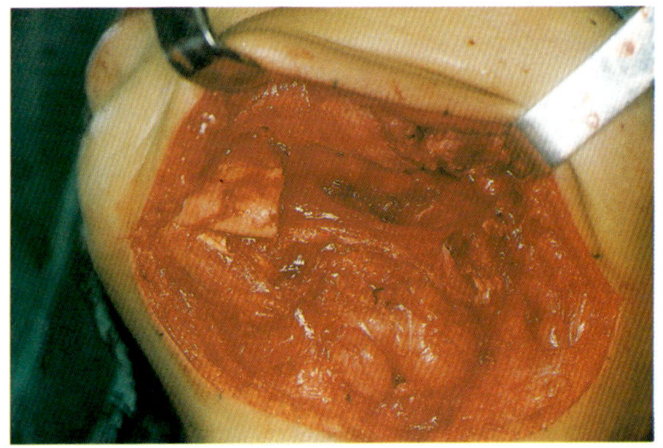

图 432

**图 431** 继用骨膜剥离器分离附着于髁状突部的关节囊，仔细将附着于髁状突颈部前上内分的翼外肌止端分离后，即可将一侧下颌骨完全游离摘除。

**图 432** 结扎活跃出血点，间断缝合口腔粘膜；然后用生理盐水反复冲洗创腔，再作一粘膜下缝合。在剩余下颌骨断端处分上下两排钻孔。

**Fig. 431** The mandible is then rotated outward and its remaining attachments, the pterygoid muscles, are divided. It is better to clamp these muscles proximal to their point of division to avoid troublesome bleeding from the pterygoid plexus.

**Fig. 432** Following removal of the mandible, the oral cavity is closed with mucosal sutures of 4 – 0 silk with the knots tied in the mouth. The resected end of the remaining mandible is driven into several holes drilled in the bone.

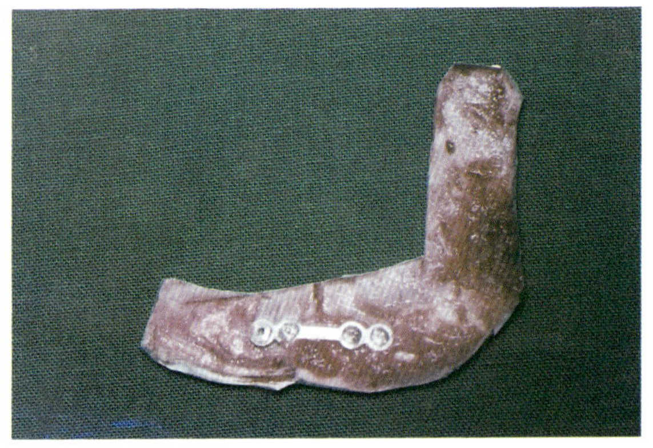

图 433

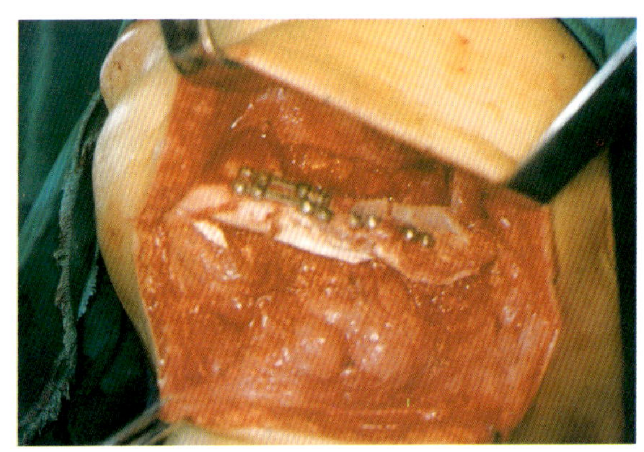

图 434

**图 433, 434** 髂骨或肋骨可以被作为骨移植体来重建切除的下颌骨，在移植体被固定于剩余的下颌骨切除端之前，必须对骨移植体进行塑形。下颌骨移植体的塑形从下颌角的形成开始，当下颌升支和髁状突骨段已用微型夹板固定之后，注意力应集中于将被变为下颌骨体的移植体的邻近部位上了。如果下颌骨截骨没有达下颌骨正中线的话，在行移植体的塑形时仅做一次切骨就可以了，如果达下颌骨中线的话，在行下颌移植体塑形时就必须在中线附近行第二次切骨以增加移植体的弯曲度。在对移植体塑形并用微型夹板固定之后，将骨移植体与剩余下颌骨断端用微型夹板固定。

**Fig. 433, 434** A bone graft of rib or iliac crest may be used to bridge the mandibular defect. Before the graft is fixed to the bone end of the resected mandible with miniplates, the shaping of the graft must be made. The shaping of lateral graft begins by forming the angle of the mandible. After the ramus and condyle segment had been fixed with miniplates, attention is turned to shaping the adjacent portion of the graft which will become the body of the mandible. The process begins by determining where upon the length of the graft an osteotomy is needed to reproduce the curve in the body. Only one osteotomy is usually necessary in the case of a typical lateral resection that does not extend as far as the midline. This osteotomy is made in two planes because the native mandible not only has a change in the degree of its curve but also usually angles either upward or downward at this transition point. Lateral grafts that extend to the midline usually require a second osteotomy to increase the curve near the midline. It is always better to leave the graft long after the first osteotomy and perform the second osteotomy at the time of graft insetting. After placement of miniplates and graft shaping is complete, graft is fixed to the resected end of the remaining mandible with the two miniplates.

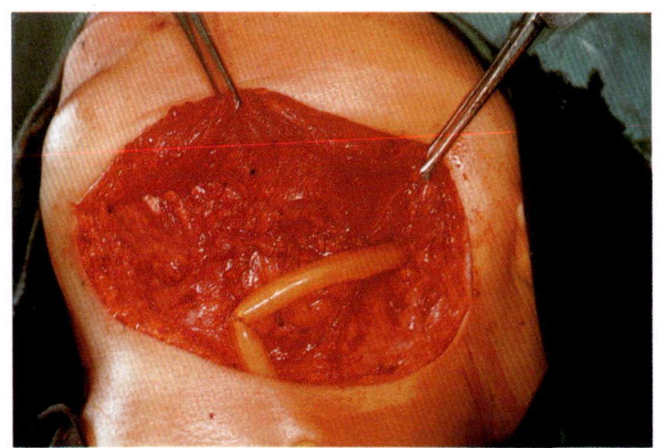

图 435

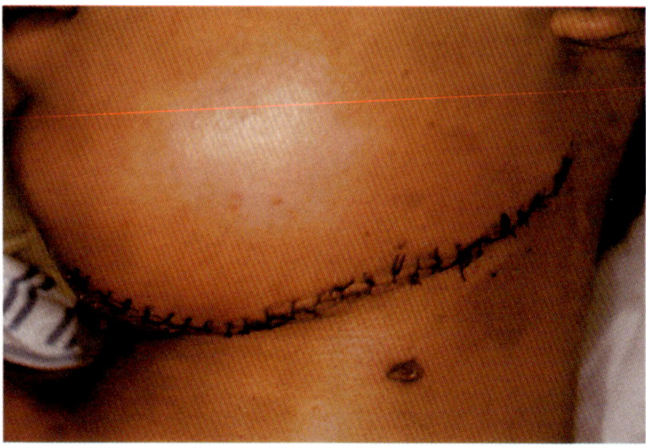

图 436

**图 435** 用细肠线缝合数针，方法是分别自植入骨的下缘进针，穿过其内侧的软组织，再由植入骨上面穿出，将每针缝线之两端包绕骨块后打结固定。最后，于植骨的上下方，再间断缝合数针，以封闭剩余之间隙，增强固位，消灭死腔。

**图 436** 对位分层缝合下颌骨骨膜、肌肉、皮下组织及皮肤。根据情况安置引流管。

**Fig. 435** The soft tissues are approximated around the graft with fine chromic sutures. The underlying dead space is obliterated by numerous sutures of 3 – 0 chromic catgut.

**Fig. 436** The skin and platysma are approximated around a drain which is left in place for 48 hours.

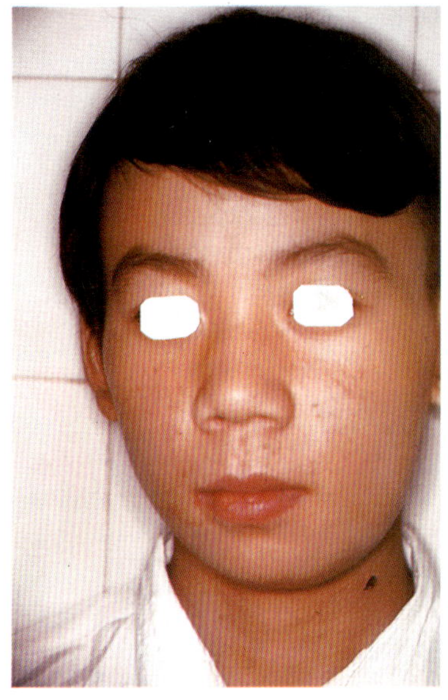

图 437

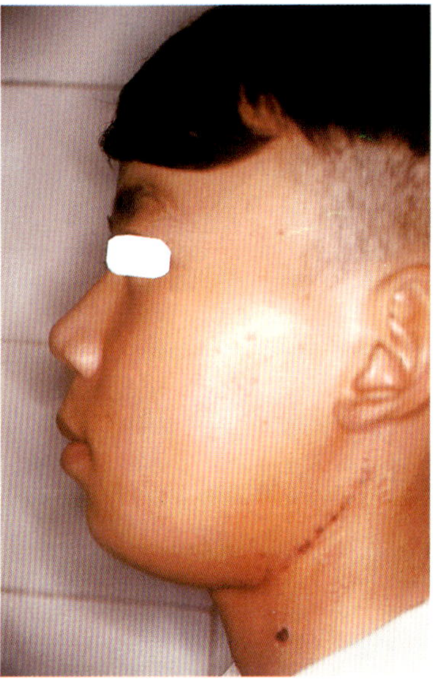

图 438

图 437，438 手术后的结果：术后 10 天正面观显示左侧面部较右侧稍大，侧面观显示创口愈合良好。

Fig. 437, 438 Postoperative results: frontal view 10 days after surgery shows the left face slightly larger compared with the right face and lateral view shows the wound healing is normal 10 days after operation.

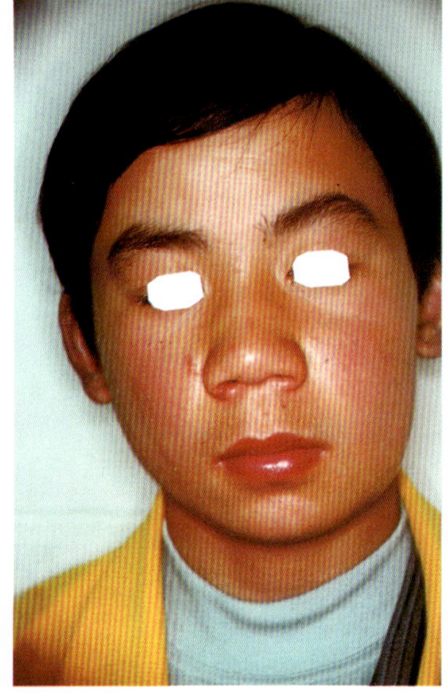

图 439

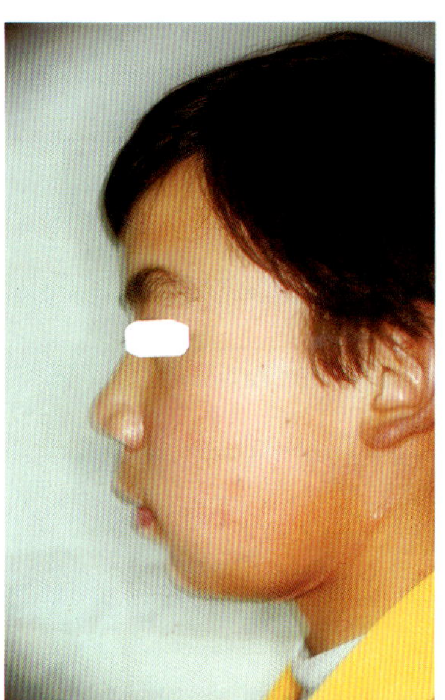

图 440

图 439, 440 患者术后 6 个月正、侧面观显示被重建后的脸部外形。

Fig. 439, 440 Frontal and lateral views show his facial configuration following a typical lateral reconstruction.

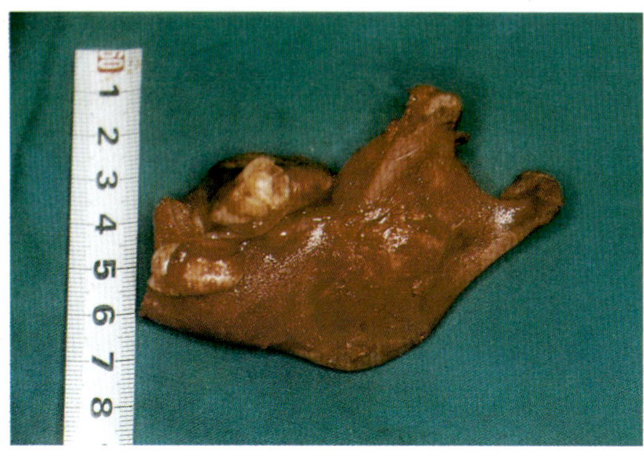
图 441

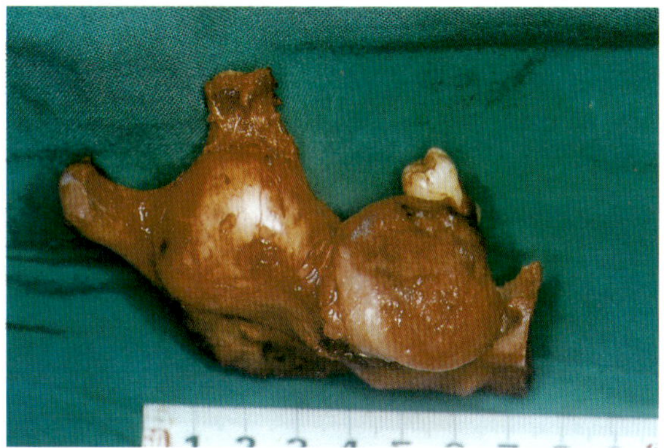
图 442

图 441, 442 被切除下颌骨的外侧和内侧面观显示下颌体和升支部明显膨隆。

Fig. 441, 442 External and internal surface views of resected mandible show expansion of the body and the ramus of the mandible.

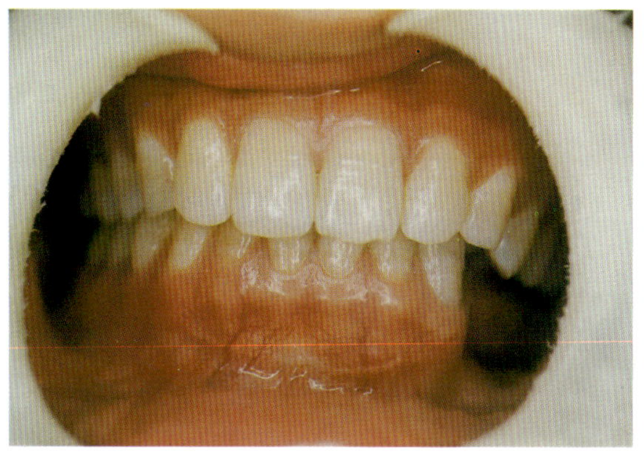
图 443

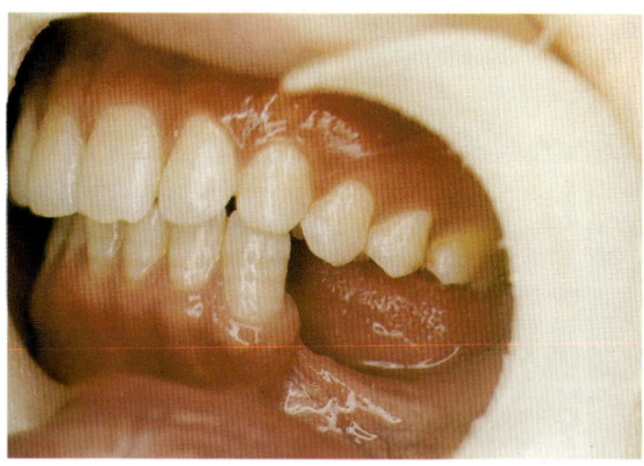
图 444

图 443, 444 患者术后 1 年咬殆关系情况的正、侧面观。

Fig. 443, 444 Frontal and lateral views of the patient 1 year after operation showing exact occlusal relationship.

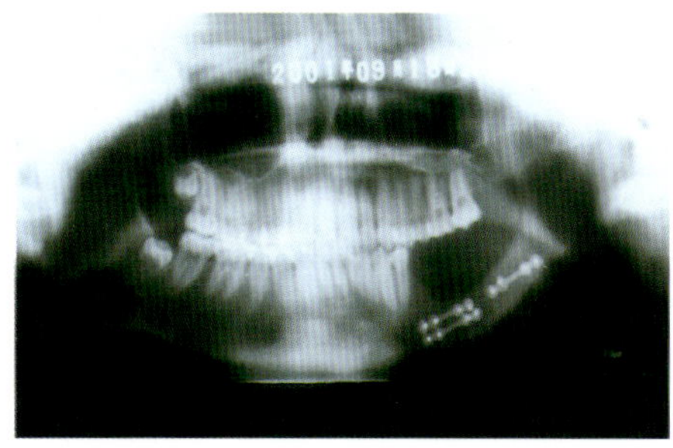
图 445

图 445 植骨后 X 光片显示愈合良好。

Fig. 445 The radiograph after bone implantation shows that healing is fine.

# 29. 改良 Barbosa 进路手术治疗下颌骨升支造釉细胞瘤

# 29. Surgical treatment of the recurrent ameloblastoma in the mandibular ramus by the modifing Barbosa approach

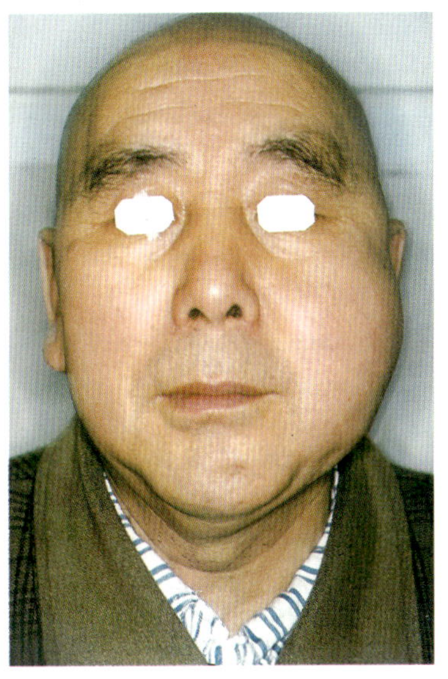

图 446

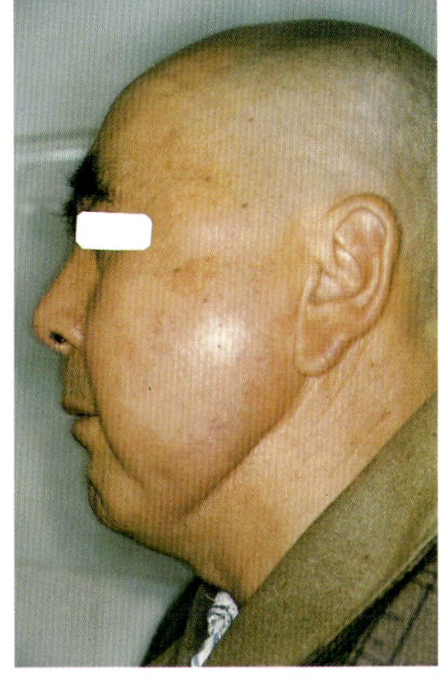

图 447

**图 446, 447** 一患左下颌骨升支复发性造釉细胞瘤的 61 岁男性患者的正、侧面观。正面观左侧面部明显膨隆，表面皮肤正常。侧面观见左颞面部膨隆明显。

Fig. 446, 447 The frontal and lateral views of a 61-year-old male patient with a recurrent ameloblastoma in the left mandibular ramus. The frontal view shows the left facial expansion and the skin on the left face is normal. The left lateral view shows expansion of the left temporofacial region.

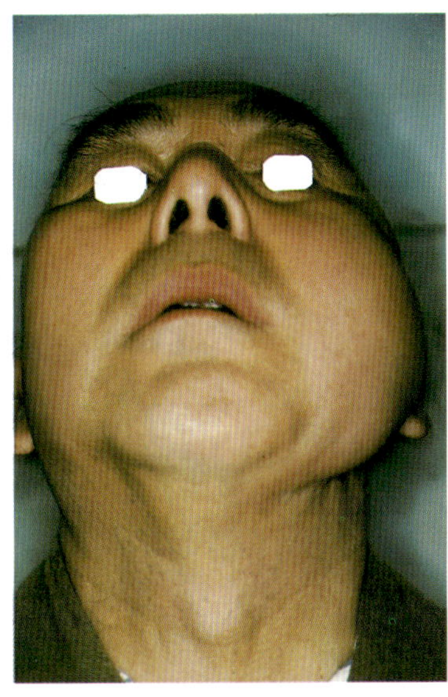

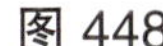

图 448

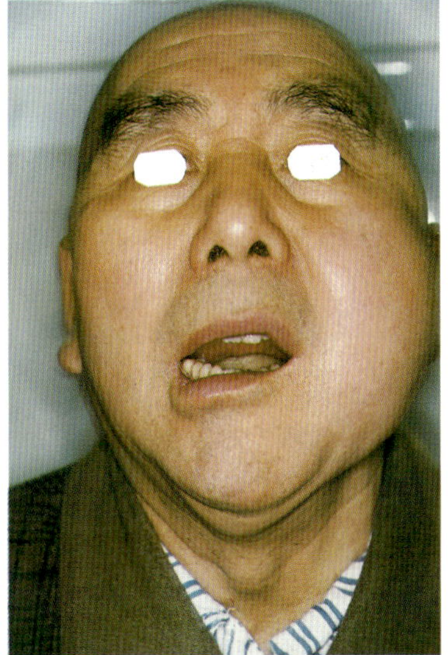

图 449

**图 448** 患者仰面观见两侧颞面部不对称，左侧明显膨隆。

**图 449** 显示张口受限。

Fig. 448 The Patient's submental view shows that both temporofacial regions are asymmetrical and the expansion of the left temporofacial region is obvious.

Fig. 449 This figure shows that patient's opening mouth is limited.

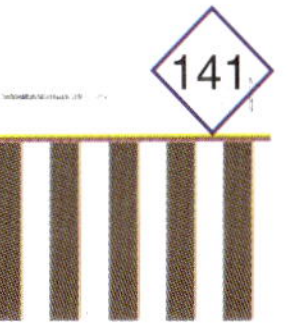

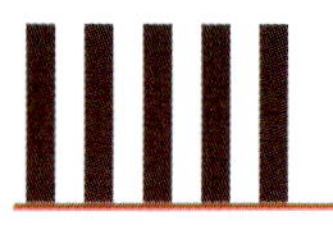



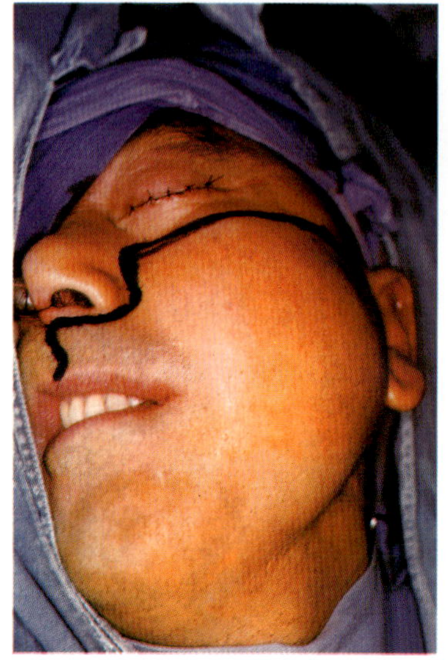

图 450

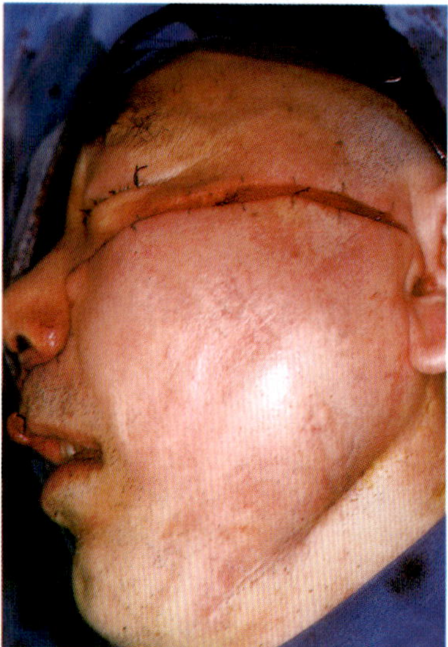

图 451

**图 450, 451** 切口设计如图 450 所示。切口从上唇正中开始，过鼻棘下绕鼻翼至眶下缘下，向外侧延伸达患侧耳屏前区域。然后在患侧的上颌龈颊沟由正中向后达磨牙后区做切口，另一切口是沿受累侧的下颌龈颊沟从尖牙开始向后达磨牙后区切开。

**Fig. 450, 451** A incision is made as Figure450 shows. The first incision divides the upper lip in the midline, passes under the nasal pyramid and extends laterally, reaching the level of the temporomandibular joint. An incision is then made along the maxillary buccogingival fold on the involved side, running from the midline to the retromolar area. Another incision is made along the mandibular buccogingival fold on the involved side, running from canine to retromolar area.

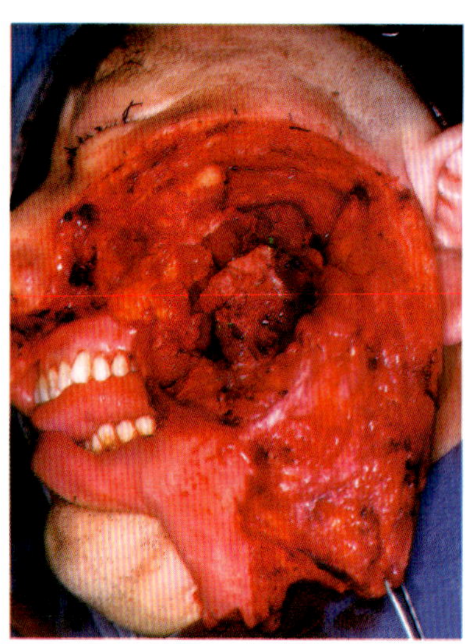

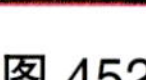

图 452

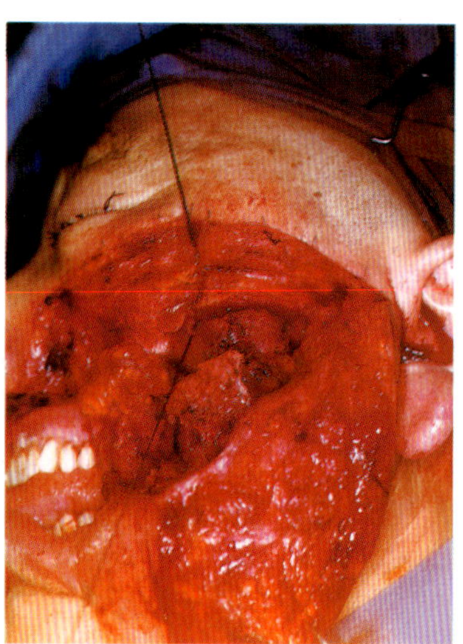

图 453

**图 452, 453** 用电刀在表情肌表面翻起组织瓣，将其瓣翻转使上颌骨的前面、眶缘以下、颞肌的下部、颞颌关节的外侧面及嚼肌和下颌骨升支有足够的暴露。在颧弓下缘切断嚼肌上缘，在颧弓上缘切断颞肌下段，用线锯锯断颧弓并将其移去。

**Fig. 452, 453** A large flap is raised at the level of the mimetic muscles with an electrosurgical knife. This flap is reflected to yield adequate exposure of the anterior aspect of the maxilla, the inferior half of the orbital rim, the inferior portion of the temporalis muscle, the zygomatic bone, zygomatic arch, the external aspect of the temporomandibular joint, the masseter and the mandibular ramus. The masseter muscle is sectioned with an electrosurgical knife a little below the zygomatic arch and temporalis muscle is sectioned a little above the zygomatic arch. The zygomatic arch is cut at both ends with a Gigli saw and is removed.

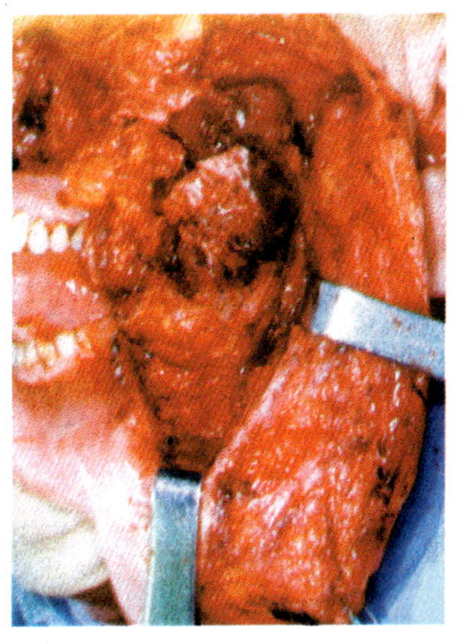

图 454

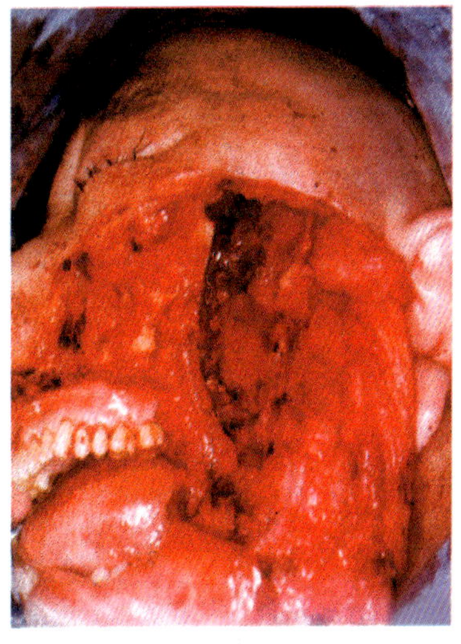

图 455

**图 454, 455** 在肿瘤的外侧约 1cm 处用线锯锯断下颌骨升支，止血后在骨膜外向上分离下颌骨升支，在下颌孔处分离下牙槽神经血管束，将其钳夹后切断、结扎。继续向上分离肿瘤前方，内侧面、后面达颞颌关节结节处，用电刀切断颞颌关节周围组织的附着。将肿瘤组织全部移去后彻底止血。

**Fig. 454, 455** The mandibular ramus is divided in about 1 cm of the outer side of the tumor with a Gigli saw. The bone is then grasped with a bone-holding forceps and rotated outward to facilitate disarticulation. The temporalis muscle which is located at its insertion on the coronoid process is severed with strong curved scissors. The condyle is then freed by incision of its attachments at the temporomandibular joint. It is often simpler to divide the neck of the mandible just below the condyle with large rib-cutting forceps. The pterygoid muscles are divided. It is better to clamp these muscles proximal to their point of division to avoid trouble some bleeding from the pterygoid plexus. The mandible and tumor are removed.

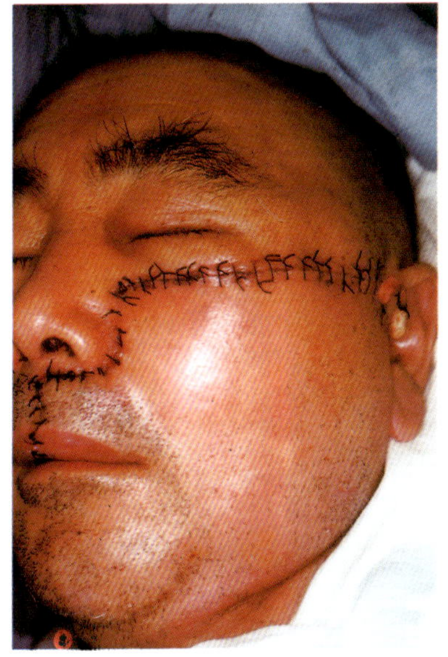

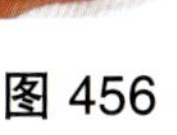

图 456

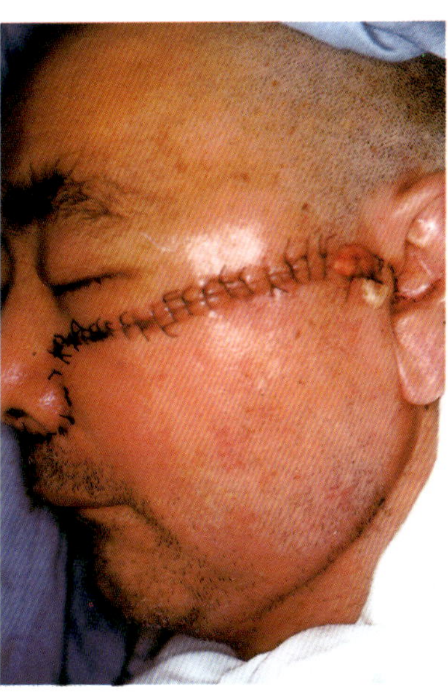

图 457

**图 456, 457** 将颞肌下端与嚼肌上端相缝合。然后将大块组织瓣还回原处后缝合肌层、皮下组织及皮肤，在缝合上述各层之前，先缝合口腔内上下颌龈颊沟粘膜。缝合完毕后局部加压包扎。

**Fig. 456, 457** The inferior end of the temporalis muscle and the superior end of the masseter muscle are sutured each other with silk. Closure is completed anteriorly by approximating the mucosa in the gingivobuccal gutter with fine silk. A cheek flap is then sutured back in place with numerous interrupted sutures of fine silk.

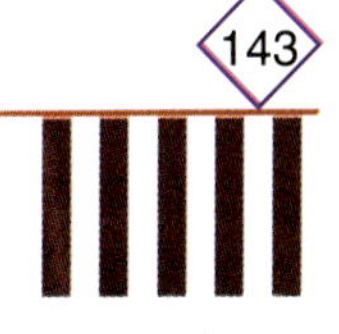

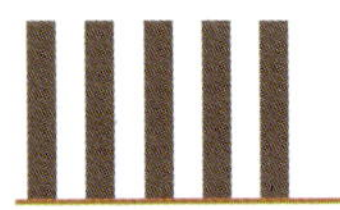



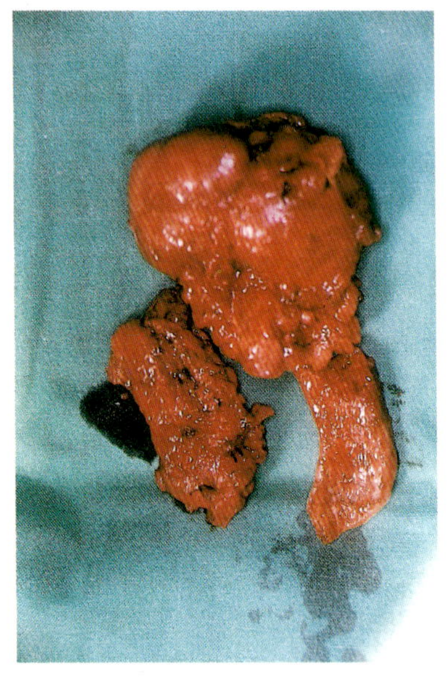

图 458

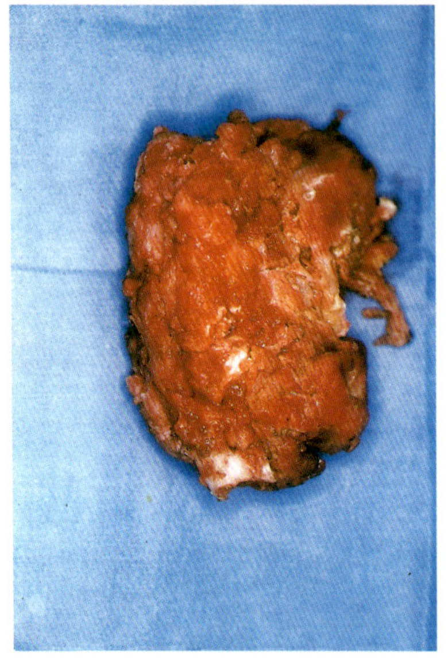

图 459

图 458，459 术后的标本正面及反面观。

Fig. 458, 459 The external and internal surfacial views of the postoperative specimen.

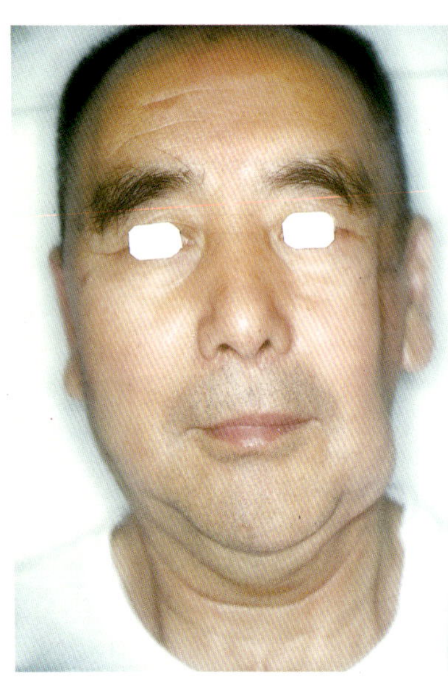

图 460

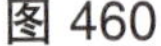

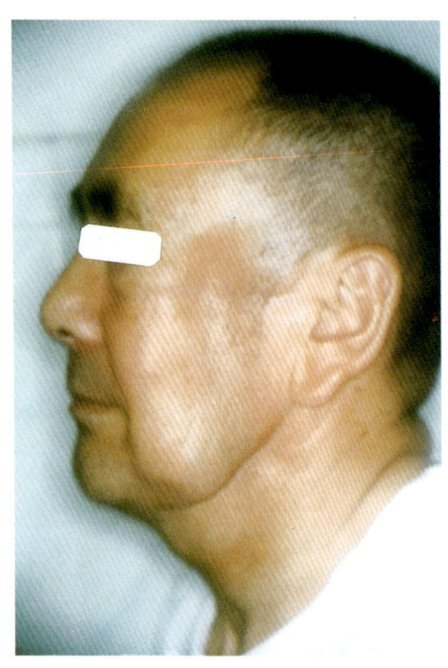

图 461

图 460，461 患者术后 2 年的正面及侧面观。正面观见两侧面颊部稍不对称，左侧稍凹陷。侧面观未见明显的切口瘢痕及皮肤异常。肿瘤无复发。

Fig. 460, 461 The frontal and lateral views of the patient 2 years postoperatively. The frontal view shows that patient's cheek is asymmetrical and the left side is slightly depressed. The lateral view shows that scar is not obvious and the tumor is no recurrent.

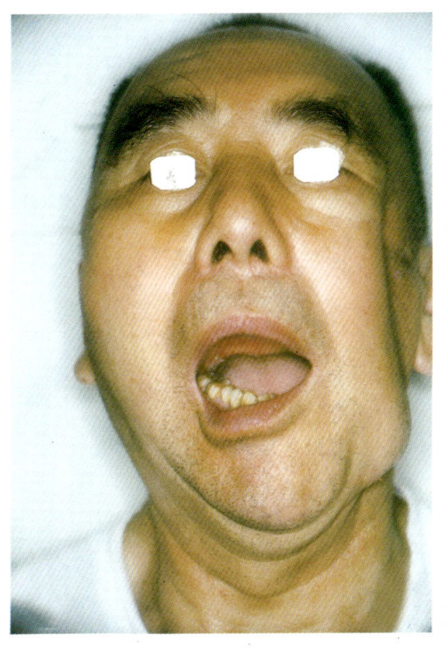

图 462

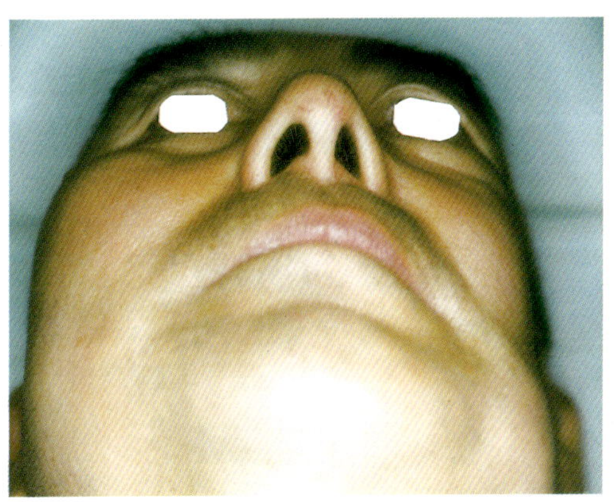

图 463

**图 462, 463** 术后 2 年患者的张口度正常。但开口型稍偏左侧。仰面观见左侧面颊部稍小于右侧。

**Fig. 462, 463** The mouth opening of the patient is normal 2 years post-operatively. Note no trismus but slight lateral sway on full opening. Submental view shows that the left facial and buccal regions are slight small than those of the right.

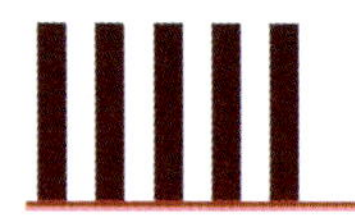



# 30. 半侧下颌骨切除肋骨移植下颌骨重建术

# 30. Rib graft for the reconstruction after hemimandibulectomy

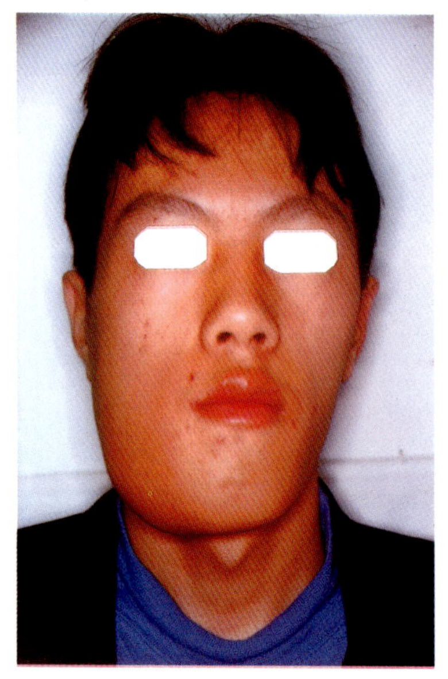

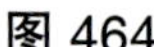

图 464

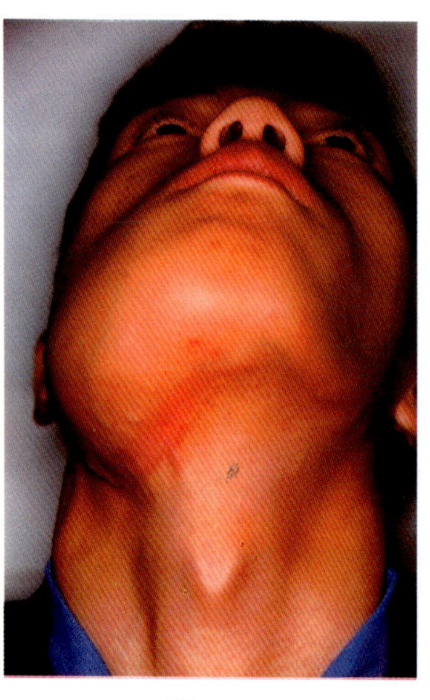

图 465

**图 464，465** 一患右下颌骨纤维异常增殖症 17 岁男性患者正、仰面显示右侧面部不对称。

**Fig. 464，465** Frontal and submental views of a 17-year-old male patient with fibrous dysplasia of the mandible show facial asymmetry and the right mandible is expansion obviously.

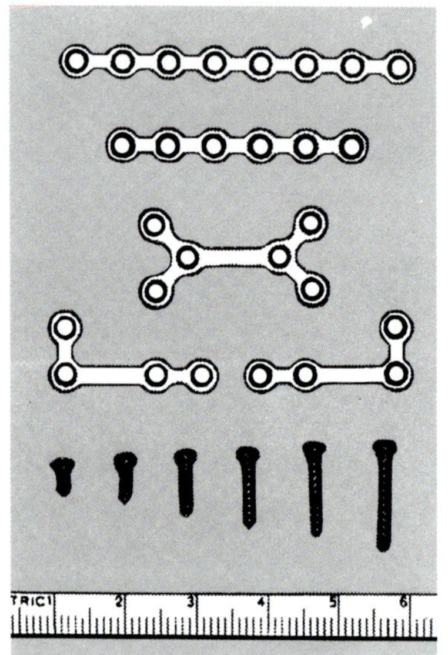

图 466

**图 466** 移植体的固定：微型夹板在移植体的塑形和固定中具有独特的优点。微型夹板使用方便、容易塑形、需要的夹板少，由于螺丝有自攻的特性而使得需要的手术器械很少。因为它能被放在移植体的外表面和移植体的下缘，为移植体塑形的保持提供了方便。

**Fig. 466** Miniplates have many advantages in graft fixation. It is only necessary to remove some of the miniplates in patients who are candidates for osseointegrated implant placement. Furthermore, miniplates are strong and easy to use. They can be shaped easily and only a minimum number of plate and screw types are required. The self-tapping native of the screws limits the amount of precision possible in graft shaping and insetting because of these properties. Miniplates are usually placed in two perpendicular planes to provide maximum rigidity against torsional stress applied across a multiply osteotomized graft. They are placed along the outer surface of the graft and along its inferior border.

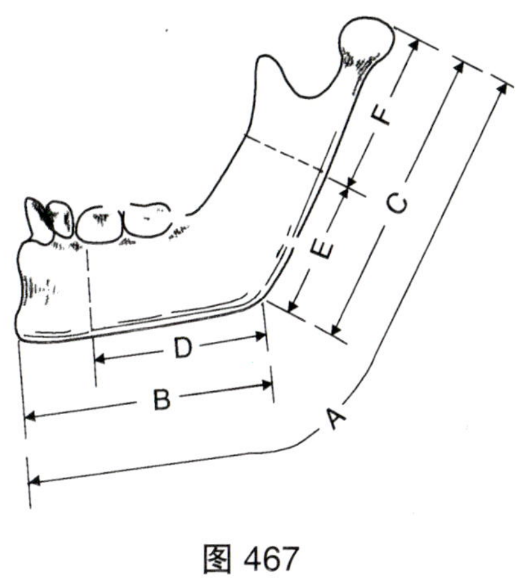


图 467

下颌侧位标本标示的关键测量点：A－标本的总长度；B－下颌体的总长度；C－下颌升支的后部总高度；D－从角到截骨处的下颌体部长度；E、F－下颌升支和髁状突的长度。

**图 467** 面后的高度是由下颌升支和髁状突的总高度来决定的，而且必须将其复制在移植体上。如果未将下颌髁状突及部分升支切除的话，就必须对外科手术标本下颌升支丧失的长度进行测量。

A typical lateral specimen is shown with key measurements indicated by A－F. Total specimen length is represented by A, total body length by B, total posterior height by C, body length from the angle to the osteotomy site which will impart curve to the body by D, and the ramus and condyle lengths by E and F.

**Fig. 467** Posterior facial height is determined by the total height of the ramus and condyle and must be duplicated on the graft. If the resection has left the condyle and proximal ramus in situ, then the length of the ramus on the surgical specimen is measured to determine the missing length.

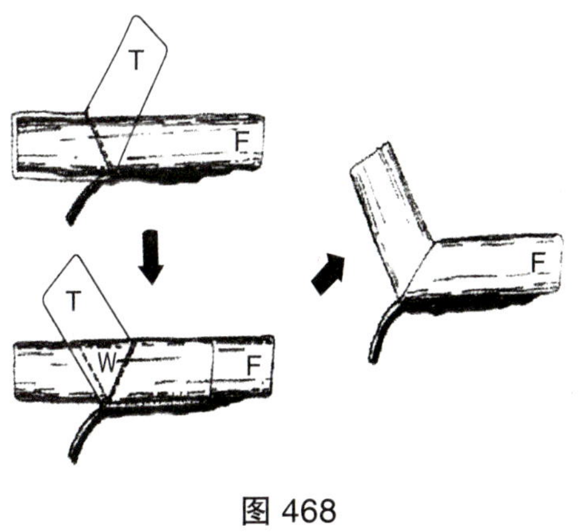


图 468

**图 468** 下颌骨移植体下颌角的塑形。

注意将透明模板（T）平放于骨移植体上，将下颌角的分角线由透明模板转移到移植体上（虚线），其下的线显示透明模板已被旋转以便于它的体部与移植体平行，将透明板上同样的线再次转移到移植体上。现在在骨上显示了一个楔形（W），用锯将其去除后将两端互相靠拢，此时下颌角形成。

**Fig. 468** The shaping of lateral grafts forming the angle of the mandible.

Note that the ramus portion of the transparent template (T) has been placed parallel to the graft (G) and the line bisecting the angle of the mandible transferred from the template to the bone (dotted line). The drawing below shows that the template has been rotated so that its body portion is parallel to graft. The same line on the template is transferred to the bone again. A wedge of bone (W) is now indicated which is removed with the saw. The graft is then put together and the angle that the ramus makes with the body now matches precisely that of the template.

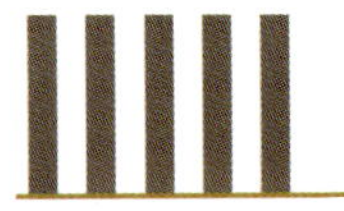


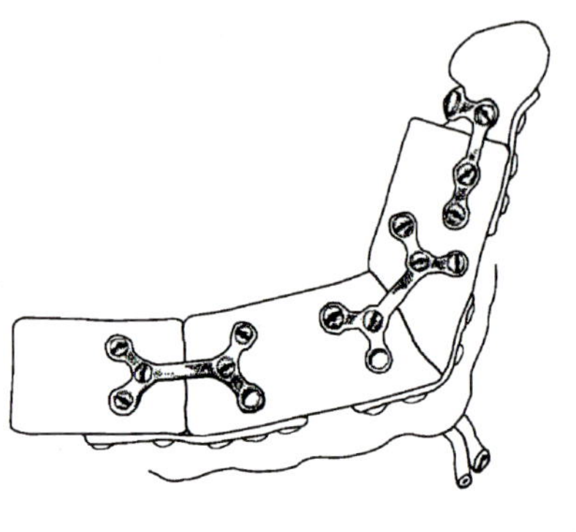

图 469

**图 469** 半侧下颌移植体的塑形与固定。

目前有观点认为应将髁突从标本上切除下来接在移植体上来恢复颞颌关节的功能及后面高的高度。方法是在把髁状突从标本上切下来之前，应对下颌升支及髁状突的高度进行测量，然后将髁状突取下并对其骨段的长度进行测量。对移植体的升支段进行测量，应使移植体升支加上髁状突的总长度等于原下颌骨的高度。

在移植体的升支和髁状突骨段已经用微型夹板固定好后，对切除下颌骨体部达中线者通常需要将移植体进行二次切断后用微型夹板固定以使移植体与原下颌骨体的曲度相似。

**Fig. 469** The shaping of lateral grafts.

In the case where the condyle is removed with the specimen. It has been shown that the condyle can be resected from the surgical specimen and mounted onto the bony flap as a nonvascularized graft. This practice restores tandem temporomandibular joint function and facilitates the accurate restoration of posterior facial height. The technique is that before removing the condyle from the specimen, the height of the ramus and condyle should be measured. The condyle is then removed and the length of the condyle segment is measured. The ramus end of the graft is then cut, taking this latter measurement into account so that the total measurement of the graft ramus plus the condyle graft equals the original overall measurement.

After the ramus and condyle segment has been fixed with miniplates, lateral graft that extend to the midline usually require a second osteotomy to increase the curve near the midline. It is always better to leave the graft long after the first osteotomy and perform the second osteotomy at the time of graft insetting.

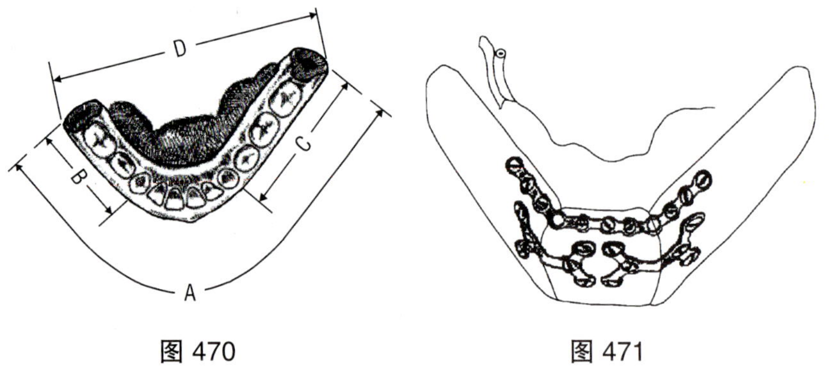


图 470　　图 471

**图 470, 471** 下颌前部移植体的塑形与固定。

在中段骨移植体的每侧做一个截骨，这种在两个平面上截骨以使移植骨段在向后和向上均呈角形，这就维持着中央骨段前面部的方向与一旦被嵌入的移植体的额平面平行，前骨段的这个方向与自然下颌骨的形态一致，这也是骨融合种植体需要的理想方向。

**Fig. 470, 471** The shaping and fixation of anterior grafts of the mandible.

An osteotomy is performed on each end of the central segment. This osteotomy is made in two planes so that the body segments are angled both posteriorly and upward. This maintains the orientation of the anterior face of the central segment parallel to the frontal plane once the graft is inset. This orientation of the anterior segment stimulates the native mandible shape most closely. It is also the ideal orientation for osseointegrated implants because the thickest dimension of the bone will remain parallel to the axis of the implants. It is important that the body segments rise upward away from the central segment at the same angle. This will avoid a twist in the graft which would become manifest as a cant of the central segment following insetting.

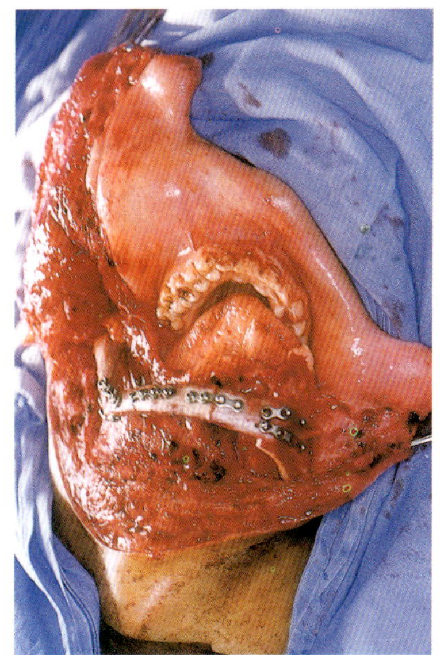

图 472

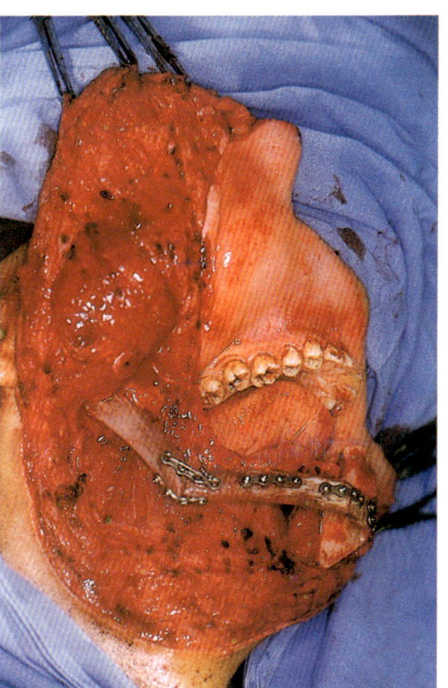

图 473

**图 472，473** 按在 24 节中所述的方法行半侧下颌骨切除术。下颌骨被切除之后，对切取的植入体进行塑形，将塑形完成后的移植体与剩余下颌骨断端用微型钛板固定，缝合口腔粘膜及粘膜下组织，消灭死腔。分层缝合肌层、皮下组织及皮肤。

**Fig. 472, 473** Hemimandibulotomy is performed as mentioned technique in the section 24. After the resection of the mandible has been completed, the shaping of grafts is made. The angle of divergence between the body segments should be checked with the transverse template and the surgical specimen. This should be corrected, if necessary, before final fixation of the osteotomy sites with miniplates. The body segments are usually different lengths. It is better to leave the body segments at least 1 cm longer than needed and make the final length adjustments during insetting. The graft is fixed to the bone end of the remaining mandible with the miniplates through holes drilled in the bone. The underlying dead space is obliterated by numerous sutures of 3 – 0 chromic catgut. The skin and platysma are approximated around a drain which is left in place for 48 hours.

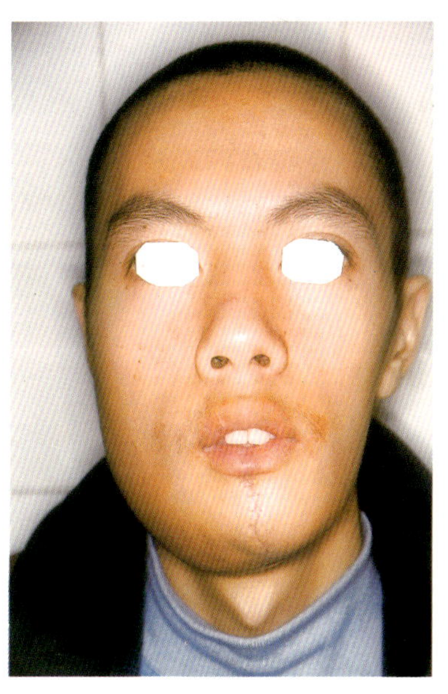

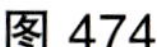

图 474

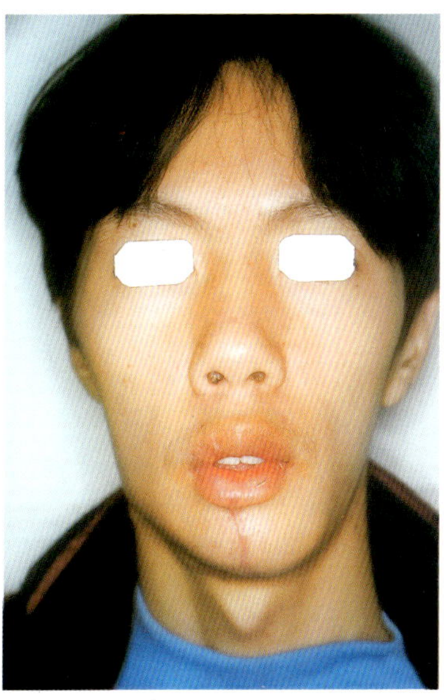

图 475

**图 474, 475** 手术后 10 天和 6 个月后的正面观。

**Fig. 474, 475** Frontal view of a 16-year-old male patient 10 days and 6 months after surgery.

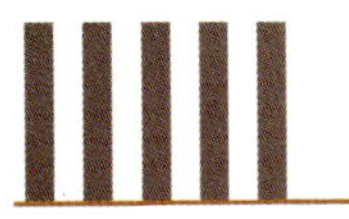



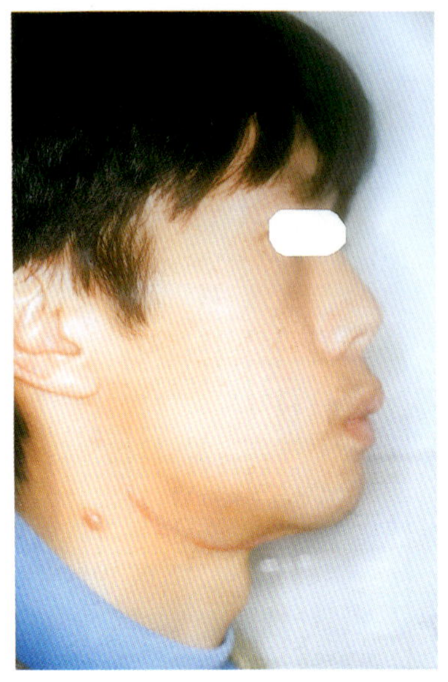

图 476

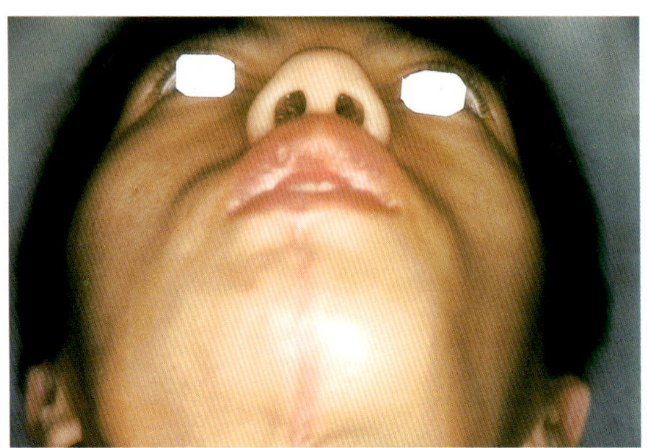

图 477

图 476, 477 半侧下颌骨切除重建后的侧面及仰面观。

Fig. 476, 477 Lateral and submental views after hemimandibular reconstruction of hemimandibulotomy.

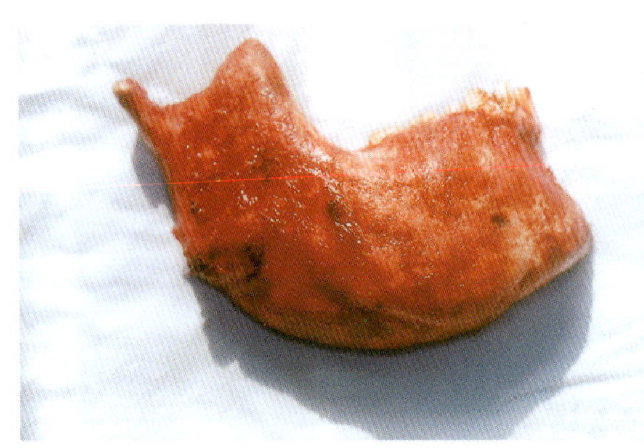

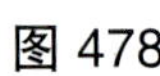

图 478

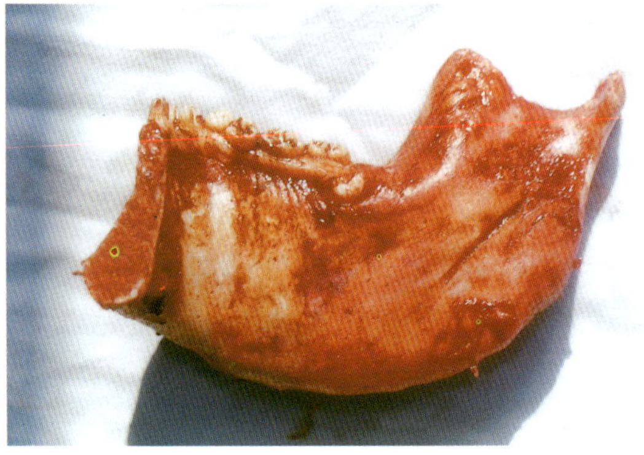

图 479

图 478, 479 手术标本的外侧和内侧面观。

Fig. 478, 479 External and internal surface views of postoperative specimen.

# 31. 下颌磨牙后区鳞状细胞癌的颌颈联合根治术

# 31. Combined operation of radical neck dissection with resection of mandible for the carcinoma arising in the mandibular retromolar trigone

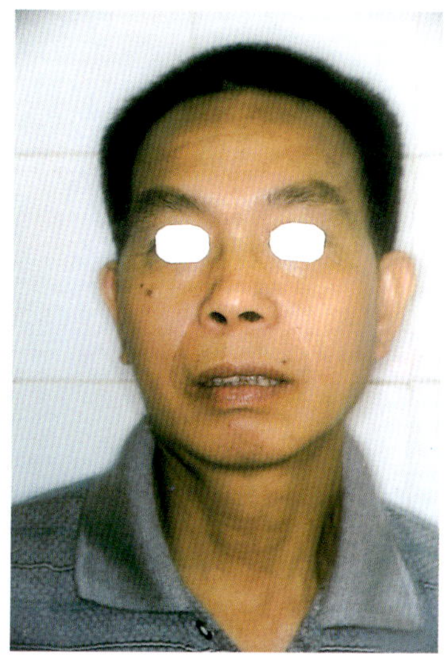

图 480

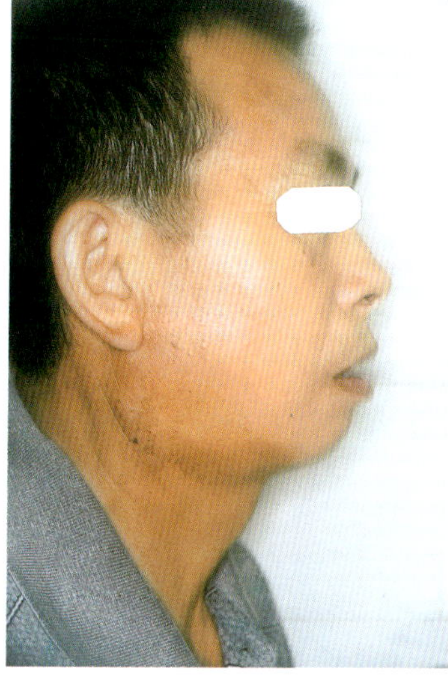

图 481

**图 480, 481** 患右下颌磨牙后三角区鳞状细胞癌患者的正面及右侧面观。

正面观见右颌下区淋巴结增大,侧面观显示右颌下区明显膨隆,为右颌下淋巴结转移。

**Fig. 480, 481** Frontal and lateral views of a 58-year-old male patient with the squamous cell carcinoma arising in the right mandibular retromolar trigone.

Frontal and lateral views show that the right submandibular nodes are involved initially.

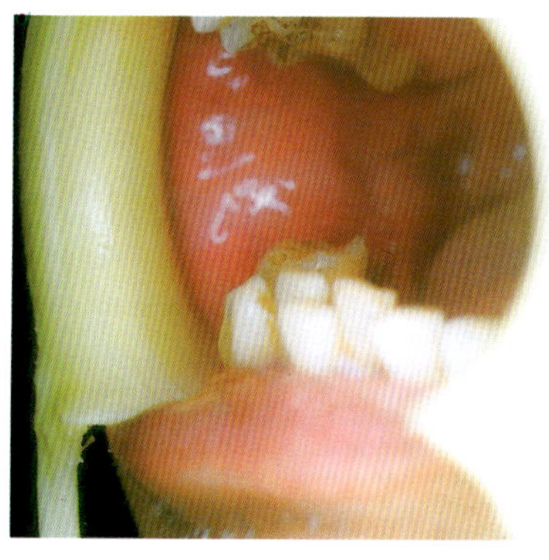

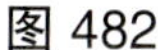

图 482

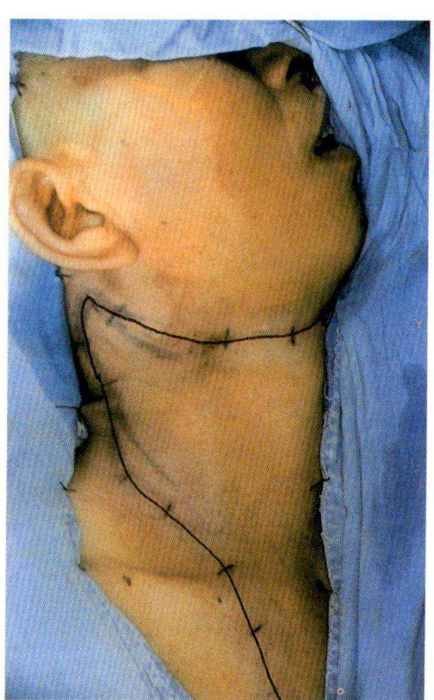

图 483

**图 482** 右下颌磨牙后三角鳞状细胞癌。

**图 483** 右侧颌颈联合根治术的颈淋巴清扫术的切口线。

**Fig. 482** Example of squamous cell carcinoma of the right mandibular retromolar trigone.

**Fig. 483** Incision line of combined operation of the mandibulo-radical neck dissection is marked out with methylene blue.

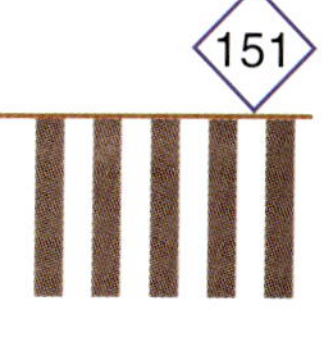

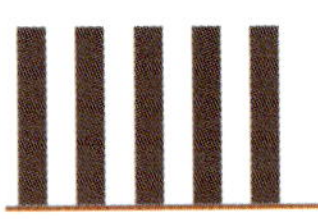



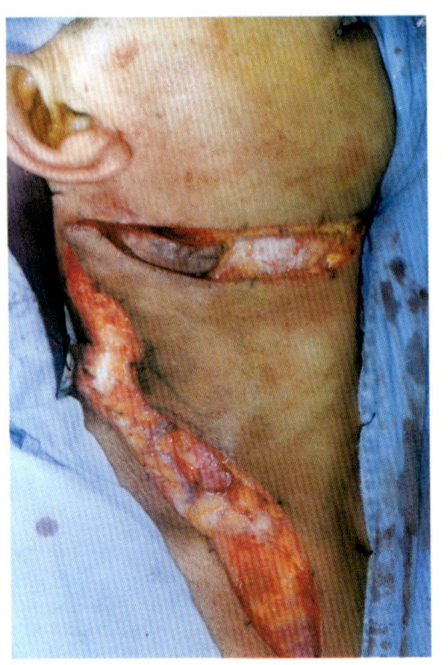

图 484

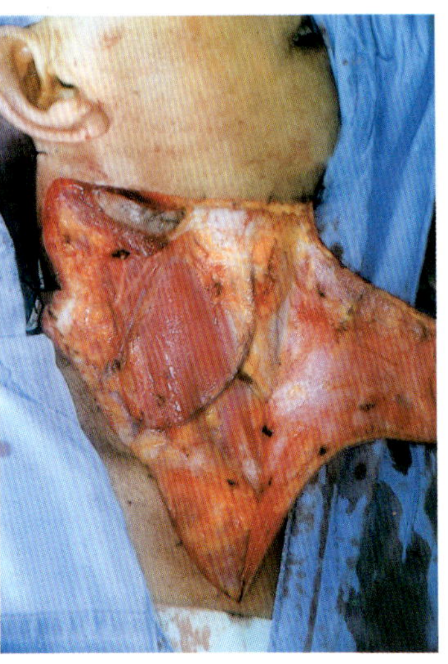

图 485

**图 484, 485** 根据根治性颈淋巴清扫术标记的切口线，切开颈部皮肤、皮下组织和颈阔肌，在颈阔肌深面由后向前掀起皮肤 - 颈阔肌瓣，上至下颌骨下缘，前至颈中线，后至斜方肌前缘，下至锁骨下。

**Fig. 484, 485** After incision line has been marked out, a rectangular incision of the radical neck dissection is made through the skin and platysma. Flap of skin and platysma is reflected anteriorly to expose the entire lateral region of the neck and the clavicle below.

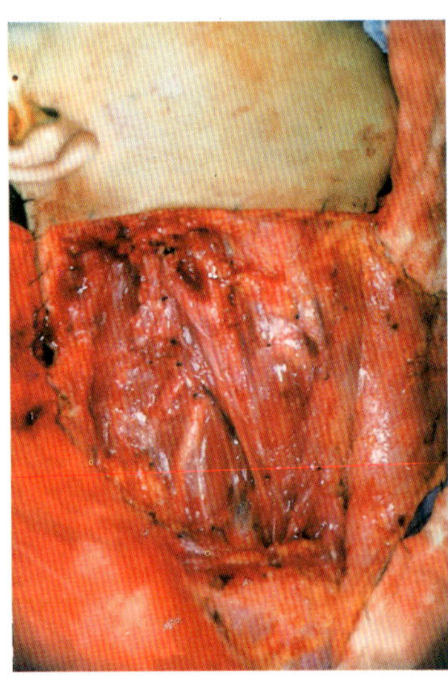

图 486

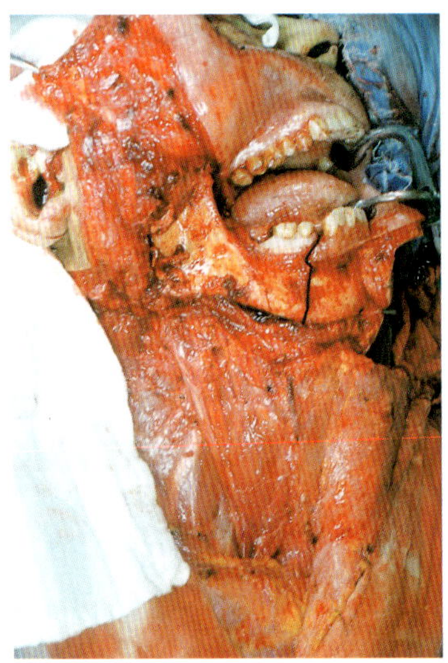

图 487

**图 486, 487** 按常规完成颈淋巴清扫术后，在下唇正中将下唇切开，然后沿口内下颌龈颊沟靠颊侧切开龈颊沟粘膜并沿下颌体部锐性解剖，掀起颊瓣，下颌骨体部被暴露。拔除4|，用线锯将右侧下颌骨体部锯开，此时下颌骨后段已游离。在肿瘤周围 1.0cm 正常粘膜内做切口，切开口底粘膜及深层肌肉，切断下颌角部外侧的嚼肌及内侧的翼外肌附着，处理下牙槽神经血管束，用弯剪刀剪断颞肌喙突附着及处理颞颌关节后将右侧下颌骨及肿瘤组织去除。

**Fig. 486, 487** After radical neck dissection has been completed, the lower lip is split in the midline and a cheek flap is elevated by an incision in the gingivobuccal gutter and dissection along the body of the mandible. The mandible is divided well anterior to the lesion with a Gigli saw. The first premolar tooth is extracted before the mandible is divided. Once the segment of mandible has been freed posteriorly, an incision is outlined around the tumor, leaving at least 1. 0 cm of normal mucosa on all its edges. The incision is carried through the deep musculature of the floor of the mouth. Posteriorly, the masseter muscle is severed at its insertion along the angle and ascending ramus. The pterygoid muscle is divided. The temporalis muscle is located by palpation at its insertion on the coronoid process and is severed with strong curved scissors. The condyle is then freed by incision of its attachments at the temporomandibular joint. The intra-oral tumor and partial mandible are removed.

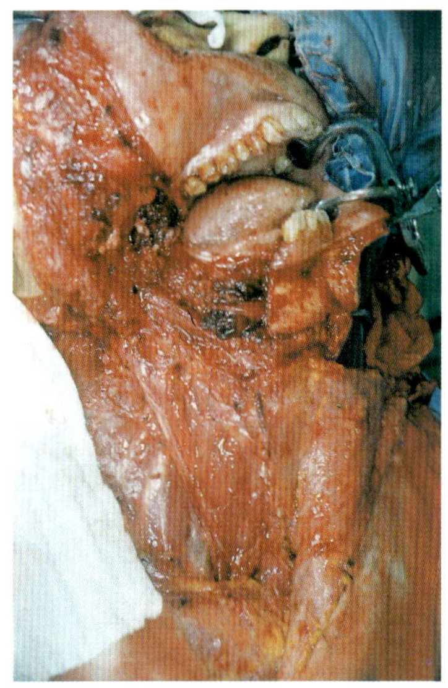

图 488

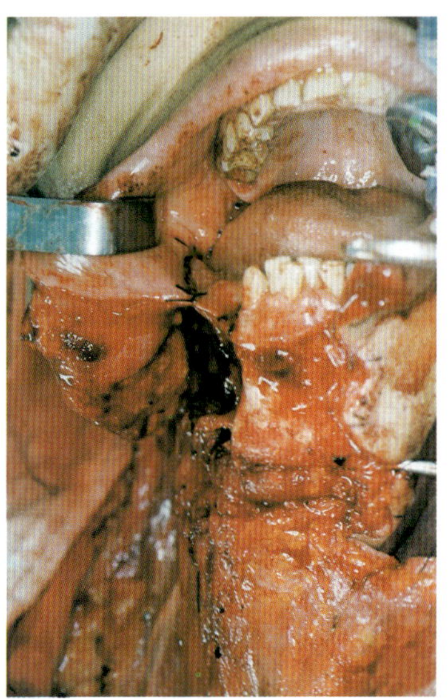

图 489

**图 488** 用生理盐水冲洗创面后将颊粘膜与口底粘膜及剩余下颌骨断端牙龈粘膜相缝合。为了防止唾液渗漏于口底创口内，在缝合的粘膜深层再将颊部肌层与口底肌层相缝合。

**图 489** 分层缝合切开的下唇及颏部组织，此时应特别注意唇红皮肤交界缘的对合。

**Fig. 488** Hemostasis is obtained by ligating all bleeding vessels with ties of fine chromic catgut, The wound is thoroughly irrigated with saline solution. The mucosal edges are joined with interrupted sutures of 4－0 silk and the knots being tied within the mouth. To prevent a leak, this suture line must be reinforced by deep sutures wherever possible. This is accomplished by suturing the muscle of the floor of the mouth to the deep surface of the cheek flap with interrupted sutures of 3－0 chromic catgut.

**Fig489** The lip is reconstructed with burried chromic sutures in the orbicularis muscle and fine silk sutures in the skin and mucosa. Care is taken to align accurately the vermilion-skin junction.

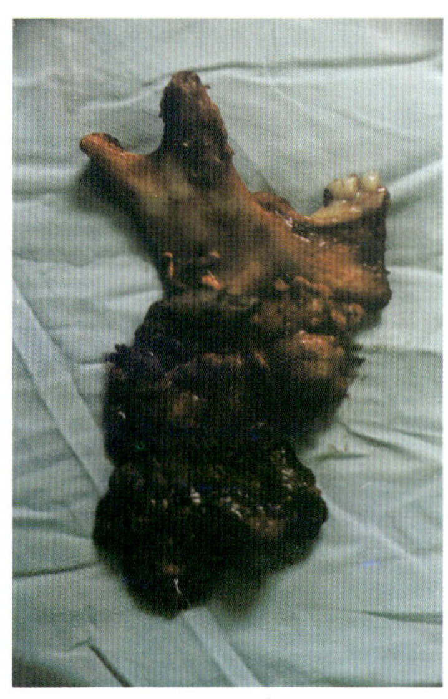

图 490

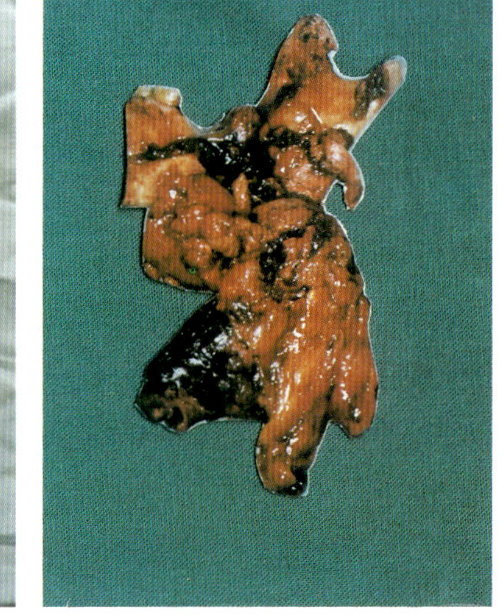

图 491

**图 490，491** 手术后标本的外侧及内侧面观。

**Fig. 490，491** External and internal views of postoperative specimen.

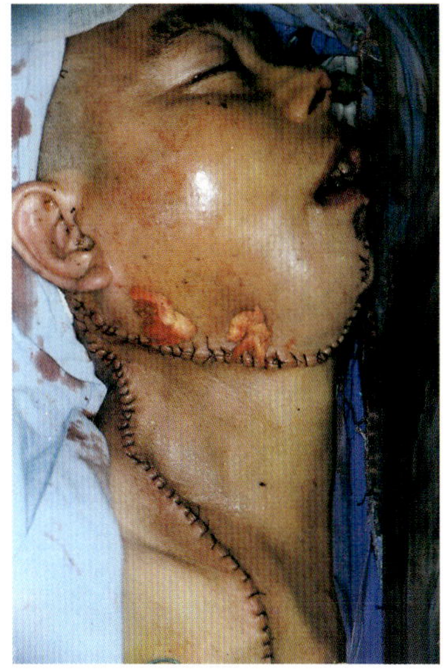

图 492

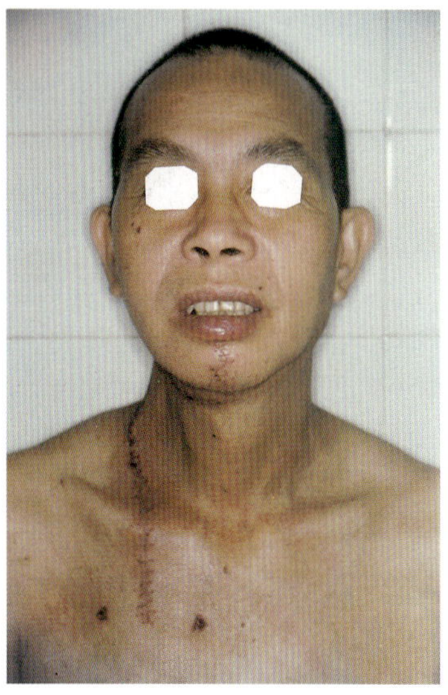

图 493

**图 492** 按常规方法在颈部创区放置橡皮引流管 2 根后分层缝合颈阔肌、皮下组织及皮肤，颈部轻加压包扎。

**图 493** 患者拆线后正面观，创口愈合良好。

**Fig. 492** The neck wound is drained and closed in the usual manner. A bulky pressure dressing is applied.

**Fig. 493** Frontal view of the patient after suture lines has been removed, the wound healing is normal.

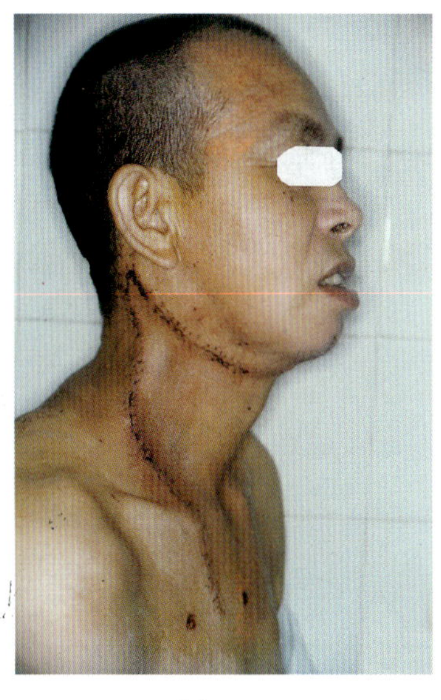

图 494

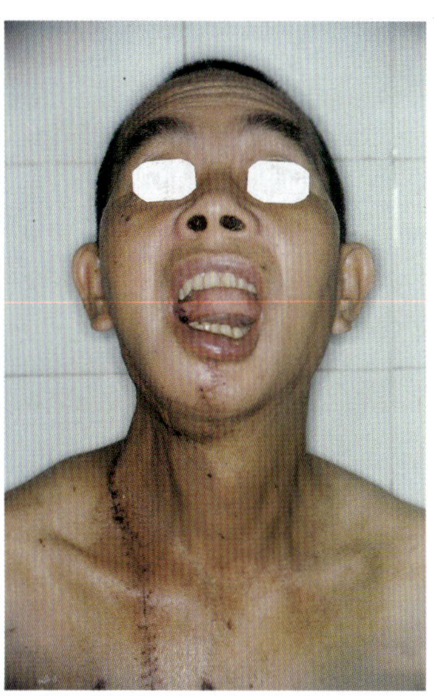

图 495

**图 494，495** 患者术后 11 天侧面观及张口情况。

**Fig. 494, 495** Lateral view and condition of the patient's openning mouth 11 days after operation.

# 32. 下颌牙龈癌切除后下颌口底缺损岛状额瓣修复

# 32. The island forehead flap reconstructing in the mandibular and the floor of the mouth after resection of the mandibular gingival carcinoma

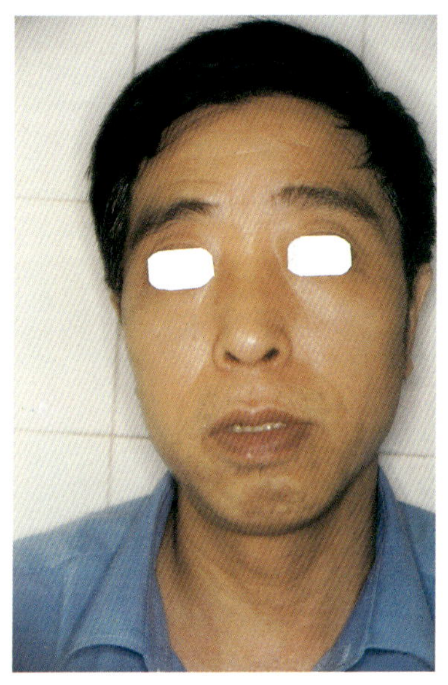

图 496

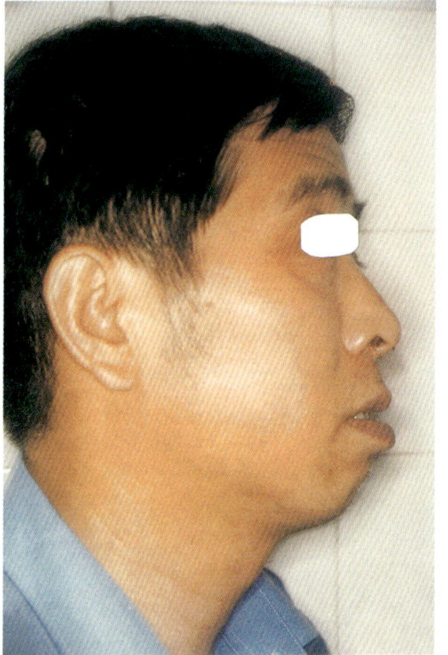

图 497

**图 496，497** 患右下颌牙龈鳞状细胞癌的一 52 岁的男性患者正、侧面观。患者右下颌前磨牙区有一溃疡性病灶，侵及下颌牙槽骨，但右颌下淋巴结肿大不明显。

**Fig. 496, 497** Frontal and lateral views of a 52-year-old male patient with the squamous cell carcinoma of the mandibular right premolar area. The patient has an ulcerative form which invade the underlying tissues and bone, but the lymph node metastases in the submandibular region has not been found.

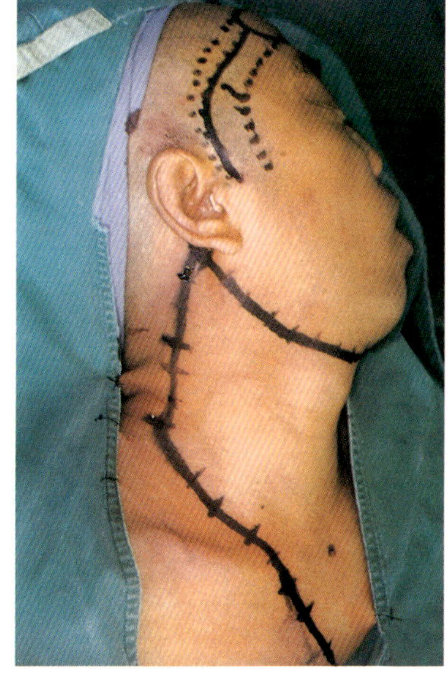

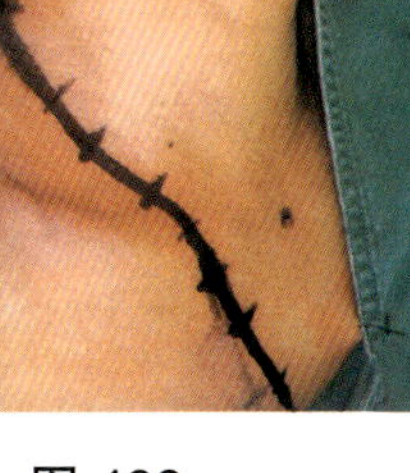

图 498

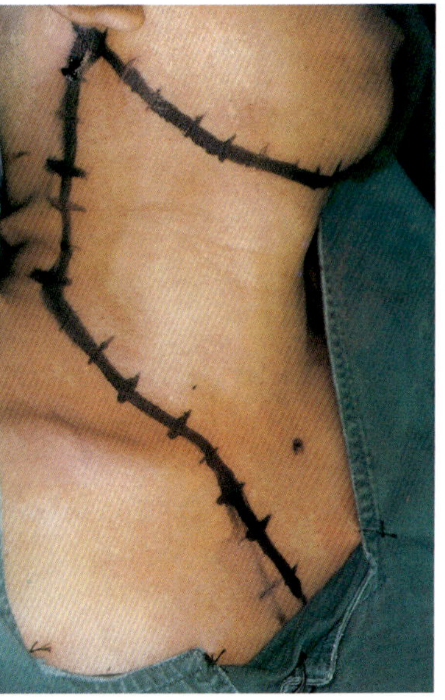

图 499

**图 498, 499** 用美蓝画出颈淋巴清扫术和岛状额瓣切口线。

**Fig. 498, 499** The incision lines of the radical neck dissection and the island forehead flap are marked out with methylene blue.

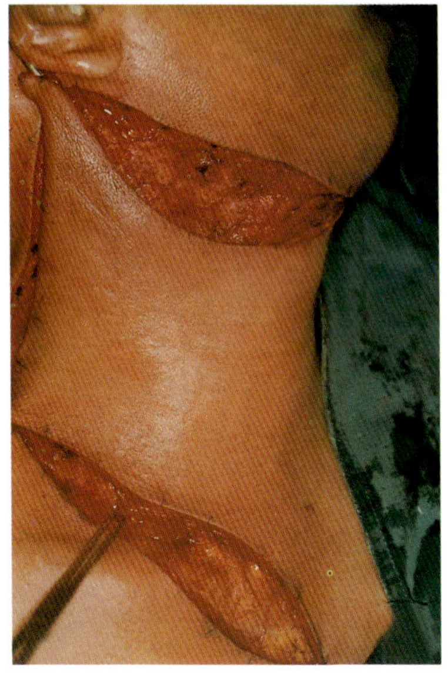

图 500

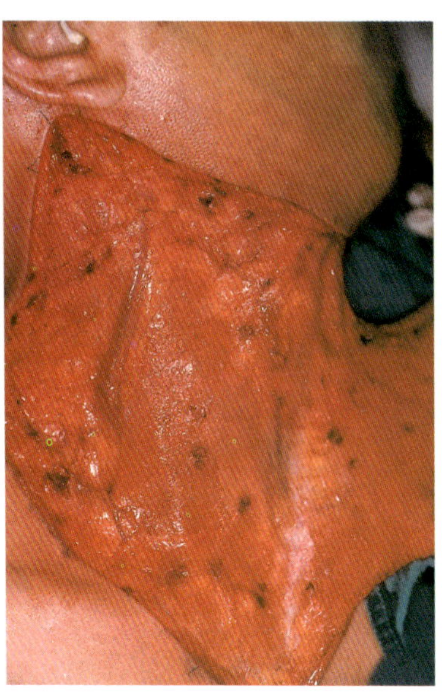

图 501

**图 500，501** 根据根治性颈淋巴清扫术标出的切口线，切开颈部皮肤、皮下组织和颈阔肌，在颈阔肌深面由后向前掀起皮肤－颈阔肌瓣，上至下颌骨下缘，前至颈中线，后至斜方肌前缘，下至锁骨下。按常规方法完成颈淋巴清扫术。

**Fig. 500, 501** After incision line has been marked out, the upper curved incision of the radical neck dissection is made through the skin and platysma. The vertical portion of the incision is made and flaps of skin and platysma are reflected anteriorly and posteriorly to expose the entire lateral region of the neck and the clavicle below. A radical neck dissection is completed in the usual manner.

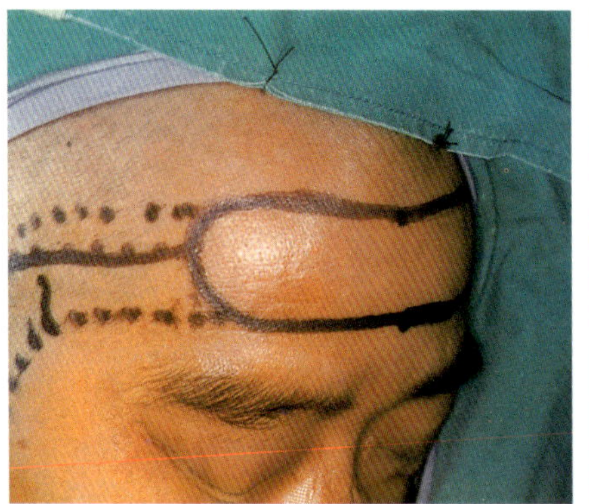

图 502

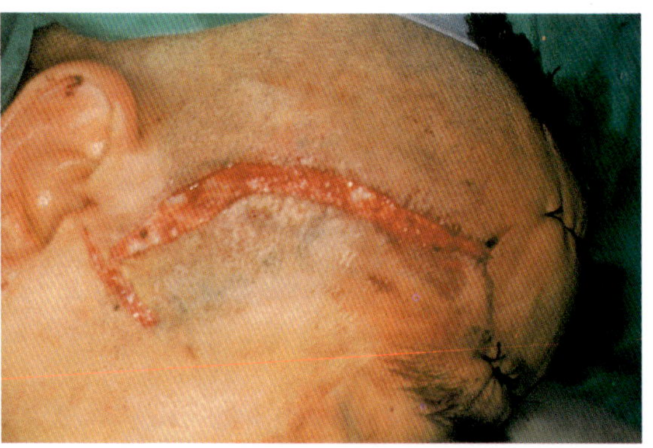

图 503

**图 502** 按全额岛状瓣设计切口线，其范围为两侧至眼外眦角，上界为发际，下界为眉弓之上，皮下蒂达患侧耳屏前区。

**图 503** 在皮下蒂的表皮上正中做切口，在毛囊下剥离表皮，注意保护皮下蒂的动、静脉。

**Fig. 502** The flap designed is outlined with methylene blue. The island forehead flap used in intraoral reconstruction is laterally based. Its base extending from the lateral border of the eyebrow to the anterior border of the pinna at approximately the level of the zygomatic arch and the flap itself curving across the hairless forehead. Its breadth is generally that of the forehead from eyebrow to hairless while its length is variable but most often extends to the hairline on the opposite temple.

**Fig. 503** A incision is made over the derma of the midline of the pedicle, the flap pedicle to the island is developed in the subfollicular plane and the vessels in the flap pedicle should be preserved.

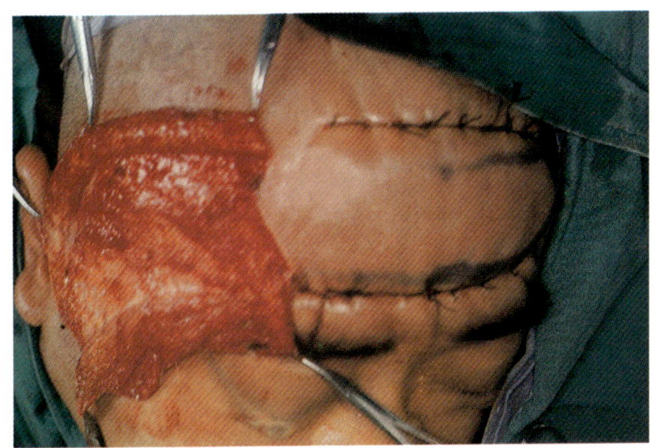

图 504

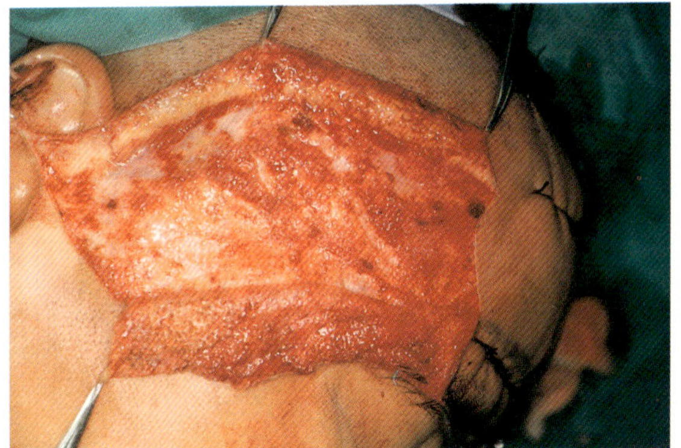

图 505

**图 504, 505** 皮下蒂的表皮被剥离完成后的正面及侧面观。

**Fig. 504, 505** Frontal and lateral views after the derma of the flap pedicle has been dissected.

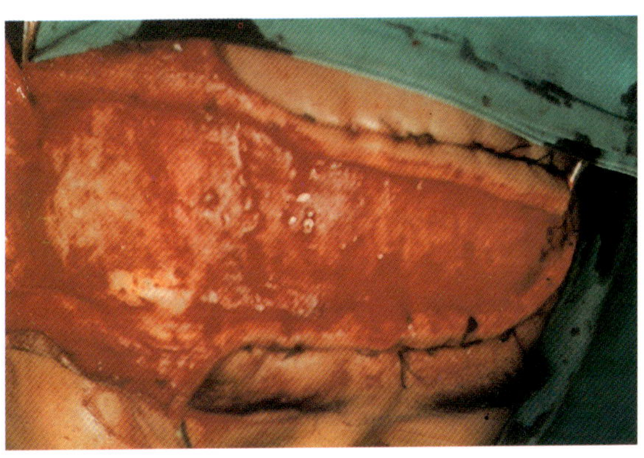

图 506

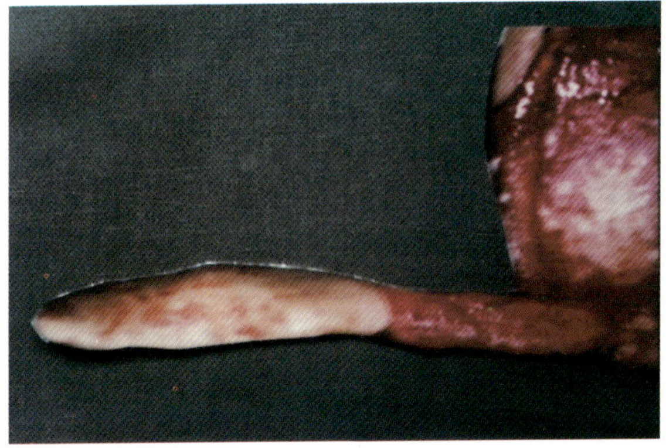

图 507

**图 506** 岛状额瓣的蒂被制备好后，由岛状额瓣远端向颧弓方向分离至颧弓上缘为止，将岛状额瓣用生理盐水纱布保护好。

**图 507** 岛状额瓣的正面观。

**Fig. 506** After the pedicle of the island forehead flap has been prepared, the whole of the forehead is raised on a unilateral pedicle. The base of the flap lies between the lateral end of the eyebrow and the upper pole of the ear and is situated just above the zygomatic arch. Elevation of flap continues until the line joining the lateral corner of the eyebrow and the superior pole of the ear is reached. The island forehead flap is preserved with saline solution gauzes.

**Fig. 507** Frontal view of the island forehead flap.

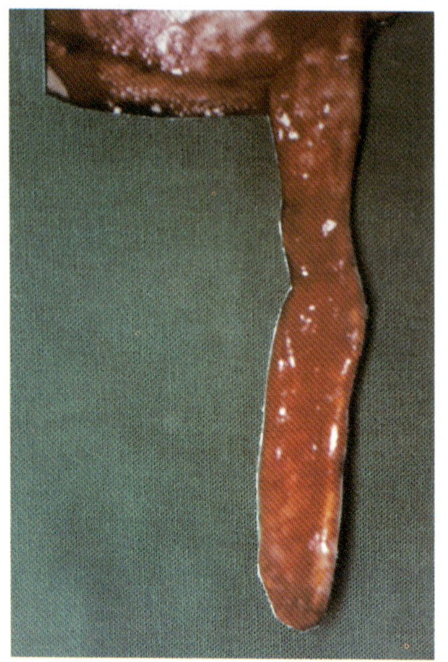
图 508

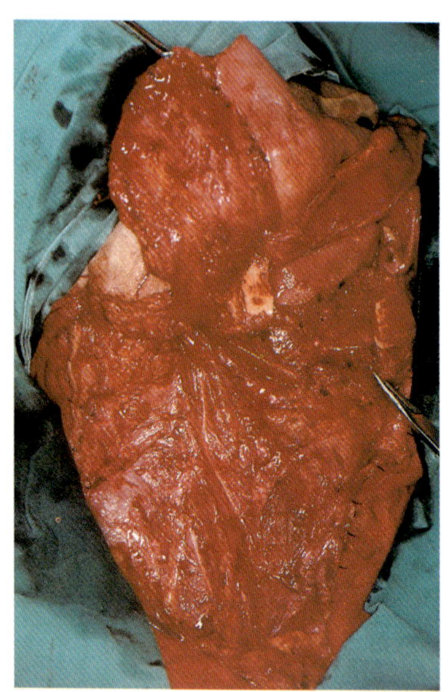
图 509

**图 508** 岛状额瓣的内侧面观。

**图 509** 在下唇正中将下唇切开，然后在下颌龈颊沟靠颊侧切开下颌龈颊沟粘膜并沿下颌体部分离将颊瓣掀起。在病变的前部用线锯锯开下颌骨，在锯开下颌骨之前，拔除3|。在下颌骨角部锯断下颌骨后部。一旦下颌骨骨段已经被游离，绕肿瘤周围的切口便可以被确定，一般在肿瘤周围正常粘膜 1.0cm 内切除。切口通过口底的深层肌肉，此时，口内的肿瘤和下颌骨已经与周围附着组织完全分离，将其去除。用细线结扎出血的血管后，创面用生理盐水冲洗。

沿额瓣蒂部切口之下缘向下内分离，切断颧弓上缘颞筋膜附着，继续向下分离至颧弓深面的翼颌间隙，咬除喙突。将岛状额瓣通过隧道转移至下颌口底缺损区。

**Fig. 508** Internal view of the island forehead flap.

**Fig. 509** The lower lip is split in the midline and a cheek flap is elevated by an incision in the gingivobuccal gutter and dissection along the body of the mandible. The mandible is divided well anterior to the lesion with a Gigli saw. The canine tooth is extracted before the mandible is divided. Posteriorly, the mandible is sectioned at the angle. Once the segment of mandible has been freed posteriorly, the incision is outlined around the tumor leaving at least 1.0 cm of normal tissue on all its edges. The incision is carried through the deep musculature of the floor of the mouth. The intra-oral tumor and mandible have now been freed from all attachments above. The intra-oral tumor, the attached segment of mandible and the neck contents are removed en masse. Hemostasis is obtained by ligating all bleeding vessels with ties of fine chromic catgut. The wound is thoroughly irrigated with saline solution.

A separate incision is made in frontal of the ear and the flap gain entry into the oral cavity through a separate incision. If a cheek flap has been elevated, as during many of our composite resection, the coronoid process of the mandible is removed after severing the inserting ligament of the temporalis muscle. This will allow the flap to seat neatly medial to the retromalor area of the mandible without the added pressure of the coronoid process.

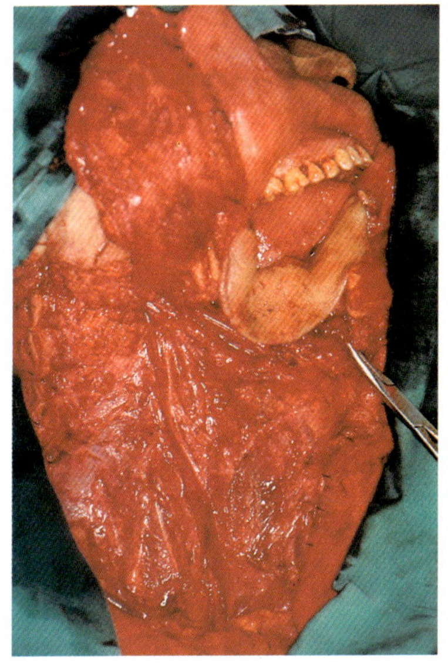

图 510

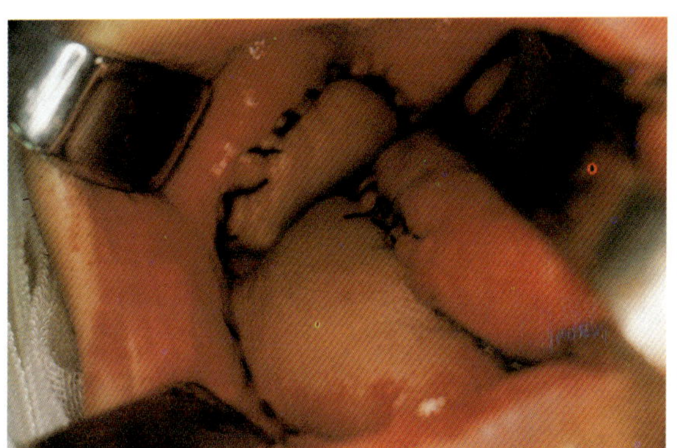

图 511

**图 510** 岛状额瓣通过隧道转移至口腔缺损区后，将穿入口内的额瓣与缺损周围粘膜缝合，将翻转之颊瓣还回原处后缝合下颌龈颊沟。

**图 511** 岛状额瓣缝合被完成后的口内观。

**Fig. 510** After the island forehead flap has reached the defective area of the oral cavity through a tunnel, the flap is then maneuvered into its bed and sutured to the surrounding mucosa with interrupted suture. The cheek flap is returned in place and closure is completed by approximating the mucosa in the gingivobuccal gutter with fine silk.

**Fig. 511** Intra-oral view after the island forehead flap is sutured to the surrounding mucosa with interrupted suture.

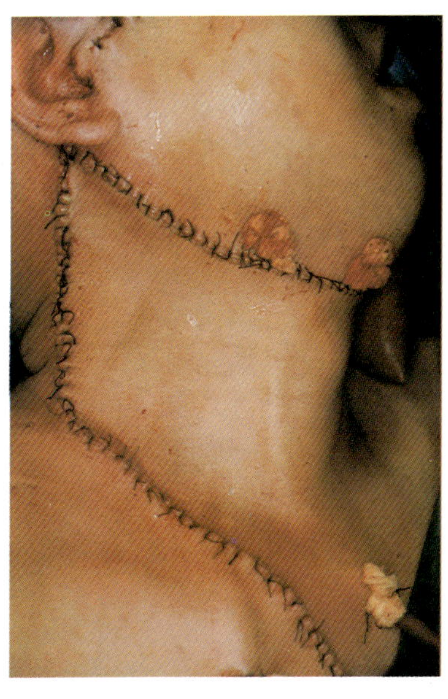

图 512

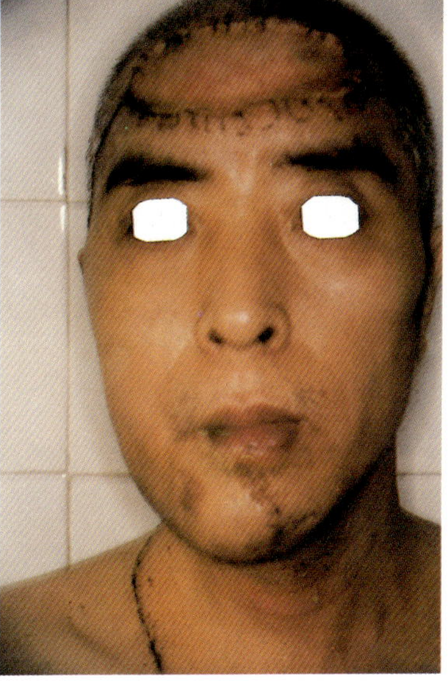

图 513

**图 512** 分层缝合下唇及颏部。生理盐水冲洗颈部创口后，置橡皮引流管 2 根，将颈部肌皮瓣还回原处后分层缝合，局部稍加压包扎。

**图 513** 患者拆线后正面观。

**Fig. 512** The lip is reconstructed with burried chromic sutures in the orbicularis muscle and fine silk sutures in the skin and mucosa. Care is taken to align accurately the vermilion-skin junction. The neck wound is drained and closed in the usual manner.

**Fig. 513** Frontal view after sutures are removed.

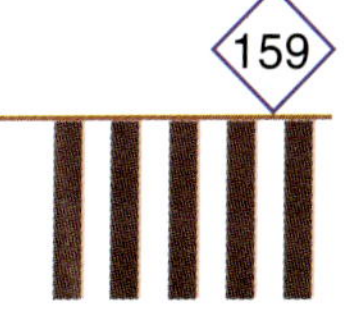

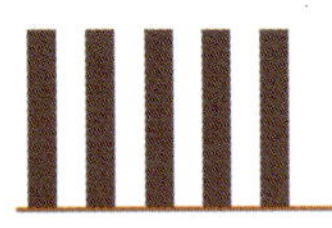



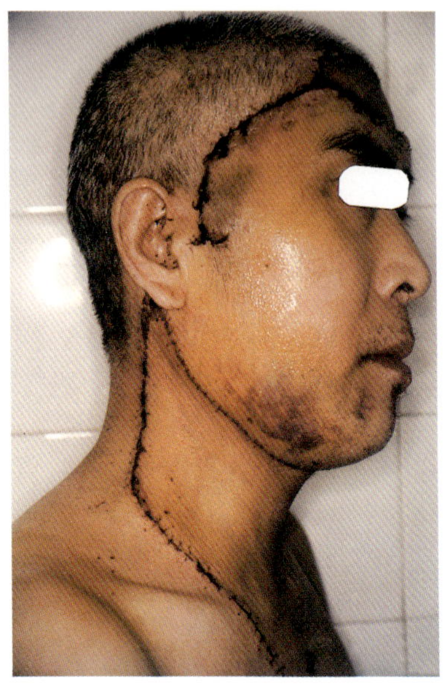

图 514

**图 514** 患者拆线后侧面观。额部及颈部创口愈合良好。

Fig. 514 Lateral view after sutures are removed. The wound healing on the forehead and the neck is fine.

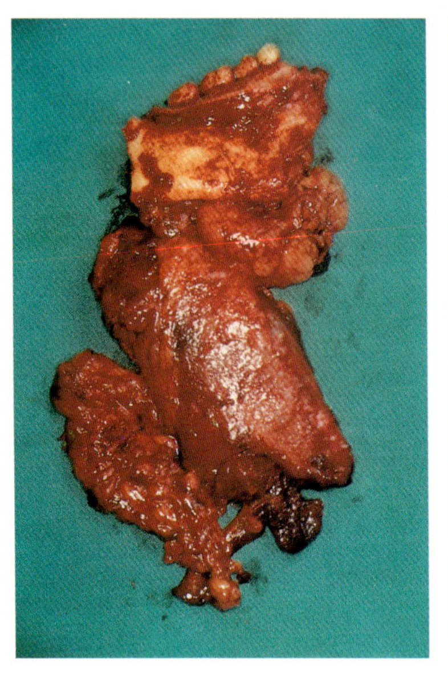

图 515

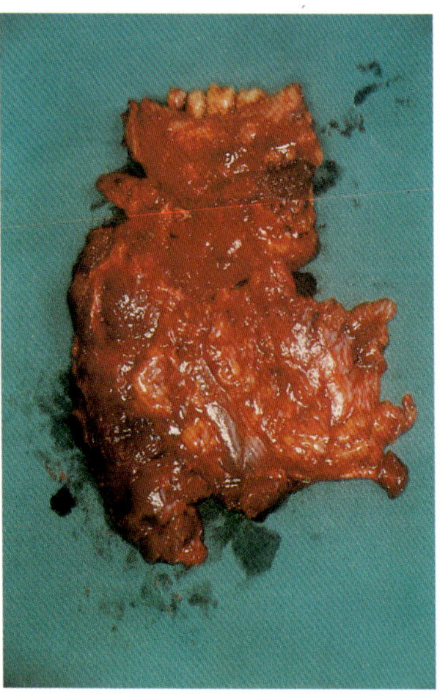

图 516

**图 515, 516** 下颌牙龈癌颌颈联合根治术的术后标本外侧面及内侧面观。

Fig. 515, 516 External surface and internal surface views after the mandibulo-neck combined operations of carcinoma of the gingiva of the lower jaw.

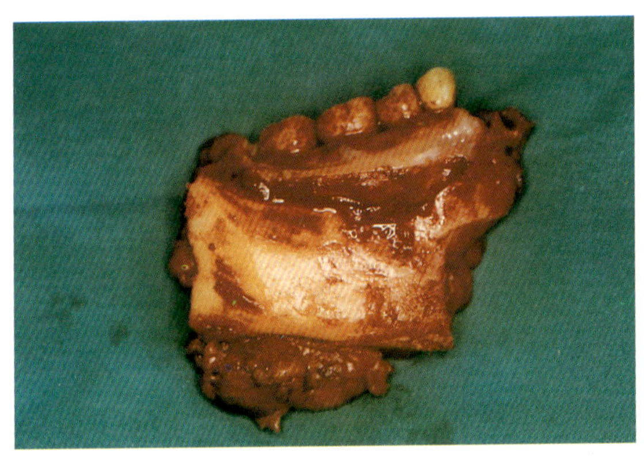
图 517

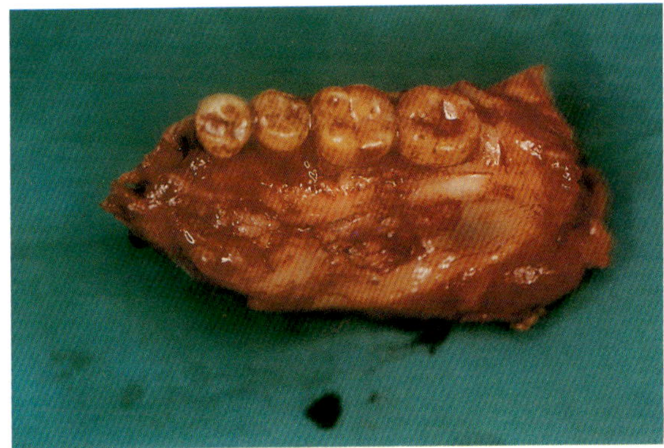
图 518

图 517, 518 被切除下颌骨段的外侧及内侧面观。

Fig. 517, 518 External surface and internal surface views of the mandibular segment resected.

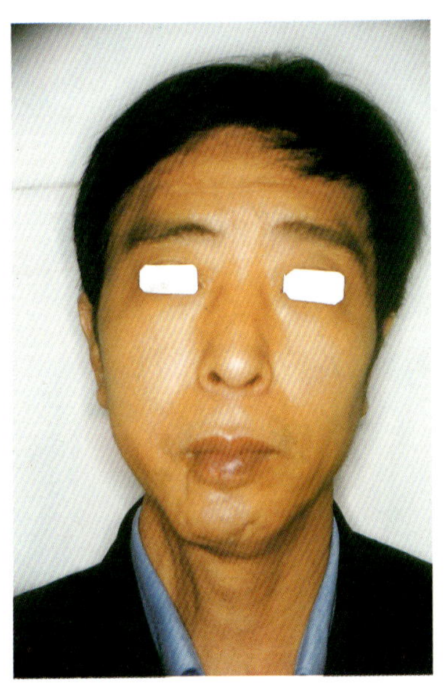
图 519

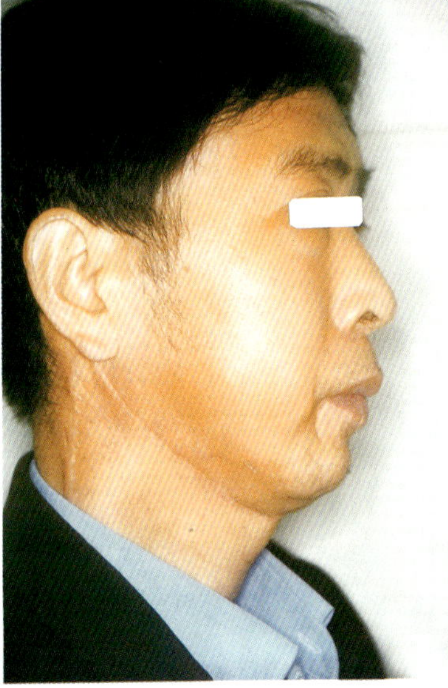
图 520

图 519, 520 患者术后 1 年的正、侧面观。

Fig. 519, 520 Frontal and lateral views of the patient with carcinoma of the right mandibular gingiva 1 year after surgery.

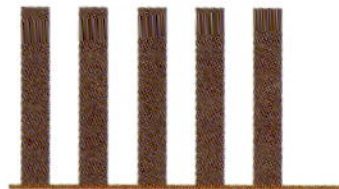



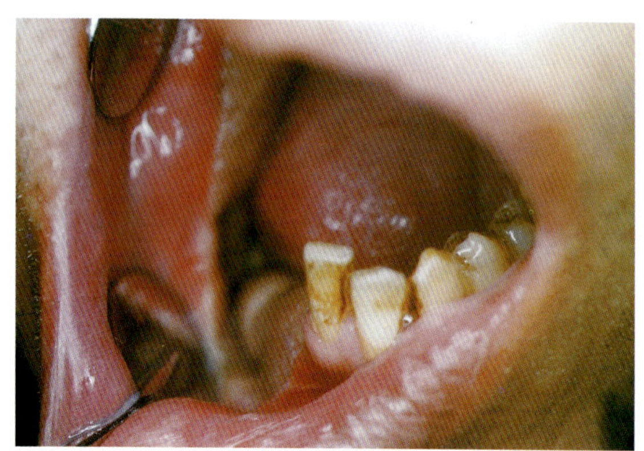

图 521

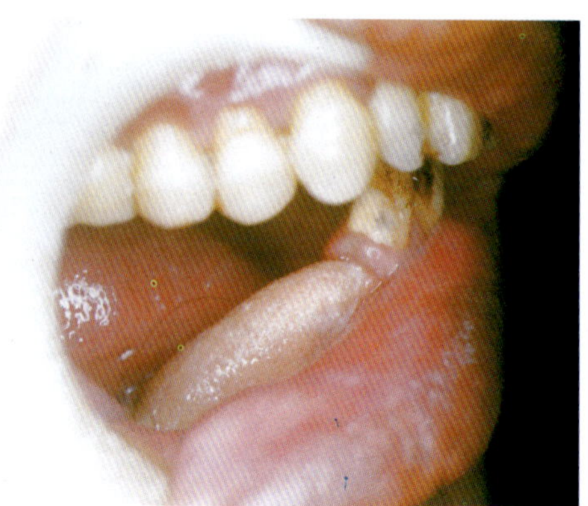

图 522

**图 521,522** 术后 1 年患者的张口度及口腔内创面的愈合情况。

Fig. 521，522 Condition of the patient's mouth openning and wound healing in the oral cavity 1 year after surgery.

# 33. 下颌牙龈癌颌颈联合根治术后下颌骨缺损金属植入体即刻下颌骨重建

# 33. Immediate metal implant for mandibular reconstruction following segmental resection of the mandible for the carcinoma of the lower gingiva

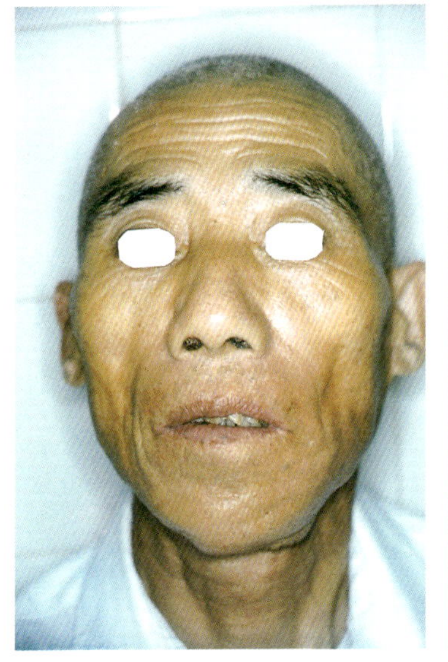

图 523

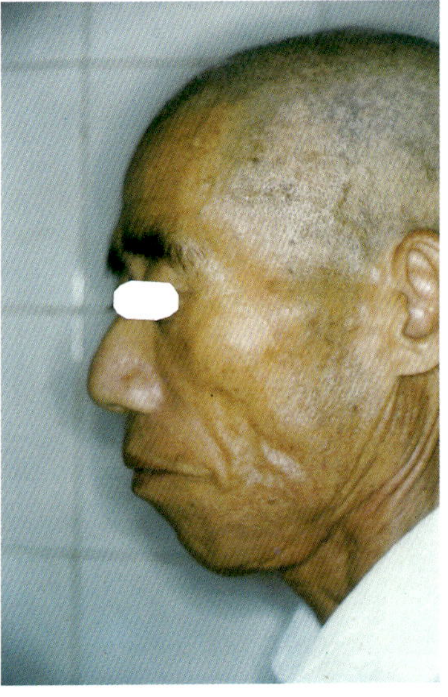

图 524

**图 523，524** 患左下颌磨牙区牙龈癌患者的正面及左侧面观。

正面观见左颌下区淋巴结增大，左侧面观见左颌下区明显膨隆，为左颌下淋巴结转移。

**Fig. 523, 524** Frontal and lateral views of a patient with squamous cell carcinoma of the left mandibular gingiva.

Frontal and lateral views show that left submandibular nodes are involved initially.

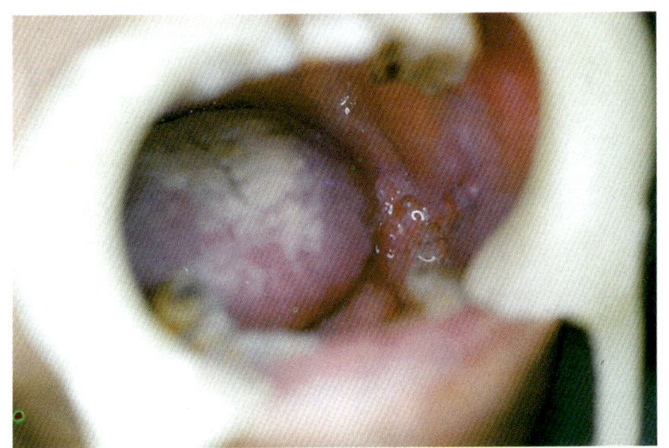

图 525

**图 525** 左下颌磨牙区牙龈癌侵犯颊部及口底。

**Fig. 525** Squamous cell carcinoma of the left mandibular molar area with marked marginal spread onto the floor of the mouth and the buccal mucosa.

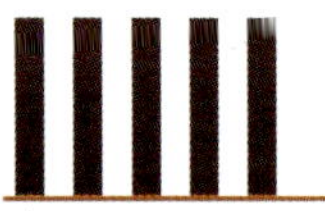



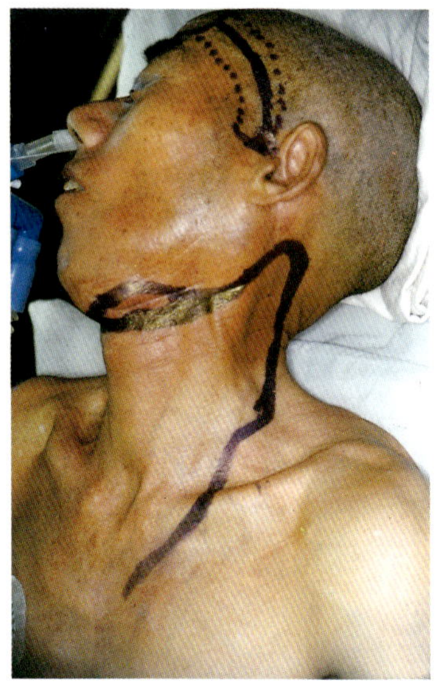

图 526

图 526 岛状额瓣及颌颈联合根治术的切口设计。

Fig. 526 Designed incision lines of the island forehead flap and combined operation of the mandibular resection and radical neck dissection.

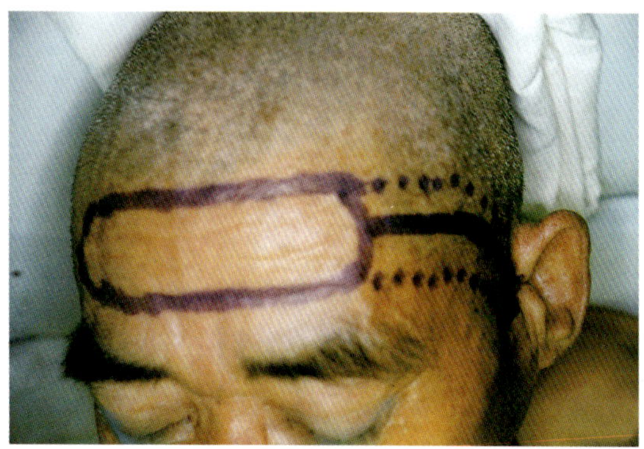

图 527

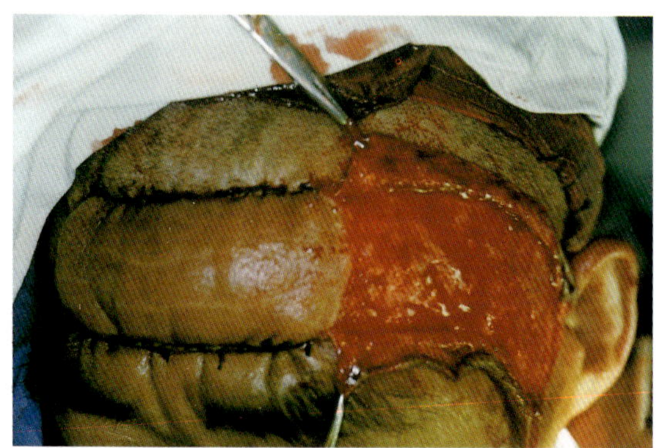

图 528

图 527 按全额岛状瓣设计切口线，其范围为两侧至眼外眦角，上界为发际，下界为眉弓之上，皮下蒂达患侧耳屏前方。

图 528 在皮下蒂的表皮上正中做切口，在毛囊下剥离表皮，注意保护皮下蒂的动、静脉。

Fig. 527 The flap designed is outlined with methylene blue. The island forehead flap used in intraoral reconstruction is laterally based. Its base extends from the lateral border of the eyebrow to the anterior border of the pinna at approximately the level of the zygomatic arch and the flap itself curving across the hairless forehead. Its breadth is generally that of the forehead from eyebrow to hairless and its length is variable but most often extends to the hairline on the opposite temple.

Fig. 528 A incision is made over the derma of the midline of the pedicle, the flap pedicle to the island is developed in the subfollicular plane and the vessels in the flap pedicle should be preserved.

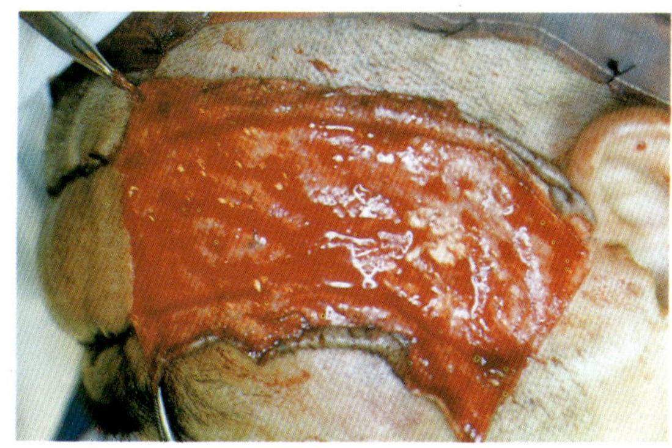

图 529

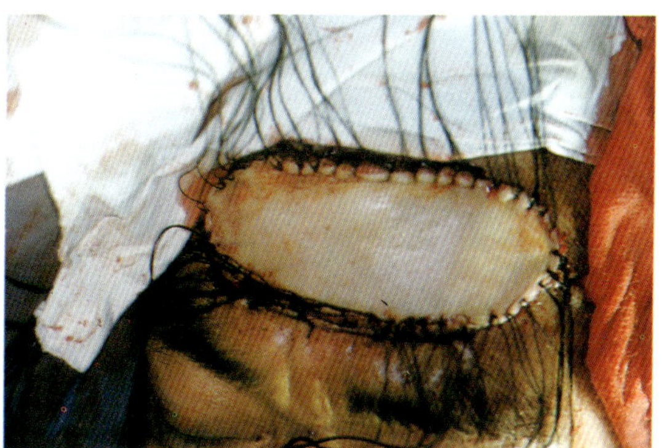

图 530

**图 529** 皮下蒂的表皮被剥离后的情形。
**图 530** 将全厚断层前臂皮片植入供区后加压包扎。

**Fig. 529** Condition after the derma of the flap pedicle has been separated from underlying pedicle.

**Fig. 530** With the whole skin graft it is usual to suture the graft edge to edge with the margins of the defect. The split-skin graft overlaps the defect, the overlap being trimmed at the first dressing.

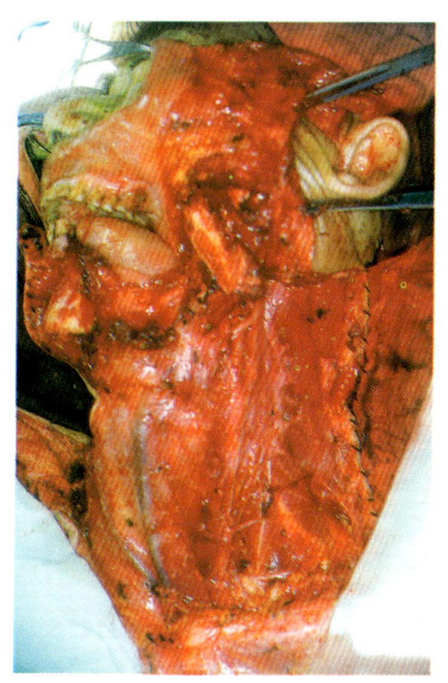

图 531

**图 531** 按常规方法完成颈淋巴清扫术后，在下唇正中将下唇切开，然后沿口内下颌龈颊沟靠颊侧切开龈颊沟粘膜并沿下颌骨体部锐性分离掀起颊瓣，下颌骨体部被暴露。拔除 ⌈2，用线锯将左下颌骨体部锯开，此时下颌骨后段被游离。在肿瘤周围 1.0cm 正常粘膜内做切口，切开口底粘膜及深层肌肉，在下颌角区切断下颌骨后段，包括咬除喙突。

**Fig. 531** The lower lip is split in the midline and a cheek flap is elevated by an incision in the gingivobuccal gutter and dissection along the body of the mandible after radical neck dissection has been completed. The mandible is divided well anterior to the lesion with a Gigli saw. The lateral incisor is extracted before the mandible is divided. Once the segment of mandible has been freed posteriorly, an incision is outlined around the tumor leaving at least 1. 0 cm of normal mucosa on all its edges. The incision is carried through the deep musculature of the floor of the mouth. Posteriorly, the mandible is sectioned at the angle and the coronoid process is removed.

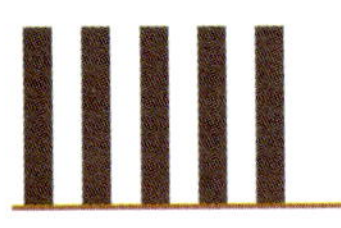



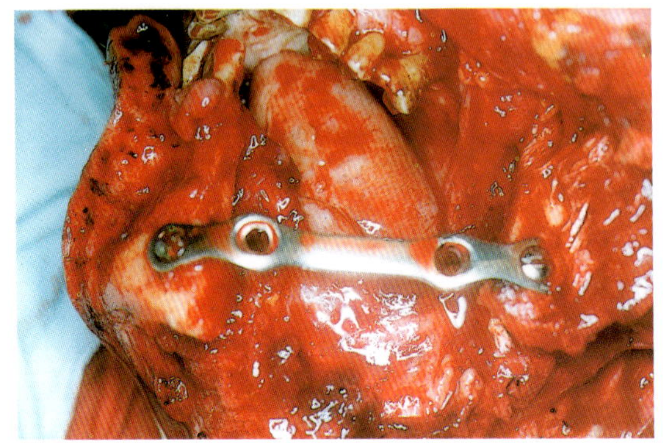

图 532

**图 532** 将岛状额瓣穿入口内后内侧与口底粘膜缝合，前端与剩余下颌骨粘骨膜缝合。在下颌骨切除两端钻孔，将钢板塑型后植入下颌骨缺损区，螺丝坚固内固定。

**Fig. 532** After the island forehead flap has reached the defective area of the oral cavity through a tunnel, the flap is then maneuvered into its bed and sutured to the surrounding mucosa with interrupted suture. A small stainless steel plate is fixed to the bone ends of the left mandibular defective region with screws through holes drilled in the bone.

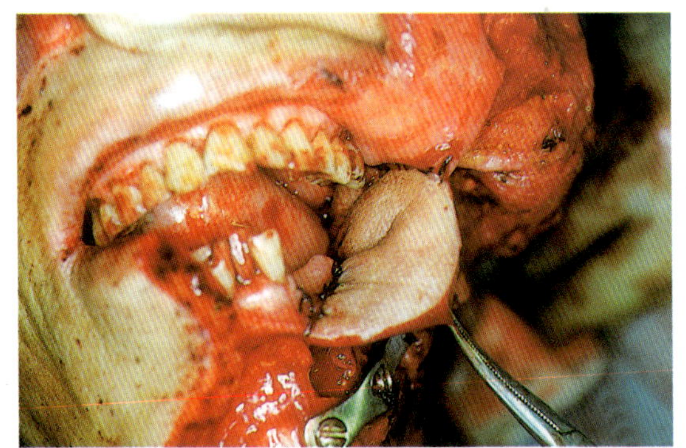

图 533

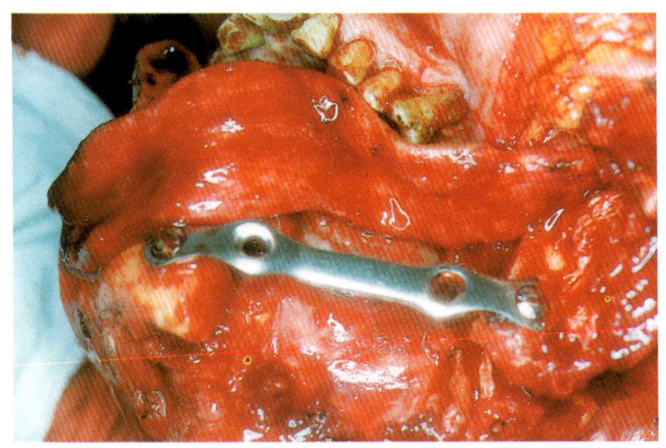

图 534

**图 533, 534** 将颊瓣还回后岛状额瓣的后端与磨牙后三角区切缘粘膜缝合，外侧缘与颊瓣粘膜切缘缝合。

**Fig. 533, 534** The cheek flap is returned in place and closure is completed by approximating the mucosa in the gingivobuccal gutter with fine silk.

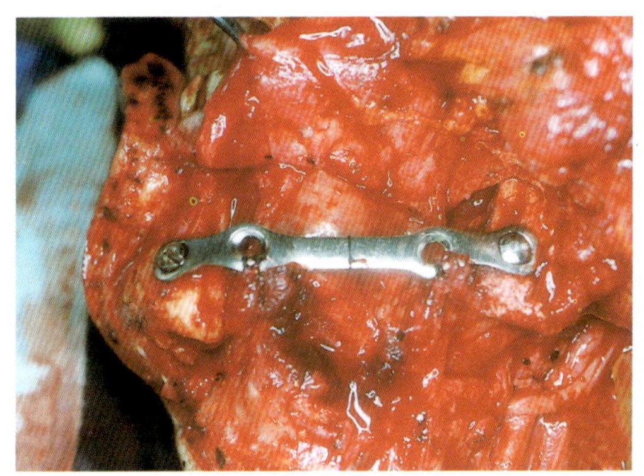

图 535

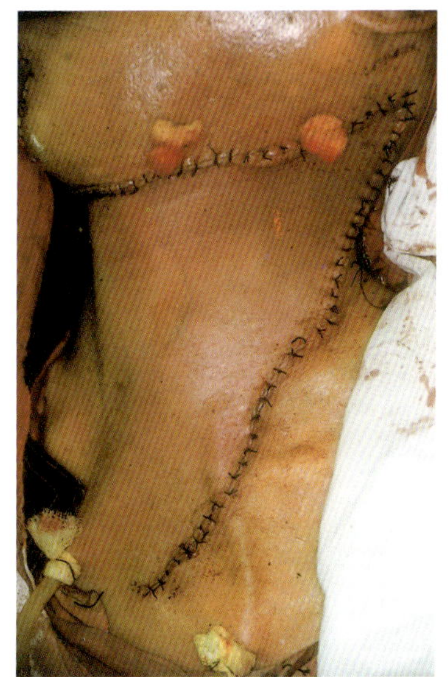

图 536

**图 535，536** 分层缝合下唇及颏部创口，颈部创面用生理盐水冲洗后置橡皮引流管 2 根后分层缝合颈部创缘。局部轻加压包扎。

**Fig. 535, 536** The lip is reconstructed with burried chromic sutures in the orbicularis muscle and fine silk sutures in the skin and mucosa. The neck wound is drained and closed in the usual manner. Pressure dressing is applied.

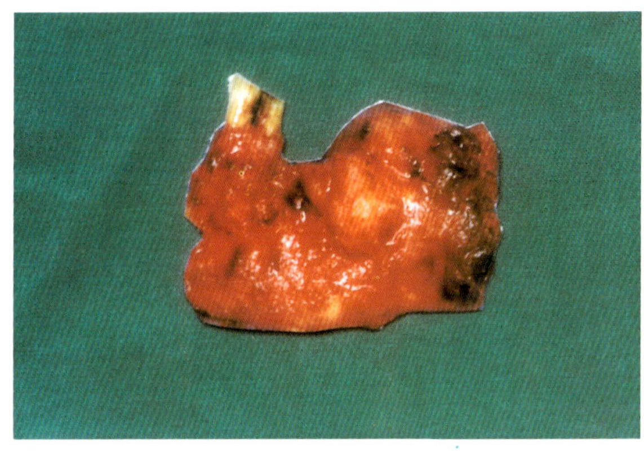

图 537

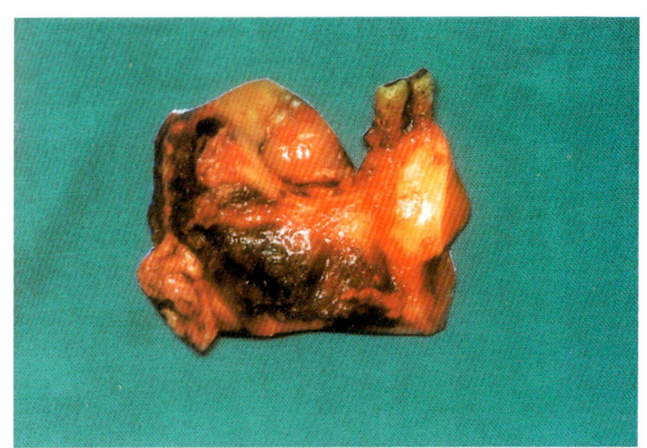

图 538

**图 537, 538** 术后下颌骨肿瘤标本的外、内侧面观。

**Fig. 537, 538** External and internal surface views of specimen of sectioned mandibular segment and the tumor.

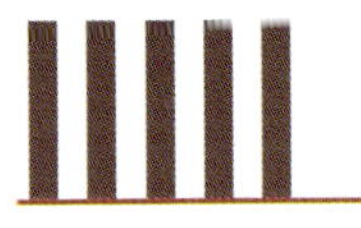


# Ⅷ. 腮腺肿瘤

34. 颊部副腮腺多形性腺瘤口内途径摘除术
35. 腮腺多形性腺瘤腮腺全切除术
36. 腮腺深叶肿瘤的手术切除术
37. 腮腺深叶肿瘤侵犯中颅窝底手术摘除术

# Ⅷ. Parotid gland tumors

34. Excision of pleomorphic adenoma in accessory parotid gland with the oral cavity approch.
35. Total parotidectomy for pleomorphic adenoma in the parotid gland
36. Surgical excision of the tumor in the deep portion of the parotid gland
37. Excision of the tumor in the deep lobe of the parotid gland involving parapharyngeal space and middle cranial base

# 34. 颊部副腮腺多形性腺瘤口内途径摘除术

# 34. Excision of pleomorphic adenoma in accessory parotid gland with the oral cavity approch

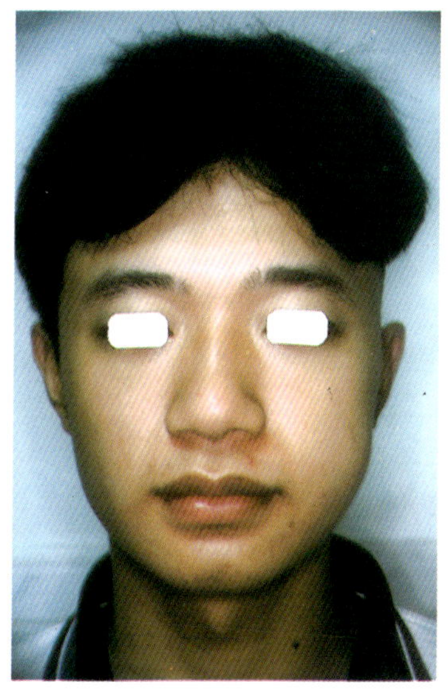

图 539

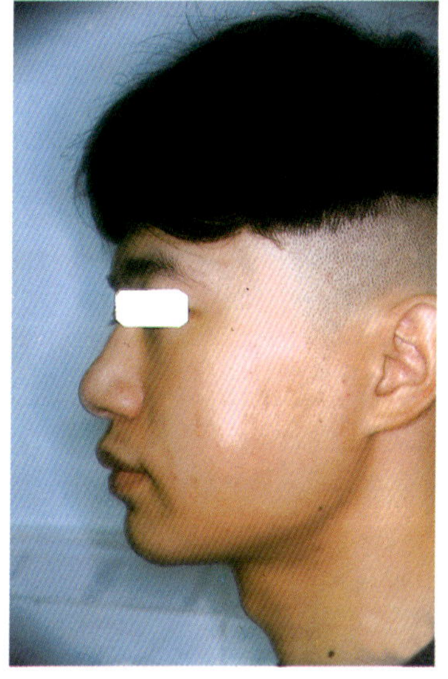

图 540

**图 539, 540** 患左侧副腮腺混合瘤的 18 岁男性患者的正、侧面观。

正面观显示左颊部膨隆，侧面观膨隆位于颊部中心区。

**Fig. 539, 540** Frontal and lateral views of a 18-year-old male patient with pleomorphic adenoma in the accessory parotid gland.

Frontal view shows expansion of the left cheek. Lateral view shows that expansion is located in the central area of the cheek.

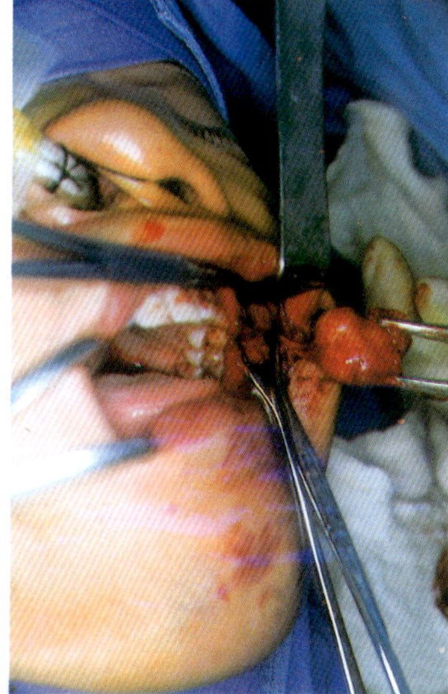

图 541

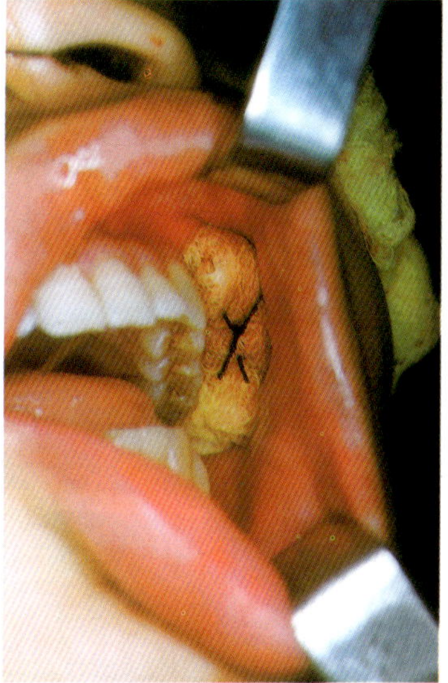

图 542

**图 541** 在左颊粘膜肿瘤之上做一小切口，切口稍大于肿瘤。然后用血管钳分离肿瘤周围组织，用组织钳夹住肿瘤包膜并将其提起，在肿瘤的基部钳夹，将肿瘤完整摘除后结扎肿瘤基部软组织。

**图 542** 将创口对合后间断缝合口腔颊部粘膜。为了防止出血，颊部往往采用“三明治”式缝合。

**Fig. 541** A small incision is made on the mucosa over the tumor of the left cheek. The incision is slight larger about 0. 5 cm than the tumors' diameter. Tumor is dissected with small forceps and the deep tissue of the tumor is clamped, divided and ligated at its attachment to the parotid duct.

**Fig. 542** The mucosa is approximated with interrupted fine silk sutures. To prevent the bleeding, the wound is covered with a small pack of fine-mesh gauze. Fixation is secured by passing sutures of silk around the pack and through the full thickness of the cheek to be tied around an external gauze stent.

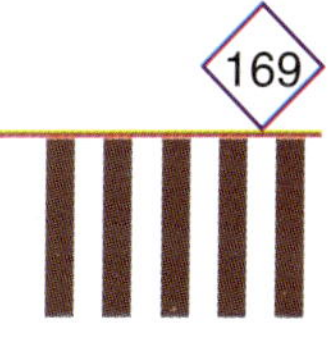

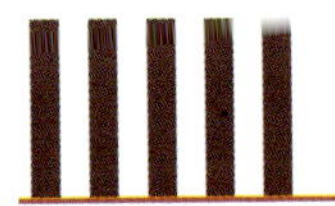



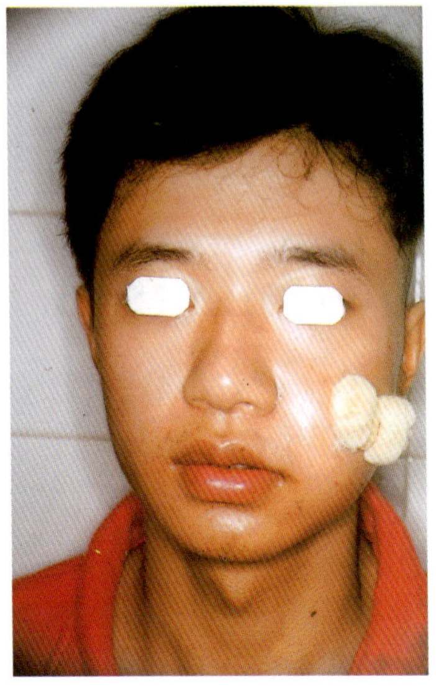

图 543

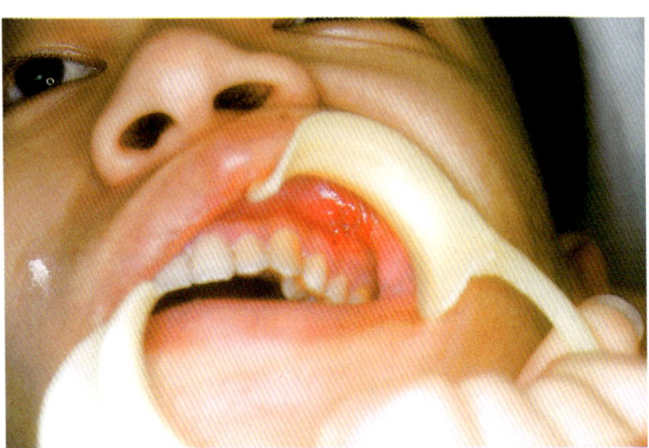

图 544

图 543 “三明治”式缝合后情景。
图 544 术后 10 天创口拆线后情景。

Fig. 543 The condition after fixation is secured by passing sutures of silk around the pack and through the full thickness of the cheek to be tied around an external gauze stent.

Fig. 544 The condition of wound healing 10 days after surgery.

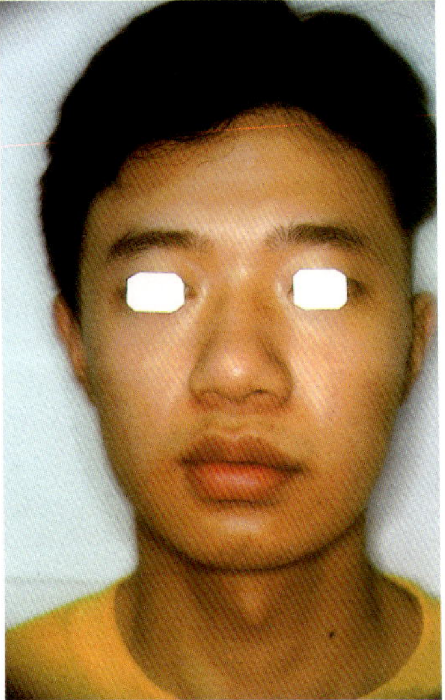

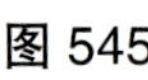

图 545

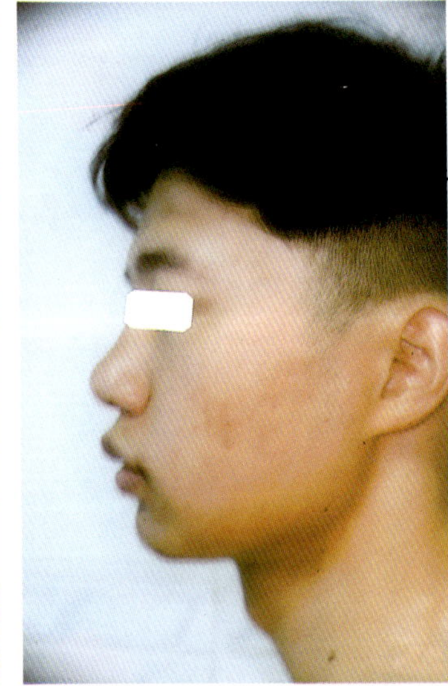

图 546

图 545, 546 术后 10 天患者的正、侧面观。

Fig. 545, 546 Frontal and lateral views of the patient 10 days after operation.

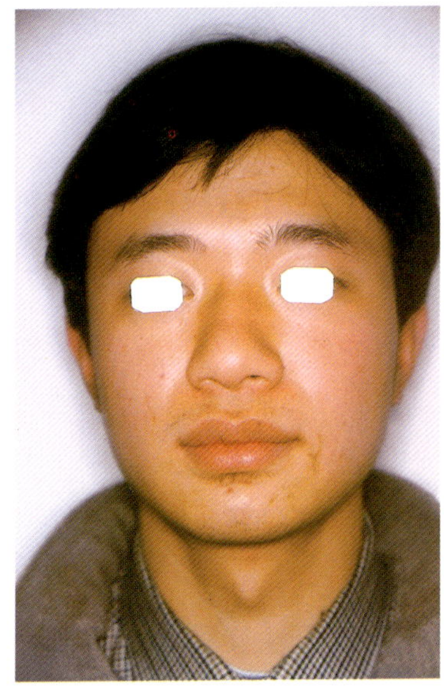

图 547

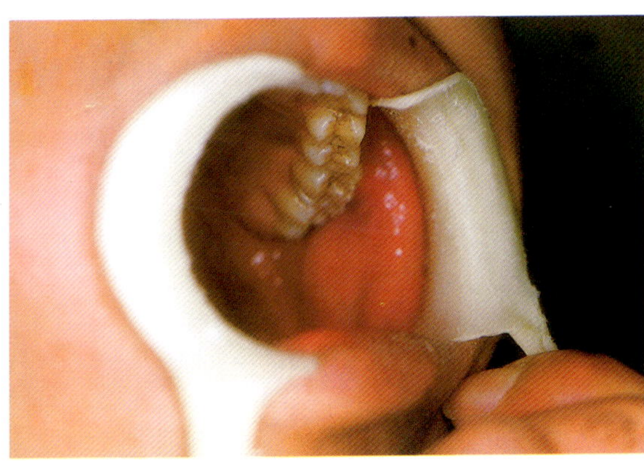

图 548

**图 547** 术后 1 年患者的正面观显示肿瘤无复发。
**图 548** 口内切口愈合良好，对张口无影响。

**Fig. 547** Frontal view of this patient shows no tumor recurrency 1 year after operation.

**Fig. 548** The wound healing is fine and the mouth opening is normal.

# 35. 腮腺多形性腺瘤腮腺全切除术

# 35. Total parotidectomy for pleomorphic adenoma in the parotid gland

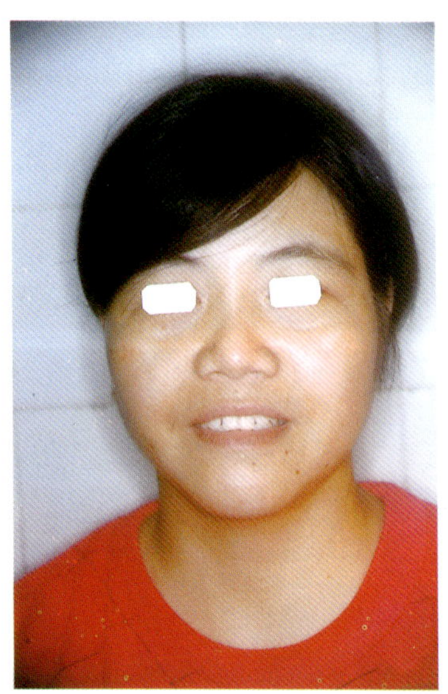

图 549

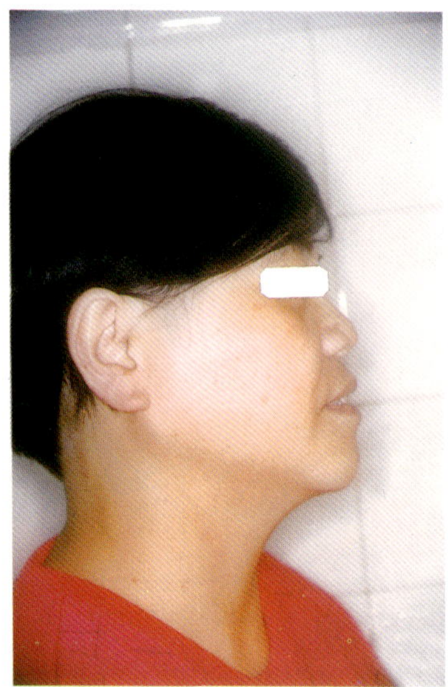

图 550

**图 549, 550** 患右腮腺多形性腺瘤的 53 岁女性患者正、侧面观。

患者 3 年前发现右腮腺区肿块，无痛，增大不明显。检查发现：肿瘤位于腮腺浅叶下极，肿瘤圆形、质硬，位于皮肤之下可活动。

**Fig. 549, 550** Frontal and lateral views of a 53-year-old female patient with pleomorphic adenoma in the right parotid gland.

Tumor grows slowly and painlessly and has been present for 3 years before the patient seeks advice. The examination found that the tumor is located in the lower third of the superficial portion of the gland in front of the lobule of the ear. The tumor is round and rubbery in consistency, painless, and nontender. The tumor lies just beneath the skin and is freely movable whereas it is actually fixed within parotid tissue.

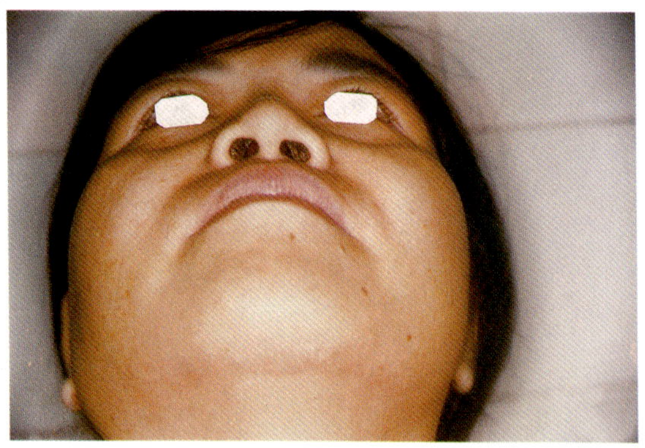

图 551

**图 551** 患者的仰面观显示双侧面部不对称，右侧明显增大。

**Fig. 551** Submental view of the patient shows that both sides of the face are asymmetry and the right face is larger than the left face obviously.

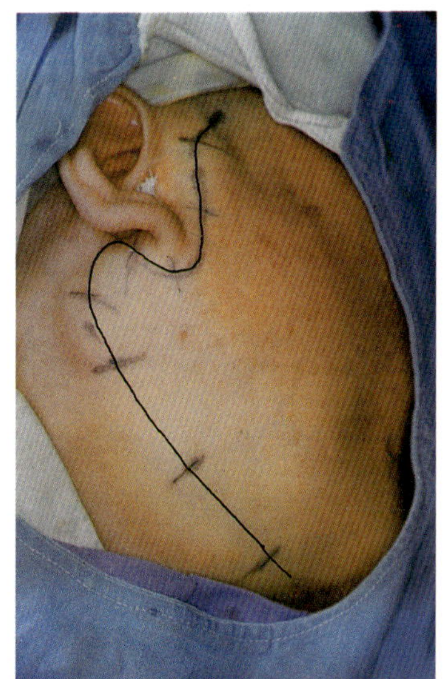

图 552

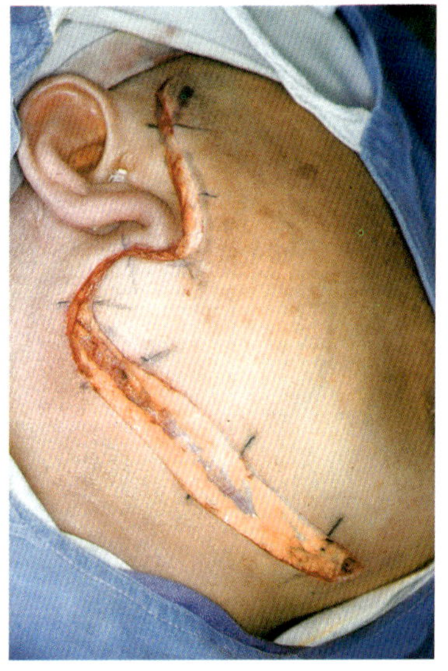

图 553

**图 552, 553** 通常采用"S"形切口，即自耳屏前方直向下行，绕耳垂下方至颞乳突尖，再转向下经颌后区，在下颌角下方 1.5～2cm 处转向前行，止于舌骨平面，切开皮肤及皮下组织与颈阔肌。

**Fig. 552, 553** A S-shaped incision is made starting just anterior to the tragus of the ear, passing down in front of the lobule, thence curving posteriorly below the lobule and passing downward and anteriorly along the angle of the mandible. This permits the elevation of a skin flap anteriorly to expose the parotid fascia overlying nearly the entire parotid gland and posteriorly to expose the mastoid tip and the sternomastoid muscle. If the tumor lies further anteriorly in the gland or in an accessory parotid gland, the surgeon may use a horizontal extension into the temporal hairline.

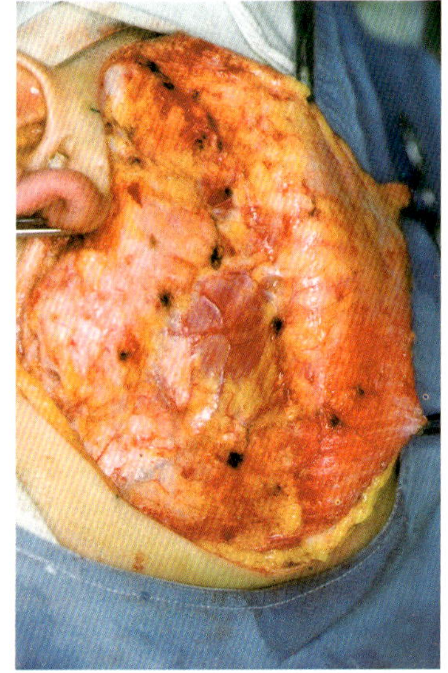

图 554

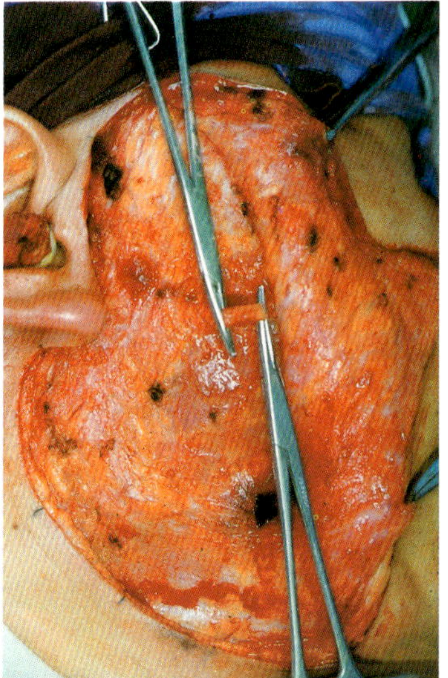

图 555

**图 554** 掀起肌皮瓣，暴露整个腮腺浅叶的表面及颈深筋膜浅层。在颈部，皮瓣的分离在颈阔肌深面进行。

**图 555** 位于腮腺前缘中部稍上找到腮腺导管将其分离、切断、结扎。

**Fig. 554** The skin flap is now elevated, exposing the entire superficial surface of the gland and the thin parotid fascia that on the neck extends through the platysma. Strong upward traction on the skin and firm downward pressure against the gland aids in separating these tissues by sharp dissection.

**Fig. 555** The parotid duct at the central portion of the anterior border of the parotid gland is seeked, ligated and divided.

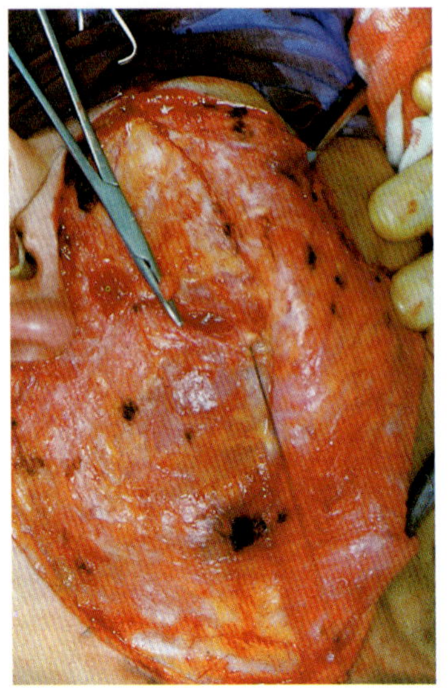
图 556

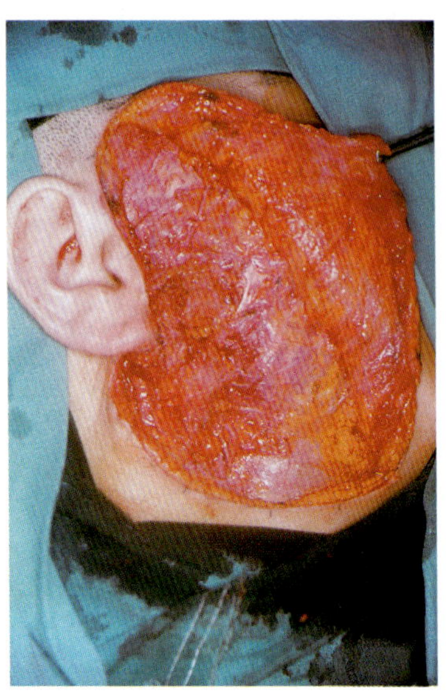
图 557

**图 556** 腮腺导管被结扎后，暴露胸锁乳突肌的上 1/3 部分和横跨其上进入腮腺的耳大神经，并将耳大神经切断。

**图 557** 掀起腮腺的下极，此时可见颈外静脉并沿其向上进入腮腺浅叶实质中。面神经的颈支位于面后神经的前支之外。发现颈支之后，沿其向后达其面神经的下颌颈干，最后达面神经的主干。

**Fig. 556** After parotid duct is ligated, the upper third of the sternocleidomastoid muscle is exposed and the great auricular nerve crossing it and entering the parotid gland is identified and divided.

**Fig. 557** The lower pole of the parotid gland is elevated. The external jugular vein is identified and traced upward into the substance of the superficial portion. The cervical branch of the facial nerve is found lying on the anterior division of the posterior facial vein. After the cervical branch is identified, it is traced back to the cervical-mandibular division and then to the main trunk of the facial nerve.

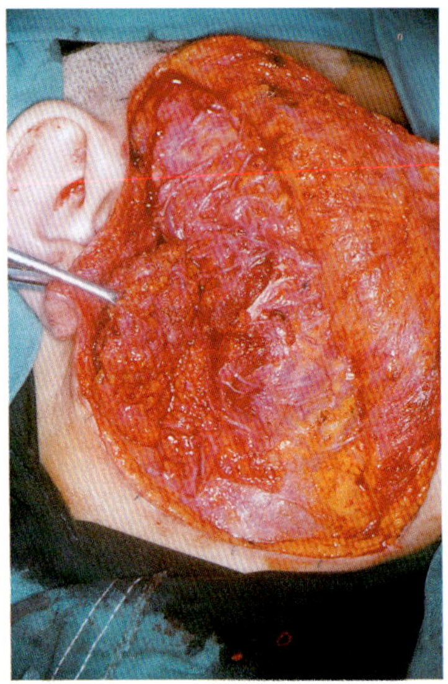
图 558

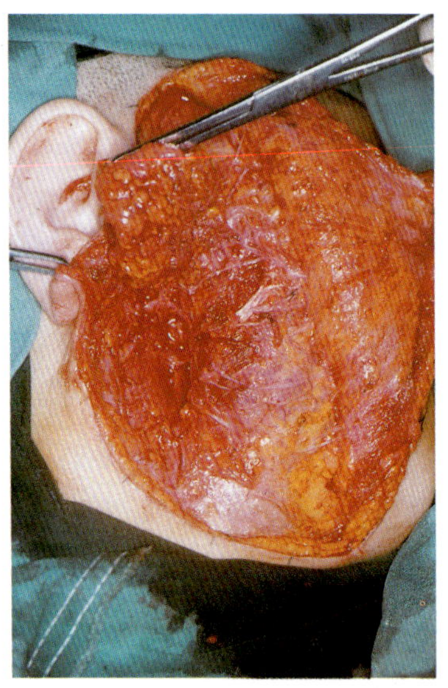
图 559

**图 558** 进一步暴露面神经的下颌颈干，向后追逆达面神经的主干，在此，也可见到面神经的颧颞干。

**图 559** 从耳软骨和颞骨的鼓板分离腮腺组织，整个过程中始终保持面神经的颧颞干于手术野中。沿该干向上追踪并保护其周围支。切除含有肿瘤的腮腺浅叶。

**Fig. 558** Further exposure of the cervical-mandibular division of the facial nerve. It is traced backward to the main trunk where the important temporozygomatic division is identified.

**Fig. 559** The parotid tissue is dissected from the cartilage of the ear and the tympanic plate of the temporal bone, keeping the temporozygomatic division of the facial nerve in view at all times. The division is traced upward and its peripheral branches are protected and preserved as the parotid tissue is divided. The superficial portion of the parotid gland containing the tumor is now removed.

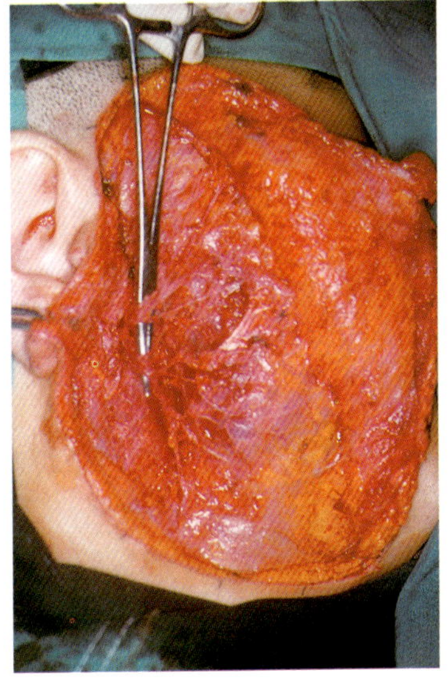

图 560

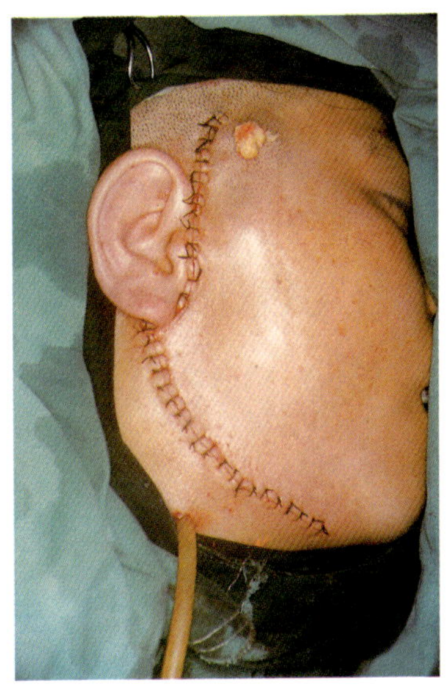

图 561

**图 560** 通过向上向外牵开面神经并在其深面解剖腮腺组织，在完全不损伤面神经的情况下去除剩余的腮腺深叶组织。可以通过牵开下颌角和下颌升支使腮腺深叶获得更好的暴露。在分离腮腺深叶时会碰到颈外动脉和它的分支，颌内和颞浅动脉。可以结扎颞浅动脉，偶尔也可结扎颌内动脉。颈内动脉和颈内静脉仅靠腮腺深叶的深面但通常不被暴露。

**图 561** 用细羊肠线缝合颈部的颈阔肌和面部的浅筋膜，用细丝线间断缝合皮肤。将一橡皮管放入腮腺床，并通过创口的下角穿出后接负压引流。

**Fig. 560** The remaining deep portion of the parotid can be removed without injury to the facial nerve by retracting the nerve upward and outward and dissecting the parotid tissue from beneath it. Adequate exposure is obtained by retracting the angle and ramus of the mandible. The external carotid artery and its terminal branches, the internal maxillary and superficial temporal arteries, are encountered. The superficial temporal artery is ligated and occasionally it is necessary to ligate the internal maxillary artery. The internal jugular vein and internal carotid artery are close to the deep portion of the gland but are usually not exposed.

**Fig. 561** The wound is closed, using fine catgut sutures for the platysma in the neck and superficial fascia on the face and interrupted silk for the skin. A catheler is placed in the parotid bed and brought out through the inferior angle of the wound.

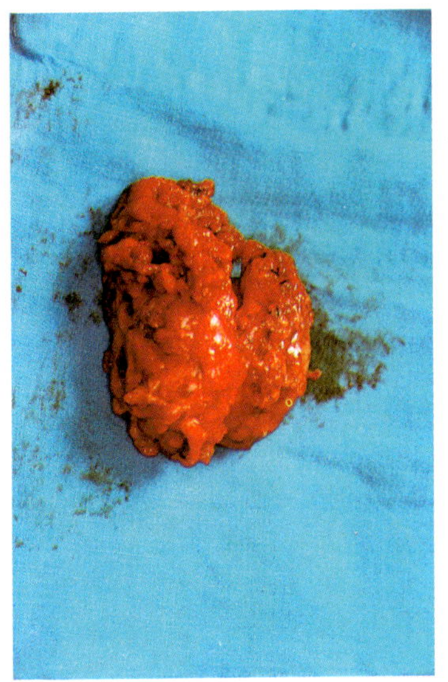

图 562

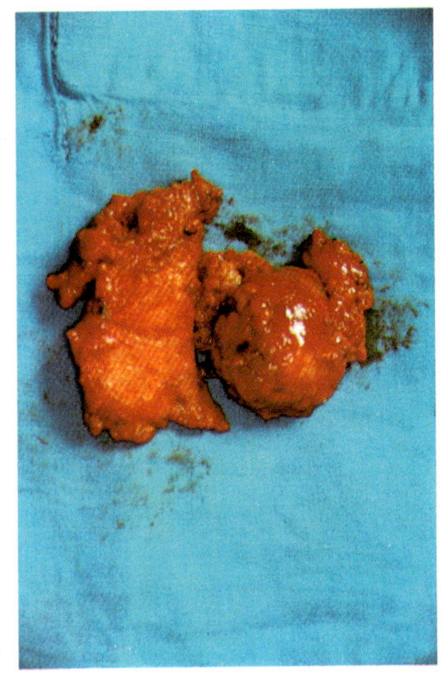

图 563

**图 562, 563** 手术标本的外、内面观。

**Fig. 562, 563** External and internal views of operative specimen.

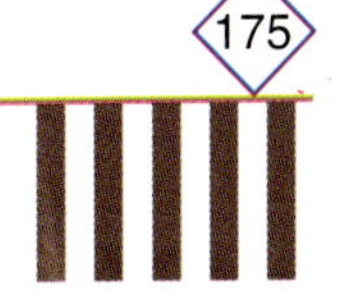

# 36. 腮腺深叶肿瘤的手术切除术

# 36. Surgical excision of the tumor in the deep portion of the parotid gland

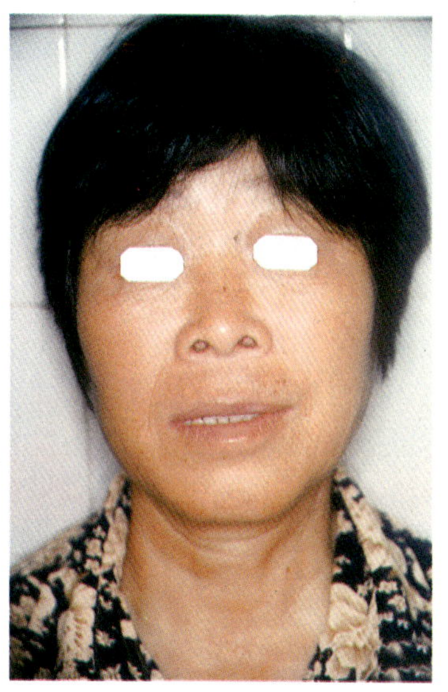
图 564

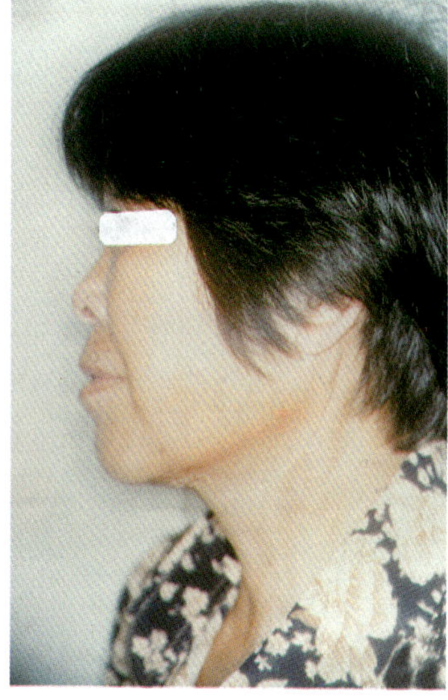
图 565

**图 564, 565** 患左腮腺深叶多形性腺瘤的一44岁女性患者正、侧面观。

发生在腮腺深叶的肿瘤常常向口咽部膨隆。通常在行咽部检查时见软腭向中线移位，甚至将腭垂推向对侧。

**Fig. 564, 565** Frontal and lateral views of a 44-year-old female patient with pleomorphic adenoma tumor in the deep portion of left parotid gland.

Retromandibular tumors arising from the deep portion of the parotid gland frequently extend into the oral pharynx. Examination of the pharynx show the tumor extending to the midline of the soft palate and at times even further displacing the uvula to the opposite side.

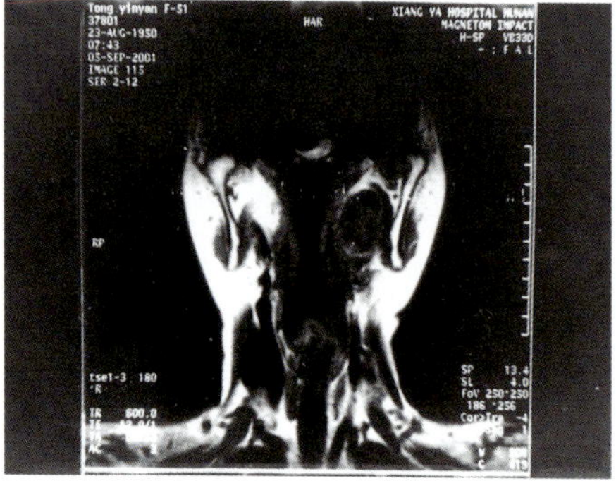
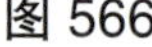
图 566

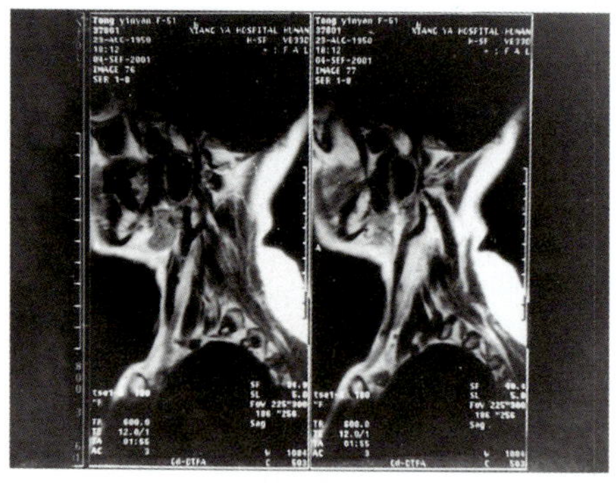
图 567

**图 566** 冠状面 MRI 片显示腮腺深叶的肿瘤。
**图 567** 矢状面 MRI 片显示腮腺深叶肿瘤与周围组织的关系。

**Fig. 566** Magnetic resonance image in coronal plane shows recurrent tumor in deep lobe of parotid gland.
**Fig. 567** Magnetic resonance image in seggital plane shows relationship around tumor tissues.

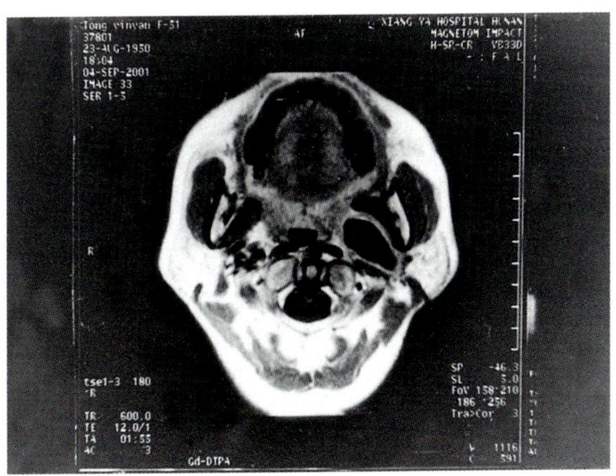


图 568

**图 568** 横断面 MRI 片示腮腺深叶肿瘤与组织的关系。

**Fig. 568** Magnetic resonance image shows extensive lateral pharyngeal involvement.

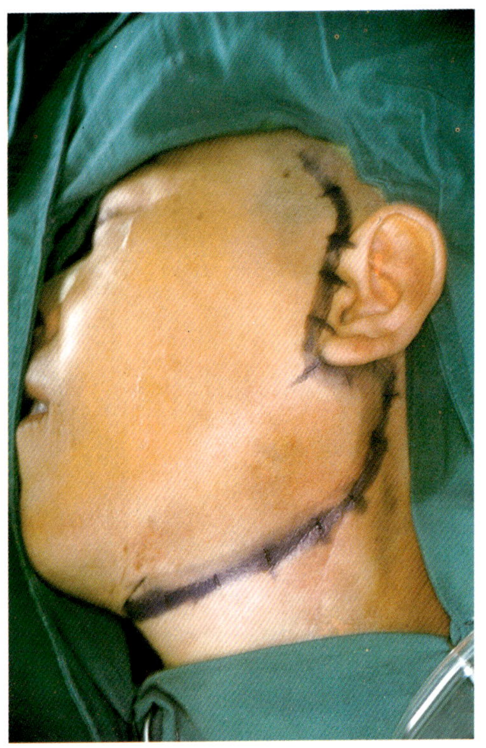

图 569

**图 569** 画出全腮腺摘除切口线。

**Fig. 569** The incision line of the parotidectomy is marked out with the methylene blue.

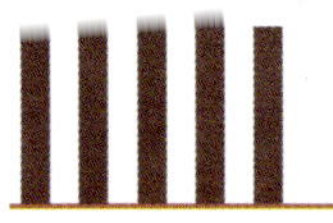



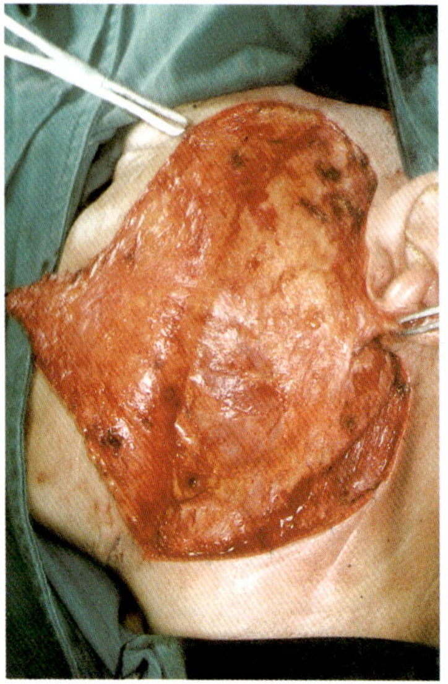

图 570

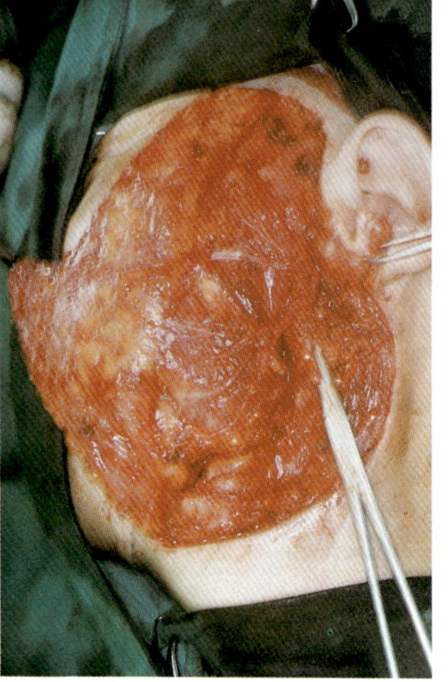

图 571

**图 570** 切除腮腺深叶肿瘤的手术按 35 节的叙述进行。在本图中,由面神经分支开始达其总干解剖面神经将腮腺浅叶摘除。

**图 571** 此时,可见腮腺深叶的肿瘤位于面神经的深面。将面神经与其下的肿瘤轻轻的分开,用组织钳抓住腮腺深叶及肿瘤向外向下牵引,可将下颌升支向前向外牵拉以增大颌后间隙,助手用手指头放入咽部向下向外施力使肿瘤向外脱出。

**Fig. 570** The operation for the removal of the deep tumor of the parotid gland follows exactly the steps described for parotidectomy. In this figure the superficial portion of the parotid gland is elevated from branches of the facial nerve to the main trunk.

**Fig. 571** The tumor is seen lying deep to the facial nerve and is pushing its main trunk and branches outward. The facial nerve and its branches are freed from the tumor by gentle dissection and retracted upward. The deep portion of the parotid gland and the tumor are now grasped by an Alis clamp and pulled outward and downward. The space between the ramus of the mandible and the mastoid process is widened by forward and outward retraction of the mandible. An assistant's finger placed in the pharynx and making downward and outward pressure aids in the delivery of the mass.

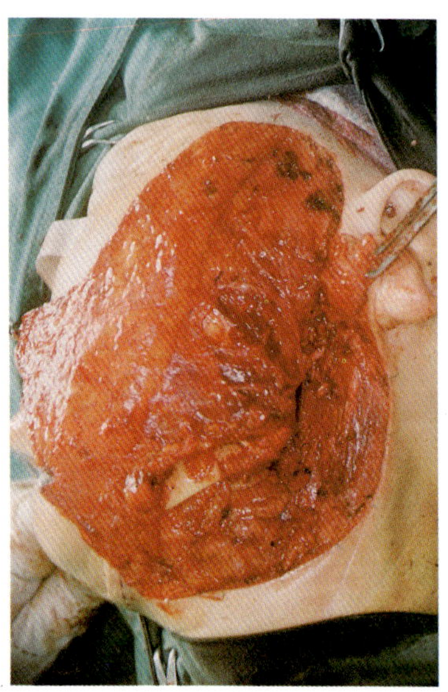

图 572

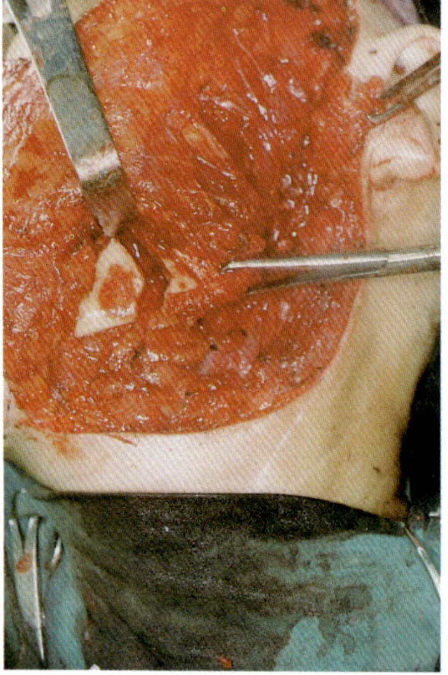

图 573

**图 572** 如不能将肿瘤完整摘除的话,可在下颌体嚼肌前缘梯形截断下颌骨。

**图 573** 下颌体部被截断之后。

**Fig. 572** If the deep portion of the parotid gland and tumor can not be removed, the body of the mandible must be divided near the masseter muscle insertion on the mandible with a Gigli saw.

**Fig. 573** The condition after the body of the mandible has been divided.

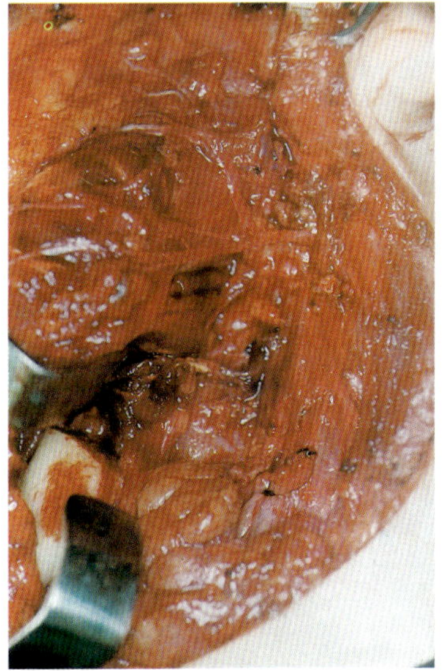

图 574

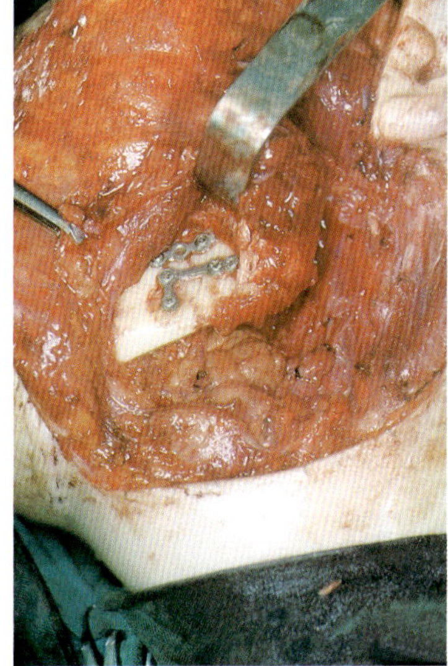

图 575

**图 574** 将下颌升支向上向前牵拉以暴露腮腺深叶及肿瘤，将腮腺与咽侧壁粘膜及翼内肌分离后将其摘除。此时可见到颌内动脉，在手术中应注意保护。有时也可将其结扎、切断，但并不是常规。

**图 575** 在下颌骨断端两端钻孔，用微型钛板坚固内固定。

**Fig. 574** The ramus of the mandible is retracted upward and forward for the exposure of the deep portion of the parotid gland and the tumor. The tumor is then separated from the pharyngeal mucosa to pterygoid muscles and removed. The internal maxillary artery is visualized and protected during this procedure. At times it is advisable to ligate and divide this artery, but this is not routinely necessary.

**Fig. 575** The mandible is fixed with small plates.

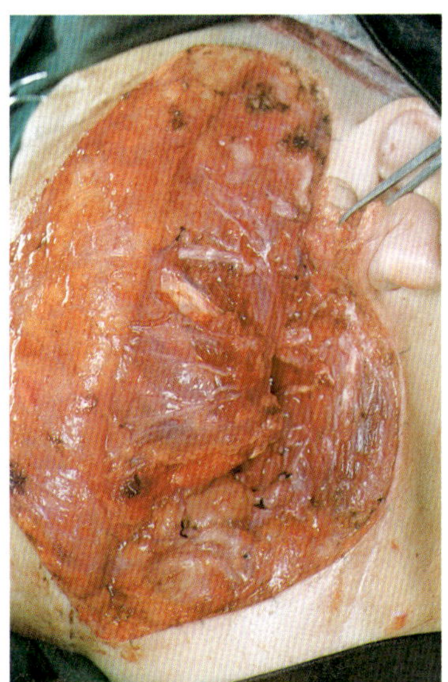

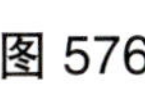

图 576

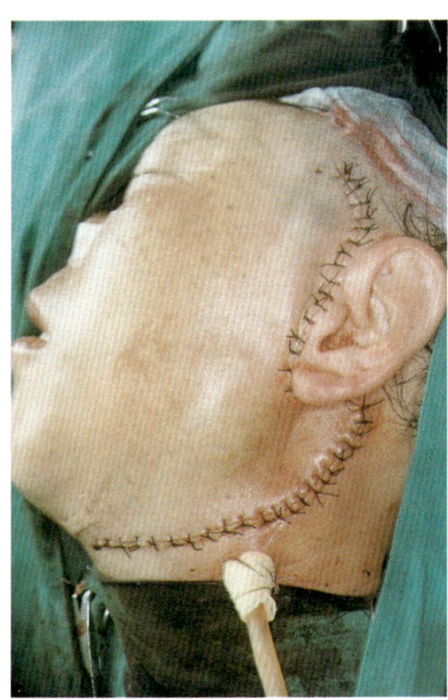

图 577

**图 576** 生理盐水冲洗创面后，缝合切开的骨膜，放引流管一根后还回颊瓣，缝合颈阔肌、皮下及皮肤。

**图 577** 缝合后情景。

**Fig. 576** The entire wound is inspected for hemostasis after which it is irrigated with saline solution. One Penrose drains are placed in the wound, one directed posteriorly. The drains may be brought out through the lower angle of the wound or through a stab wound in the lateral skin flap. The flaps are then approximated with buried sutures in the platysma and interrupted sutures of fine silk in the skin. A bulky pressure dressing is applied to the neck. Suction catheters may be used in place of Penrose drains.

**Fig. 577** The condition after suture.

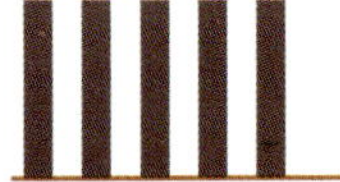



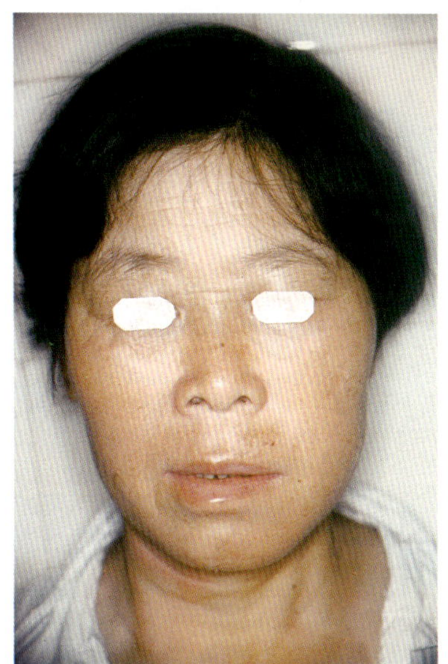

图 578

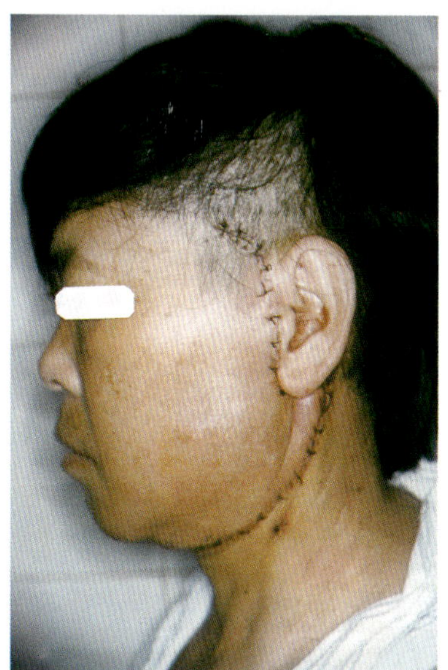

图 579

图 578, 579 术后 7 天正、侧面观。

Fig. 578, 579 Frontal and lateral views 7 days after operation.

# 37. 腮腺深叶肿瘤侵犯中颅窝底手术摘除术

## 37. Excision of the tumor in the deep lobe of the parotid gland involving parapharyngeal space and middle cranial base

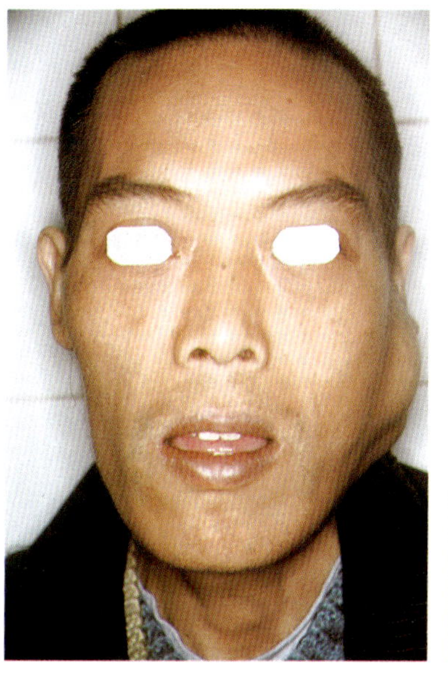

图 580

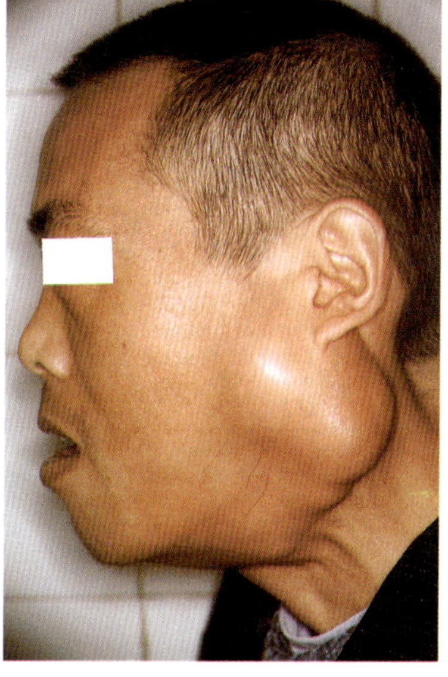

图 581

**图 580, 581** 患左颞下及咽旁间隙巨大肿瘤 48 岁男性患者的正面及侧面观。

该患者的最初临床表现主要集中在腮腺、下颌及咽旁间隙逐渐增大的肿瘤。肿块向内生长,使呼吸道变窄而需要开口呼吸。

**Fig. 580, 581** Frontal and lateral views of a 48-year-old male patient with giant tumor of the infratemporal fossa and parapharyngeal space.

The primary clinical finding in this patient is a growing mass centered principally in the parotid, mandibular region and parapharyngeal space. The growth is mainly medial in the patient causing the airway is so narrow that is necessary to open his mouth for respiration.

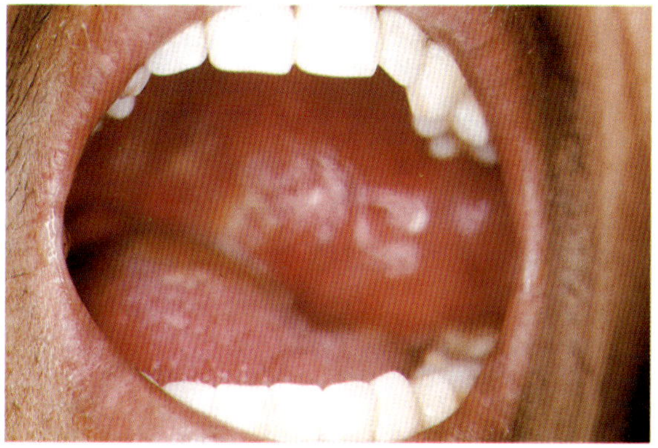

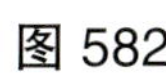

图 582

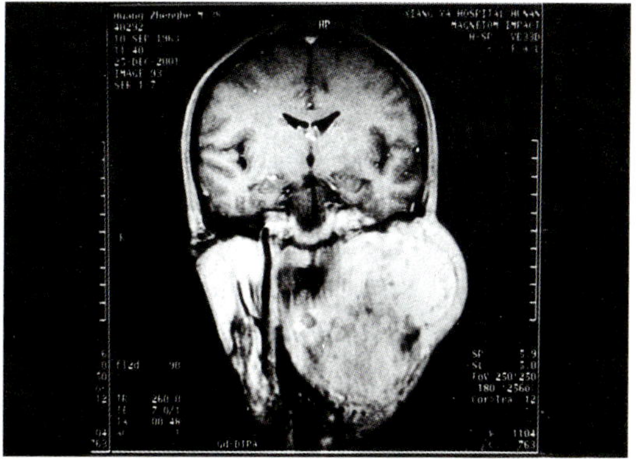

图 583

**图 582, 583** 肿瘤通过咽后间隙跨越中线,侵犯对侧的咽后间隙。

**Fig. 582, 583** The mass crossed the midline through the retropharyngeal space, invading the contralateral retropharyngeal space.

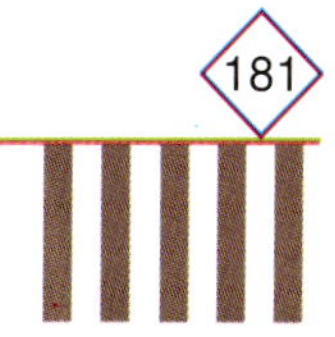

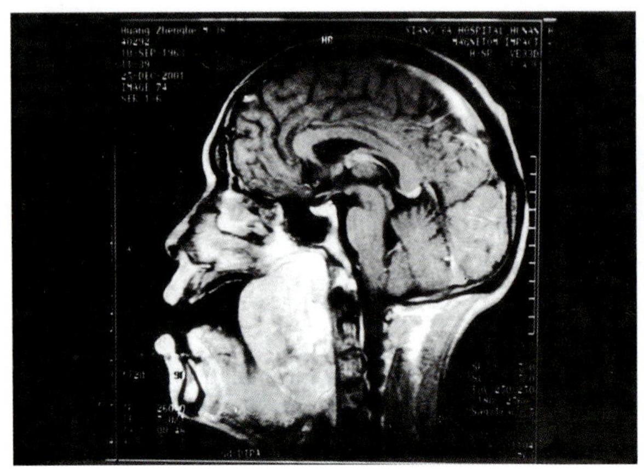

图 584

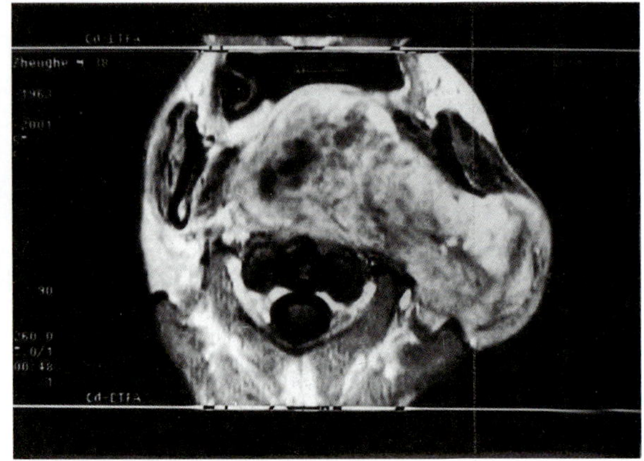

图 585

**图 584, 585** 矢状和轴性 MRI 扫描显示肿瘤侵及面部、颞下窝、咽旁间隙和中颅窝底。

Fig. 584, 585 Sagittal and axial MRI scans show that tumor invades the face, infratemporal fossa, parapharyngeal space and middle cranial base.

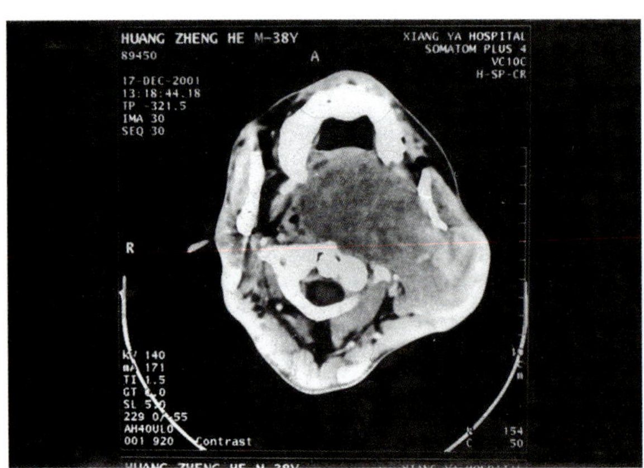


图 586

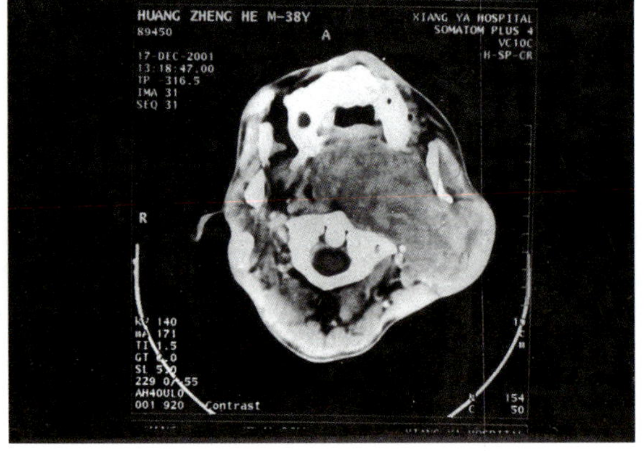


图 587

**图 586, 587** 不同层面轴性平扫显示肿瘤的大小与范围。

Fig. 586, 587 Different axial MRI scan shows the size and extent of the tumor.

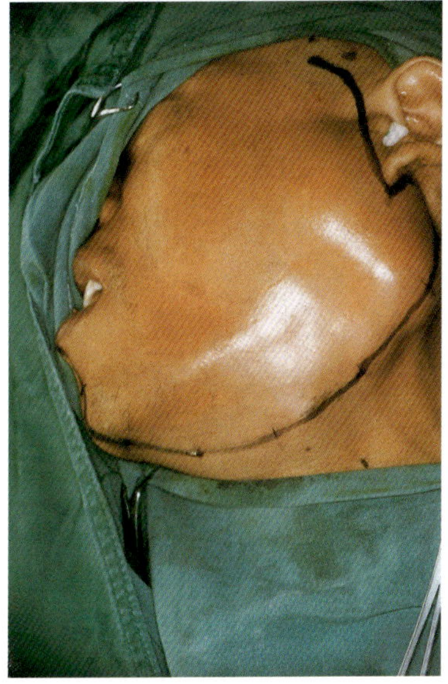

图 588

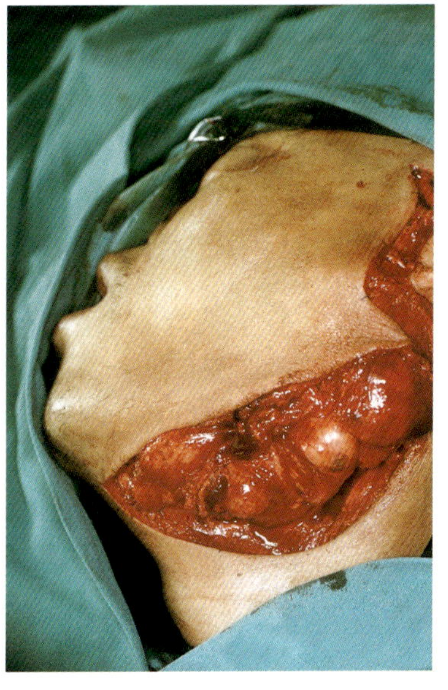

图 589

**图 588** 按腮腺深叶及咽旁间隙肿瘤手术进路设计切口线，用美蓝画出切口线，切口从耳屏前开始向下，绕耳垂下方至颞乳突尖，再转向下经颌后区，在下颌角下方 2cm 处转向前行达颏下区，然后向上达下唇红唇缘。

**图 589** 按切口线切开皮肤、皮下组织及颈阔肌，由后向前翻起肌皮瓣，暴露整个腮腺浅叶的表面及颈深筋膜浅层。在颈部，皮瓣的分离在颈阔肌深面进行。

**Fig. 588** Incision design is made to surgical approach to deep lobar tumor of the parotid gland and tumor of parapharyngeal space. A incision design is made starting just anterior to the tragus of the ear, passing down in front of the lobule, then curving posteriorly below the lobule and passing downward and anteriorly along the angle of the mandible to submental region, then a lip-splitting incision line can be made vertically through the midline.

**Fig. 589** According to designed incision line, skin, subcutaneous tissue and platysma are incised. This permits the elevation of a skin flap anteriorly to expose the parotid fascia overlying nearly the entire parotid gland and posteriorly to expose the mastoid tip and the sternomastoid muscle. The skin flap is now elevated, exposing the entire superficial surface of the gland and the thin parotid fascia that on the neck extends through the platysma.

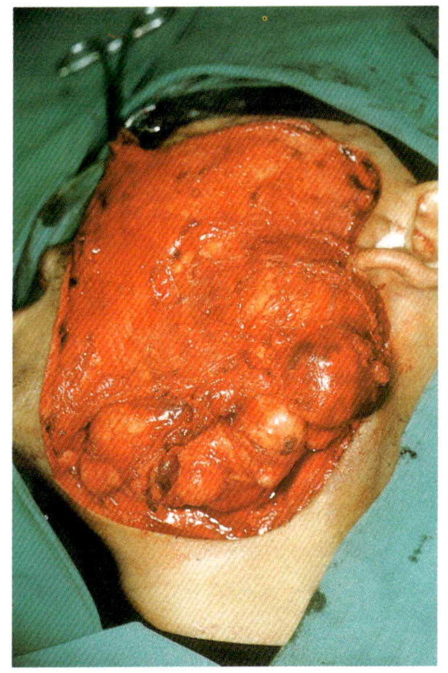

图 590

图 591

**图 590** 按腮腺摘除术的操作步骤摘除腮腺浅叶，此时，肿瘤的外表面、嚼肌及面神经分支清晰可见。

**图 591** 牵开下颌骨内侧面，将肿瘤与下颌骨内侧面分开。

**Fig. 590** According to surgical steps of parotidectomy, the superficial lobules of the parotid gland is excised. During this time, the superficial surface of the tumor, masster muscle and branches of the facial nerve may clearly be seen.

**Fig. 591** The tumor is seen lying deep to the facial nerve and the mandible. The facial nerve and its branches and internal surface of mandible are freed from the by gentle dissection and retracted upward.



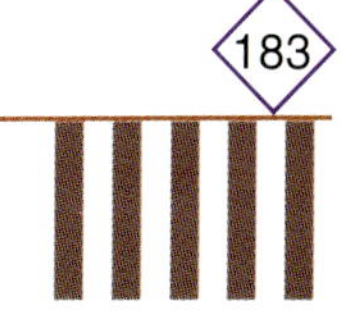

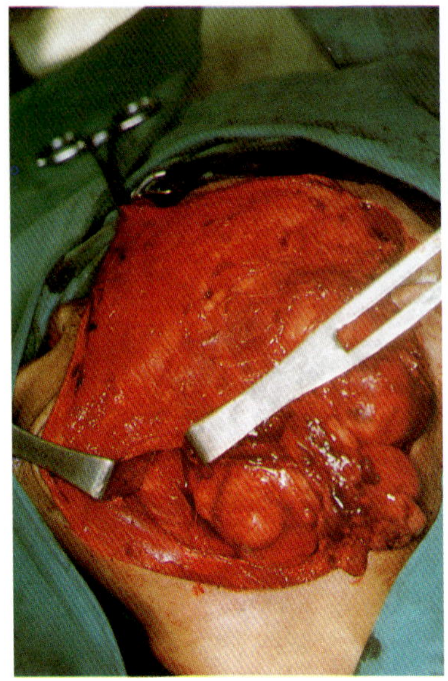
图 592

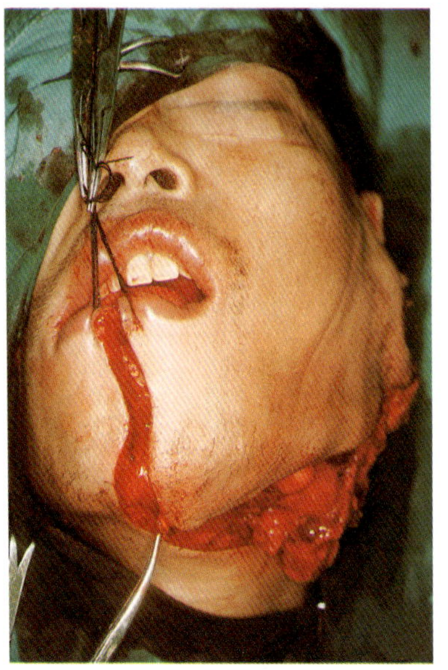
图 593

**图 592，593** 肿瘤的外表面被完全暴露之后，从颏下至下唇红唇缘切开下唇及颏部软组织。

**Fig. 592, 593** After the superficial surface of the tumor is completely exposed, the lip-splitting incision can be made vertically through the midline.

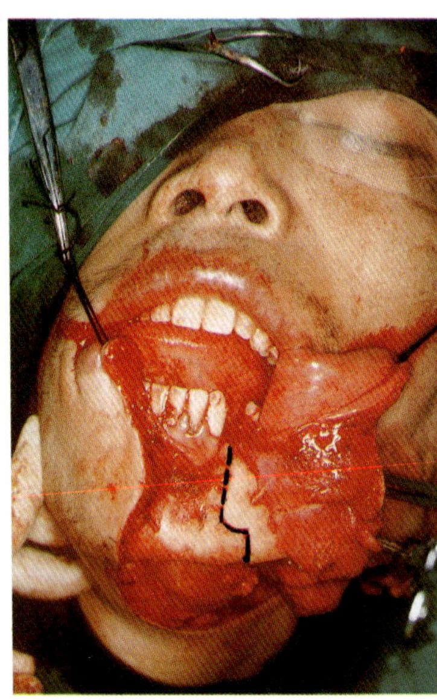
图 594

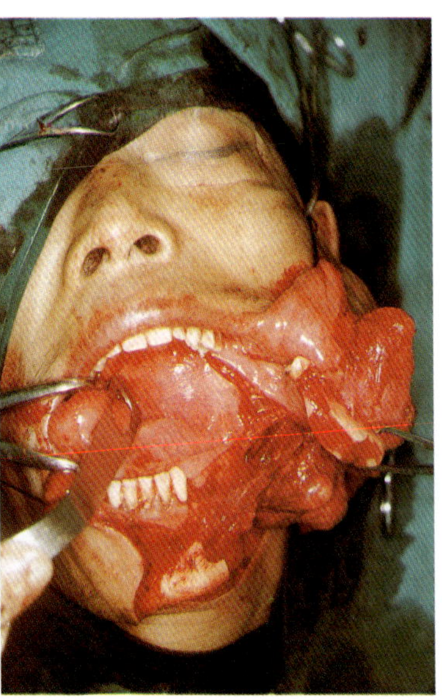
图 595

**图 594** 在下唇被切开之后，在颏孔前将骨膜切开。在保留颏神经不被损伤的情况下向前向后将骨膜掀起。此时，决定下颌骨截骨的位置。截骨的方向可以采用梯形或垂直性截骨，由于有了微型钛板，直线截骨之后，仍可使术后的下颌骨固定稳定。

**图 595** 在颏孔前截开下颌骨。在此时，在口底粘膜上由前向后达咽前柱切开粘膜，切开下颌舌骨肌和二腹肌。为了对颞下窝获得足够的视野，可以将翼外肌切断。注意：在行口底粘膜切口时，应在颌下腺导管外侧切开，以保持导管的完整性。

**Fig. 594** The lip-splitting incision is completed and the mandibular periosteum is incised anterior to the mental foramen. The periosteum is elevated anteriorly and posteriorly, ensuring that the mental nerve is not compromised. A decision now has to be made as to the optimal site and configuration of the osteotomy. The mandibulotomy may be performed in a stair-step or notched fashion to increase postoperative stability. However, with newer plating techniques, a straight vertical midline osteotomy probably yields comparable stability.

**Fig. 595** The optimal site for the osteotomy is anterior to the mental foramen. At this stage, a mucosal incision is made in the lateral floor of the mouth extending posteriorly toward the anterior tonsillar pillar. The mandible is now swung laterally by dividing the mylohyoid and digastric muscles. The mucosal incision is then progressively extended along the anterior pillar until adequate exposure is obtained. The pterygoid muscles may need to be divided to obtain adequate visualization of the infratemporal fossa. Note that the floor of mouth mucosal incision is lateral to the submandibular duct and gland which are kept intact.

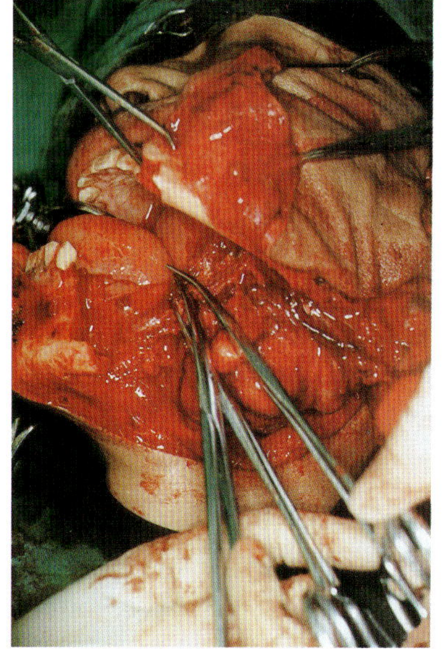
图 596

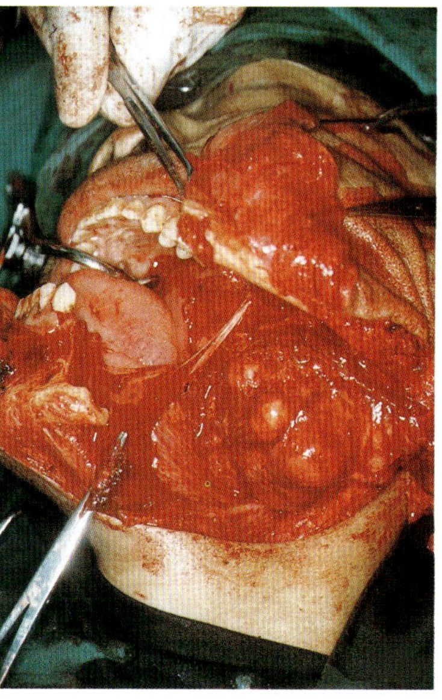
图 597

**图 596, 597** 当将下颌骨被牵开后，咽旁间隙出现在手术野中。在茎突基部将其截断并移去。向上追踪颈内动脉、颈内静脉、迷走神经、副神经、舌下神经及舌咽神经达颅底。

当继续向上解剖的时候，咽与咽鼓管软骨、腭帆提肌和腭帆张肌连为一体。假若必要的话，这些结构可以被切断，必须保护颈内动脉。将咽向内侧旋转，以暴露颅底的中室。

**Fig. 596, 597** As the mandible is retracted, the parapharyngeal space comes into view. The styloid process is fractured at its base and removed. The internal carotid artery, internal jugular vein and vagus, spinal accessory, hypoglossal, and glossopharyngeal nerves are then traced superiorly to the skull base.

As the dissection continues superiorly, the pharynx is noted to be tethered by the cartilaginous eustachian tube and levator veli palatini and tensor veli palatini muscles. These structures can then be divided if necessary with care taken to protect the internal carotid artery. The pharynx can then be rotated medially, exposing the midline compartment of the skull base.

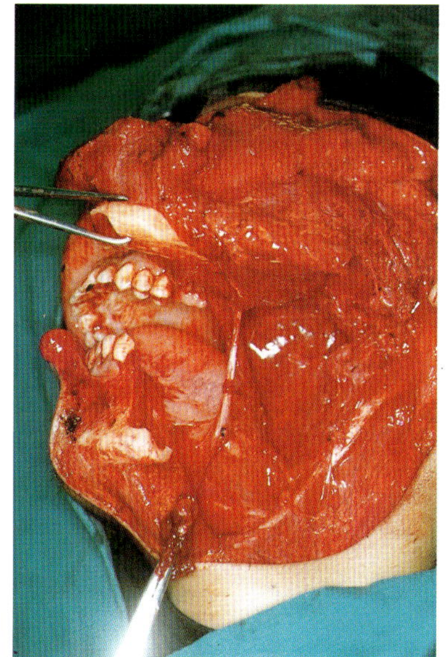
图 598

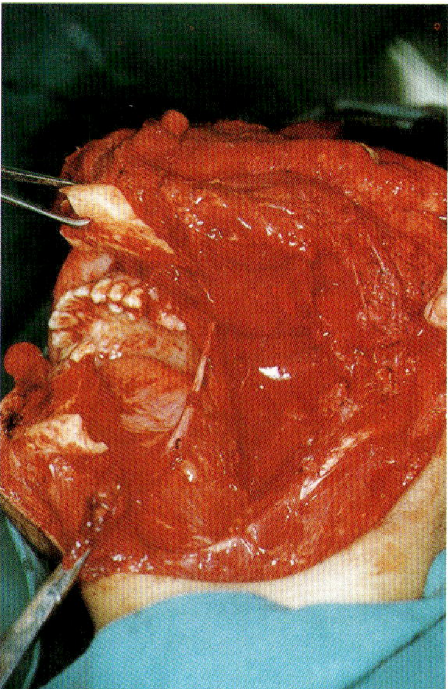
图 599

**图 598** 肿瘤被摘除后，颞下窝、咽旁间隙与颅底的中室一同暴露在手术野中。

**图 599** 颅面外科手术成功的关键是成功的关闭。如果有颅底缺损存在的话，必须考虑重建；如有硬脑膜缺损的话，可用颞肌筋膜瓣或颞肌瓣修复重建。如有咽侧壁缺损，可用胸大肌肌皮瓣或游离皮瓣修复。

**Fig. 598** After the tumor has been excised, the infratemporal fossa and parapharyngeal space together with midline compartment are exposed in the surgical field.

**Fig. 599** The key to successful craniofacial surgery is successful closure. If a significant skull base defect has been created, then this has to be meticulously reconstructed. Dura should be reconstructed and then various muscle flaps, either pericranial or temporalis, should be used to reinforce this. If a significant pharyngeal wall defect resuts, it is reconstructed using a pectoralis major myocutaneous flap or cutaneous free flap, depending on the size and site of the defect.

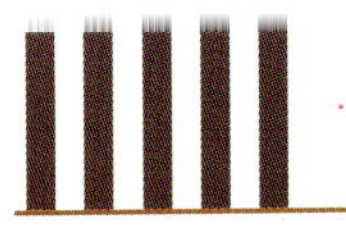

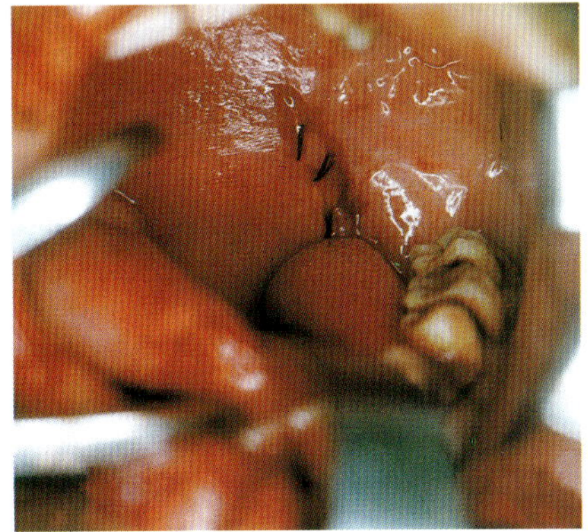

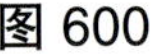

图 600

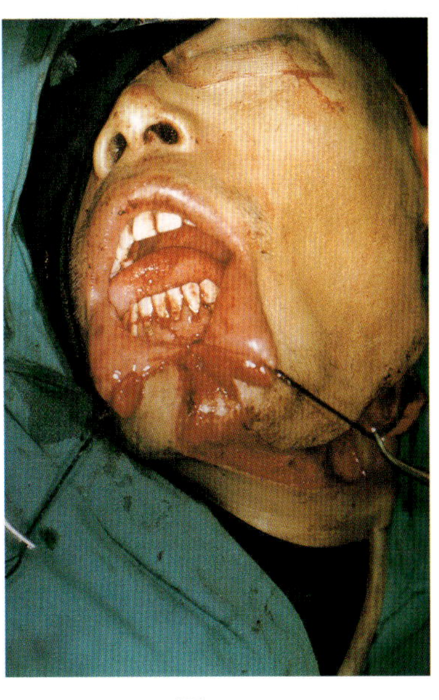

图 601

**图 600, 601** 将咽上缩肌重新缝合于颅底，咽缝于椎前筋膜上。当封闭口底切口时，重要的是不仅将口底粘膜与牙槽嵴粘膜缝合好，也应将牙槽嵴骨膜缝合。

**Fig. 600, 601** The superior constrictor muscle is then reattached to the base of the skull and the pharynx sutured to the prevertebral fascia. When closing the floor of mouth incision, it is important to suture the floor of mouth mucosa not only to the cuff of the alveolar ridge mucosa but to the alveolar ridge periosteum to prevent dehiscence.

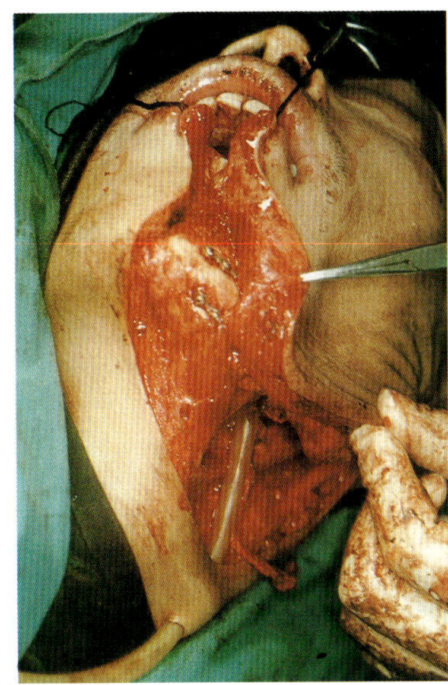

图 602

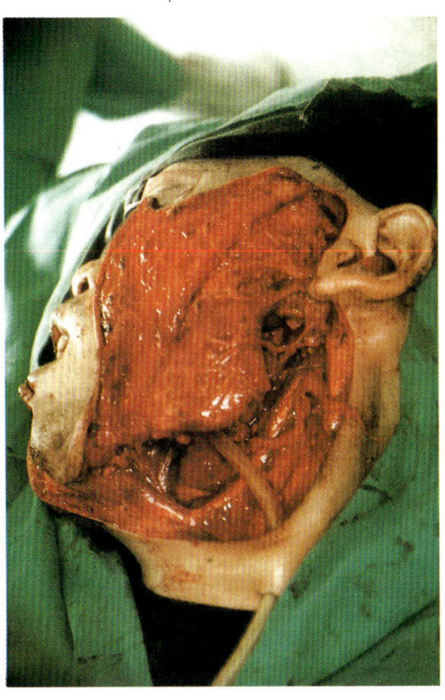

图 603

**图 602** 将截断的下颌骨用钛板固定。先缝合口轮匝肌，然后修整红唇缘。

**图 603** 分层关闭颈部切口。

**Fig. 602** The mandible is then reapproximated using plates. The lip is reapproximated by first reattaching the orbicularis oris by means of a permanent suture and then realigning the vermilion border accurately.

**Fig. 603** The neck incisions closed in layers.

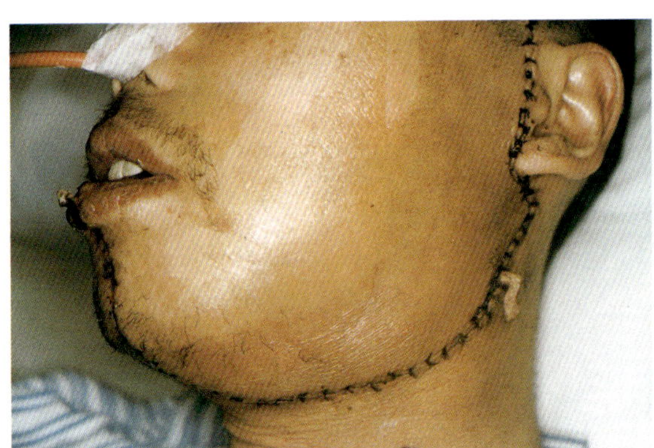

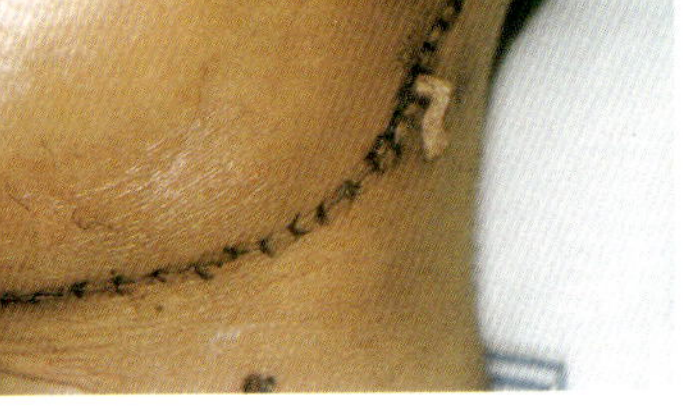

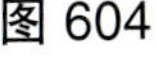

图 604

图 605

图 604, 605 鼻饲管被维持到患者能口腔进食为止。

Fig. 604, 605 A nasogastric tube is maintained until the patient can tolerate an oral diet.

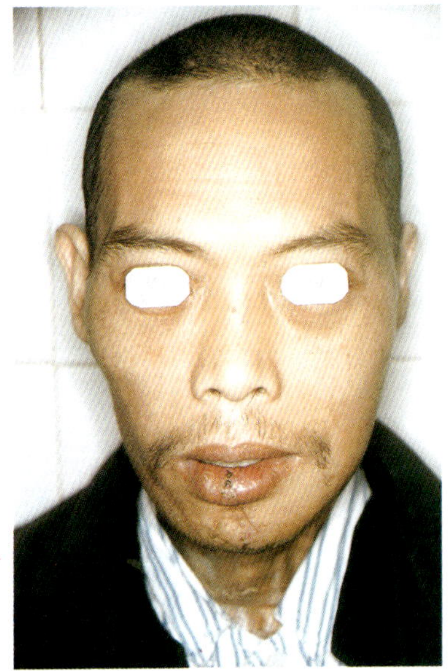

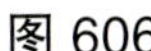

图 606

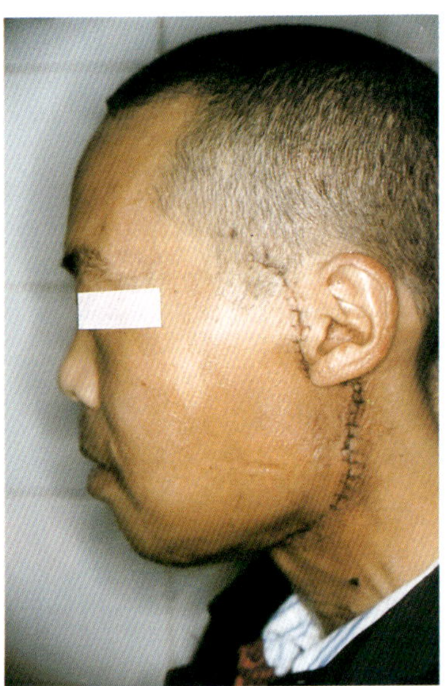

图 607

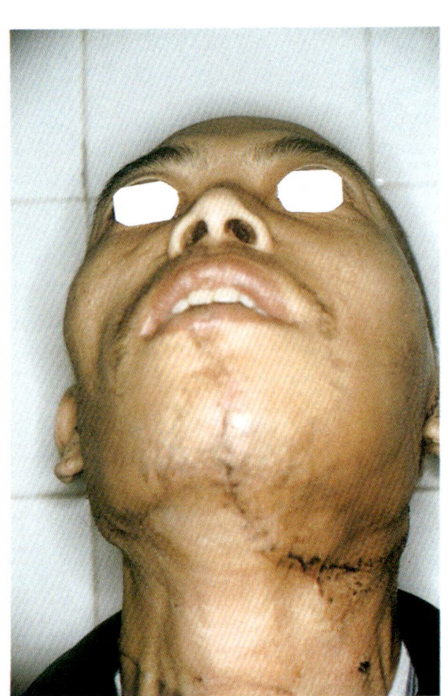

图 608

图 606－608 术后 10 天正面、侧面及仰面观。

Fig. 606－608 The patient's frontal, lateral and submental views 10 days postoperatively.

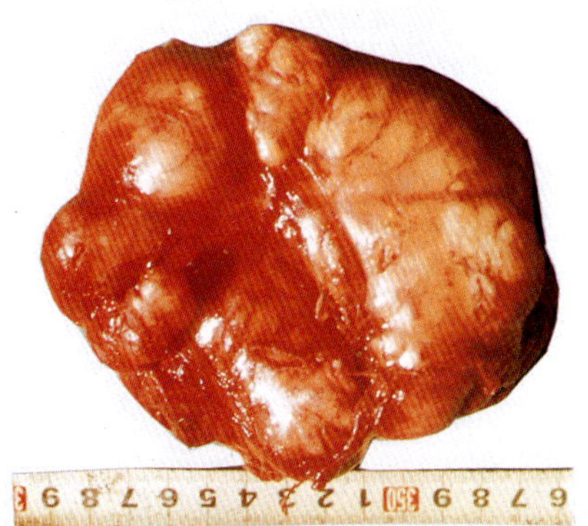
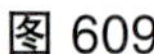

图 609

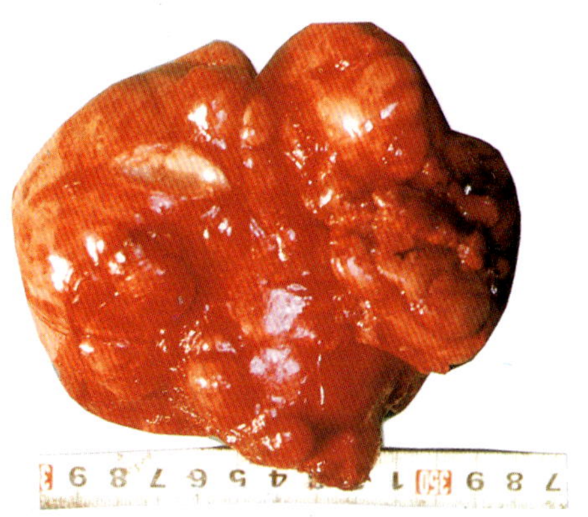

图 610

**图 609, 610** 术后肿瘤标本的内外侧观。

Fig. 609, 610 Internal and external surfacial views of tumor specimen postoperatively.

# Ⅸ. 颌下腺肿瘤

38. 颌下腺多形性腺瘤摘除术
39. 颌下腺腺样囊性癌切除术
40. 颌下腺腺样囊性癌颌颈联合根治术

# Ⅸ. Submandibular gland tumors

38. Excision of the submandibular gland and pleomorphic adenoma
39. Excision of adenoid cystic carcinoma in the submandibular gland
40. Combined operation of radical neck dissection with resection of mandible for the adenoid cystic carcinoma in the submandibular gland

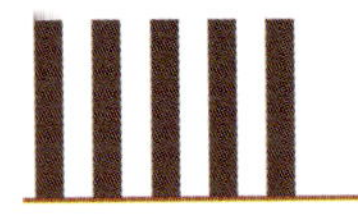



# 38. 颌下腺多形性腺瘤摘除术

# 38. Excision of the submandibular gland and pleomorphic adenoma

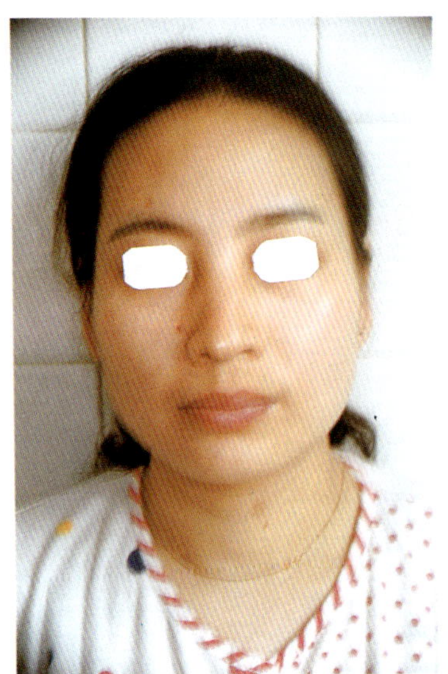

图 611

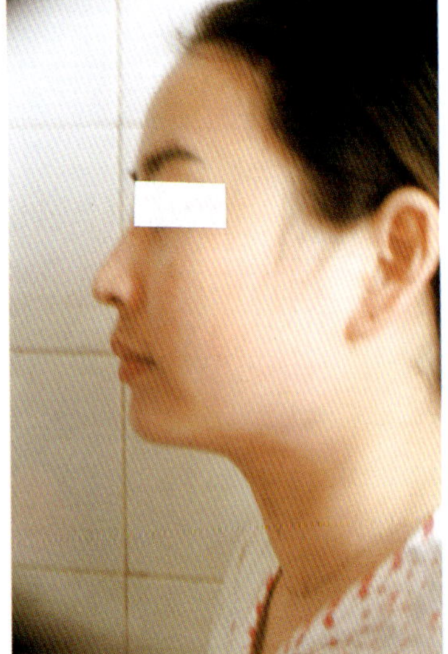

图 612

图 611, 612 患左颌下腺多形性腺瘤的 32 岁的女性患者正面及侧面观。

Fig. 611, 612 Frontal and lateral views of a 32-year-old female patient with pleomorphic adenoma of the submandibular gland.

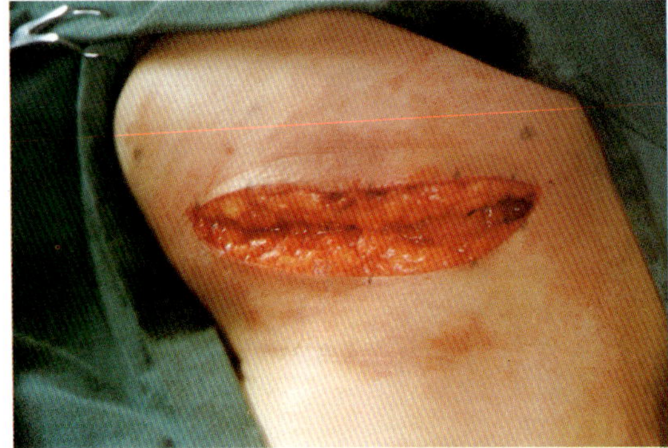

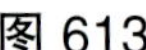

图 613

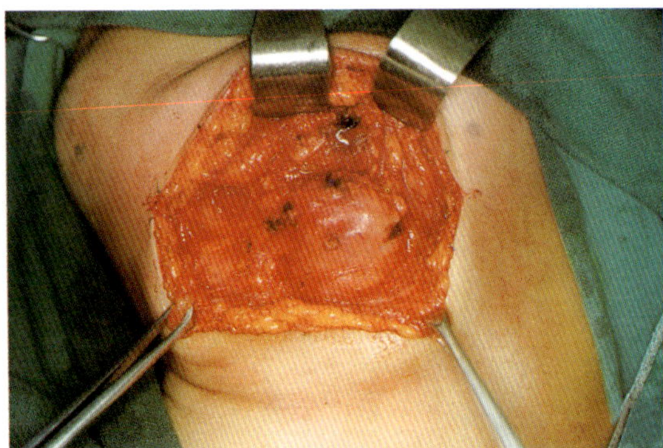

图 614

图 613 在下颌体下缘约 2cm 平下颌骨体从下颌角开始向前延伸达颏下做长约 4cm 的切口，切口深达颈阔肌之下。

图 614 在颈阔肌深面与覆盖颌下腺的颈筋膜之间的平面解剖皮瓣，识别并保护面神经的下颌缘支。此时，二腹肌的前、后腹及颌下腺的浅面被暴露在手术野中。

Fig. 613 The incision is made 4 cm below and parallel to the body of the mandible, extending from the angle of mandible forward to beneath the chin. It is deepened through the skin and platysma.

Fig. 614 The skin flaps are dissected on a plane between the undersurface of the platysma and the cervical fascia covering the gland. The upper flap need not be dissected beyond the body of the mandible. The mandibular branch of the facial nerve must be identified and protected. The anterior and posterior bellies of the digastric muscle are clearly identified and the entire superficial surface of the gland exposed.

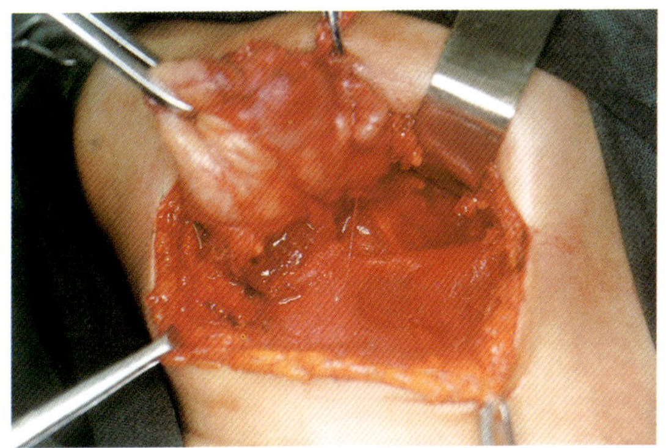

图 615

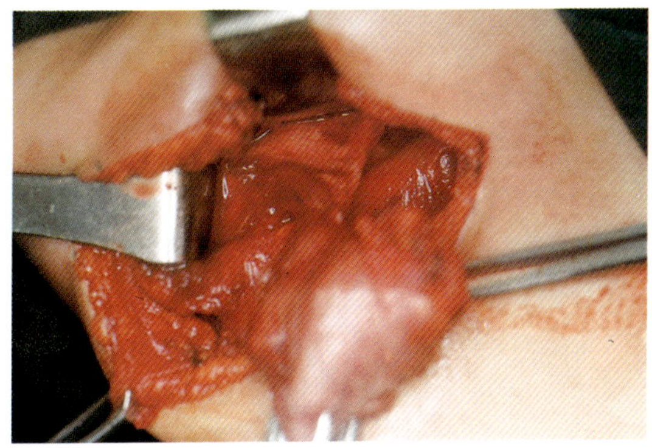

图 616

**图 615** 从颌下腺的前缘开始，由下颌舌骨肌上掀起颌下腺，向前牵开下颌舌骨肌，暴露位于舌骨舌肌浅面的舌静脉及舌下神经。用钝分离解剖颌下腺的深面和颌下腺导管。将导管结扎、切断。在腺体的后缘游离颌下腺的后极。

**图 616** 在颌下腺的后缘分离结扎颌外动脉的近心端。

**Fig. 615** Beginning at its anterior border, the submandibular gland is elevated from the mylohyoid muscle. The free edge of this muscle is retracted forward, exposing the lingual veins and the hypoglossal nerve, lying on the hyoglossus muscle. By blunt dissection, the deep surface of the gland is freed and the submandibular duct and the lingual nerve lying medial to it are identified. The duct is ligated and divided and the gland freed backward to its posterior border.

**Fig. 616** The external maxillary artery is divided at the posterior border of the gland and again at the edge of the mandible.

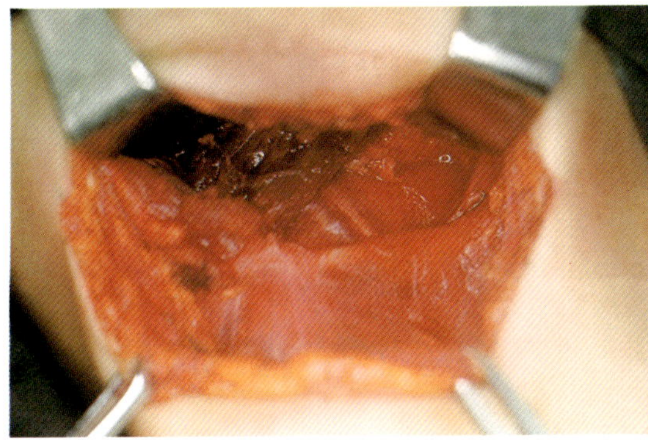

图 617

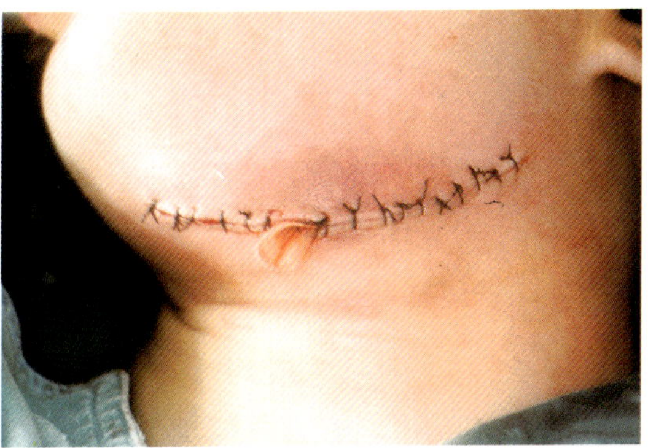

图 618

**图 617** 完全摘除颌下腺及肿瘤，可见颌外动脉和颌下腺导管的断端。舌下及舌神经被保留。

**图 618** 在颌下区内放入一橡皮引流管后用羊肠线间断缝合颈阔肌及丝线缝合皮肤。

**Fig. 617** The submandibular gland can now be removed completely. The divided ends of the external maxillary artery and the submandibular duct are shown here. The hypoglossal and lingual nerves have been preserved.

**Fig. 618** The wound is closed by approximating the platysma with interrupted fine sutures of catgut and by closing the skin with fine silk after placing a small Penrose tube drain in the submandibular bed.



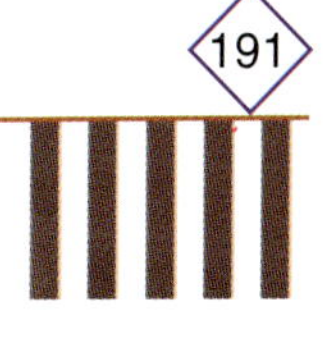

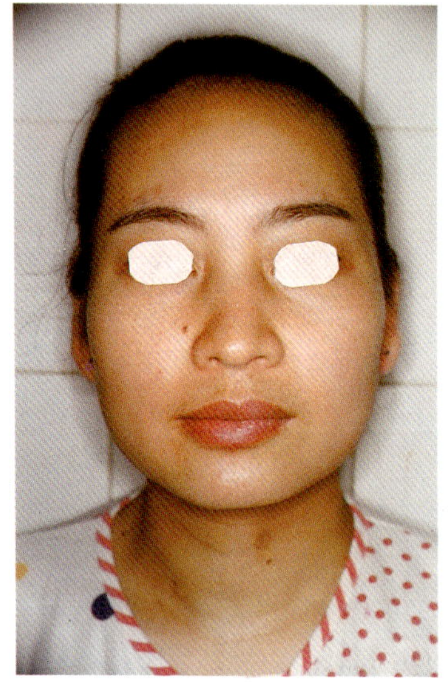

图 619

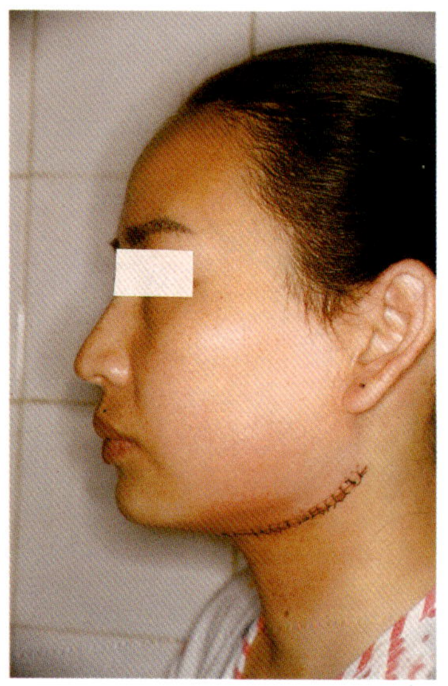

图 620

图 619, 620 术后 5 天的正、侧面观。

Fig. 619, 620 Frontal and lateral views of the patient 5 days after surgery.

# 39. 颌下腺腺样囊性癌切除术

# 39. Excision of adenoid cystic carcinoma in the submandibular gland

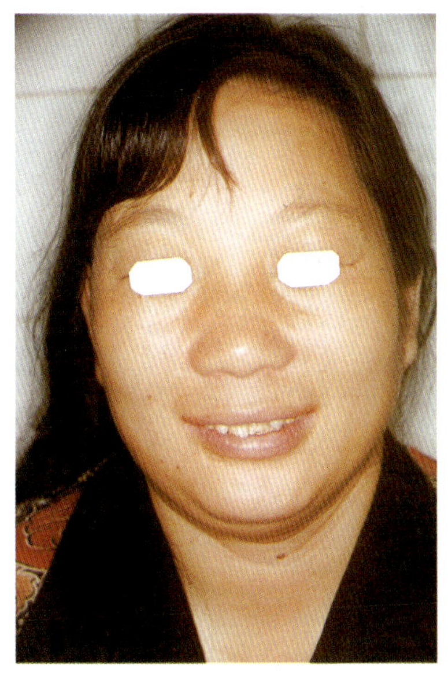

图 621

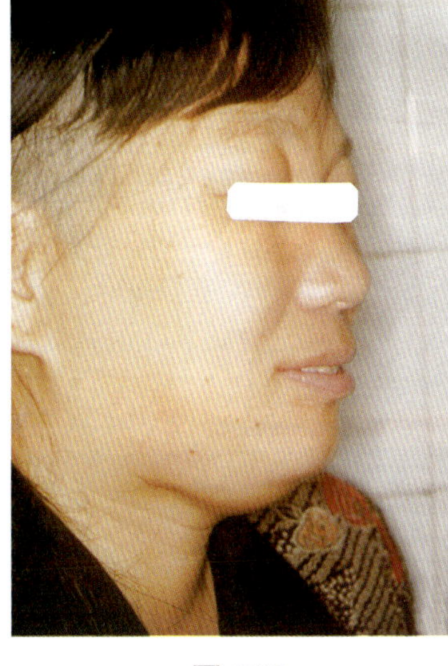

图 622

图 621, 622 一患右颌下腺腺样囊性癌患者的正面及侧面观显示右颌下区明显膨隆，表面皮肤有手术后的瘢痕，为手术切除后局部复发。

Fig. 621, 622 Frontal and lateral views of a 38-year-old female patient with adenoid cystic carcinoma in the submandibular gland show the left submandibular obvious expansion, postoperative scars on the skin may be seen and local recurrence after surgical resection.

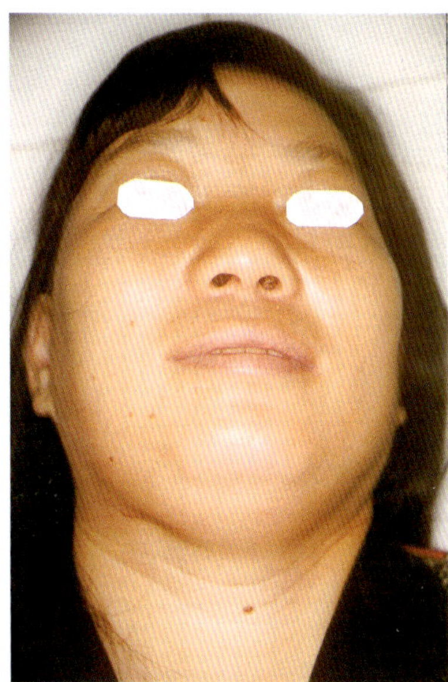

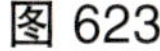

图 623

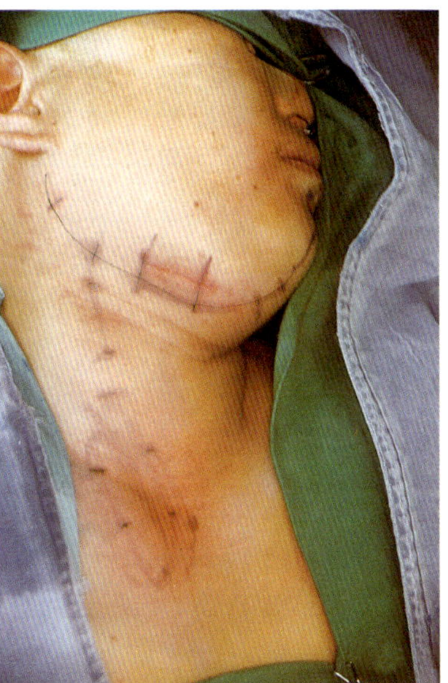

图 624

图 623 患者仰面观示两侧颌下区不对称，右侧颌下区较左侧丰满。

图 624 肿瘤切除进路切口设计。

Fig. 623 Submental view of the patient shows that both submandibular regions are asymmetry and the right submandibular region is larger than the left that.

Fig. 624 Incision design of approach to excise tumor.

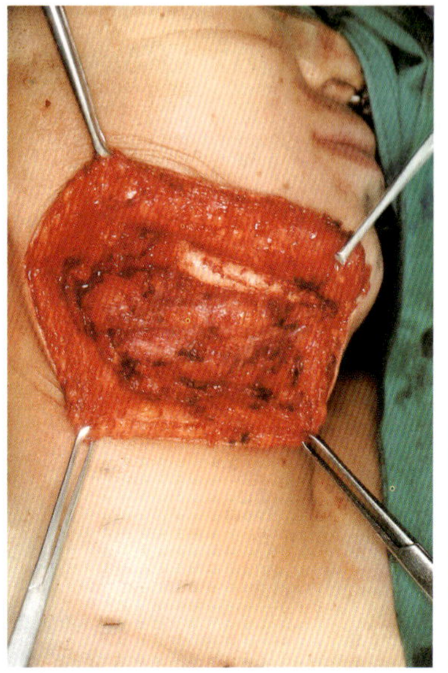
图 625

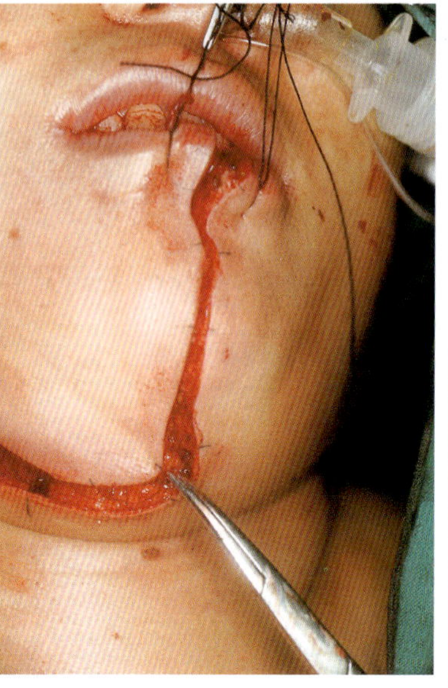
图 626

**图 625** 先在下颌下缘与下颌缘平行做切口，由后向前达颏部切开皮肤、皮下组织及颈阔肌。分离达下颌下缘后找到颌外动、静脉，将其结扎、切断。

**图 626** 在下唇正中做曲线切口达颏下并与颌下切口相连，切开下唇全层组织。

**Fig. 625** The incision is made below and parallel to the body of the mandible, extending from the lower segment of the ramus of the mandible forward to beneath the chin. It is deepened through the skin and platysma. The skin flaps are dissected on a plane of the undersurface of the platysma. The mandibular branch of the facial nerve is identified and protected. The external maxillary artery and vein are dissected at the anterior border of the masseter, divided and ligated.

**Fig. 626** The lower lip is split in the midline to under the chin and associated with the submandibular incision.

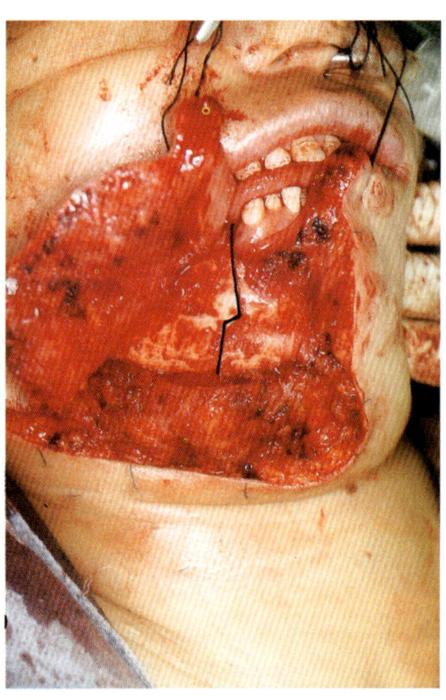
图 627

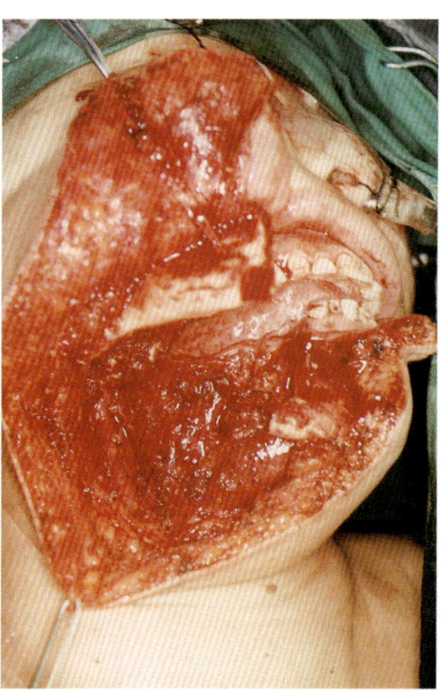
图 628

**图 627** 于下颌正中患侧唇颊沟偏颊侧由前向后切开达下颌第二前磨牙之前，于下颌下缘向上分离颊侧骨膜达颏孔之前，暴露患侧颏神经，将其保护不予切断。

**图 628** 拔除第一前磨牙，在下颌第一前磨牙区分离舌侧骨膜，穿入线锯，锯断患侧下颌骨，止血后切开舌侧口底粘膜及下颌舌骨肌达舌腭弓前缘，将下颌骨短骨段向上牵拉，暴露颌下肿瘤的外表面。

**Fig. 627** A cheek flap is elevated by an incision in the gingivobuccal gutter and dissection along the body of the mandible as far as the mental foramen and the mental nerve is protected.

**Fig. 628** After the first premolar tooth is extracted, the lingual mucoperiosteum is separated at the first premolar area and the mandible is divided with a Gigli saw. At this stage, a mucosal incision is made in the lateral floor of the mouth extending posteriorly toward the anterior tonsillar pillar. The mandible is now swung laterally by dividing the mylohyoid muscle. The external surface of the submandibular tumor is now exposed.

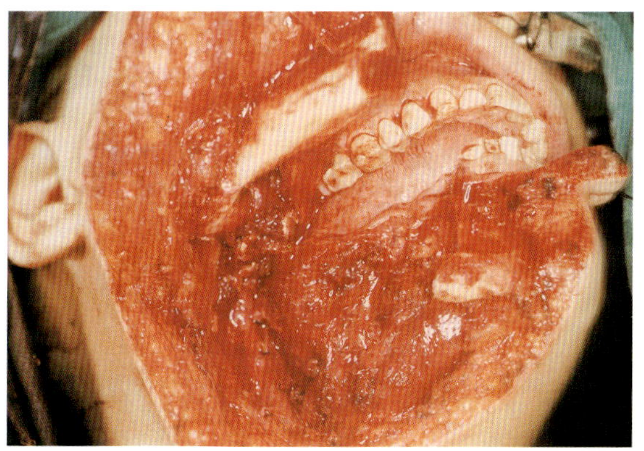

图 629

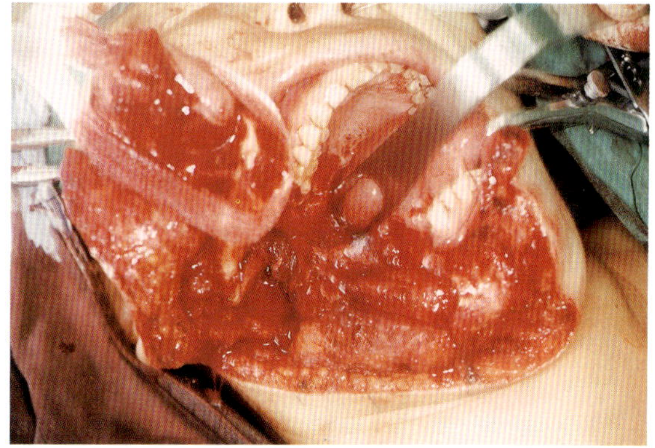

图 630

**图 629** 分离肿瘤的下极、前极和后极，分离肿瘤的深面有困难，此时应切除被肿瘤侵犯的舌下肌群，包括舌神经在内的软组织。

**图 630** 肿瘤完全被切除后的情景。

Fig. 629 The anterior, inferior and posterior poles of the tumor are separated. It is difficult to dissect the deep tissues of the tumor. The surrounding tissue involved by the tumor should be excised including lingual nerve.

Fig. 630 The condition after the tumor has been removed.

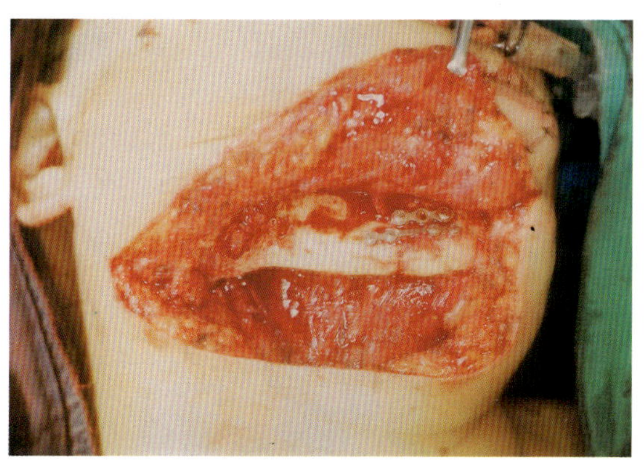

图 631

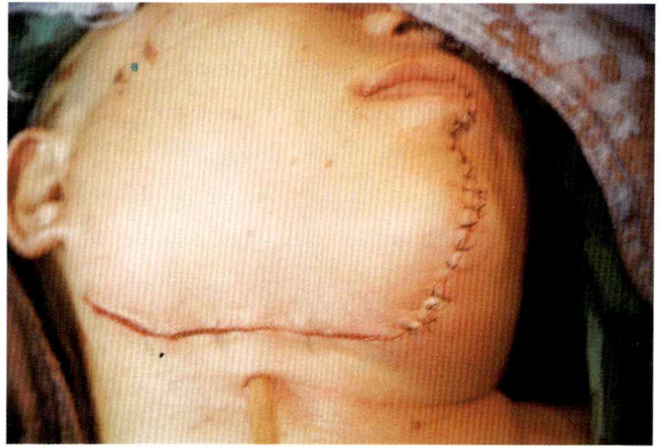

图 632

**图 631** 缝合口底切开的粘膜之后，在骨断端上钻孔，用钛板将锯断的下颌骨固定。还回颊瓣后缝合龈颊沟粘膜及下唇正中。

**图 632** 生理盐水冲洗后分层缝合颈阔肌及皮肤，放橡皮引流管一根引流 48 小时。

Fig. 631 After the incised mucosa of the floor of the mouth has been sutured, the mandibular split is fixed with miniplate through holes drilled in the bone. Closure of the gingivobuccal gutter is accomplished with interrupted mucosal sutures of fine silk. The lip is reconstructed with buried chromic sutures in the orbicularis muscle and fine silk sutures in the skin and mucosa.

Fig. 632 The wound is irrigated with saline solution and is sutured with fine silk in layers. The wound is drained with a rubber tube for 48 hours.

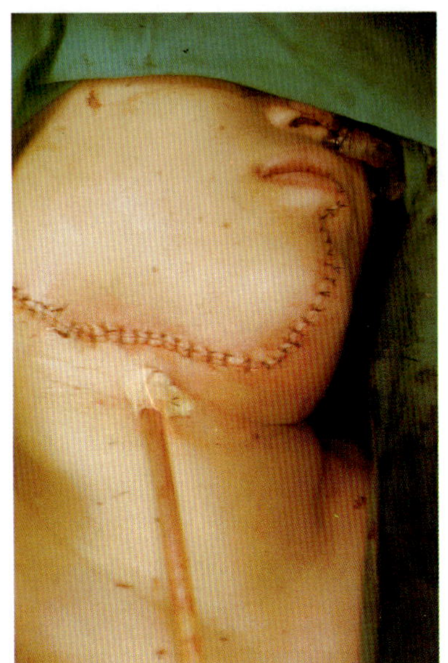

图 633

图 633 创缘缝合后情景。

Fig. 633 The condition after the wound has been sutured.

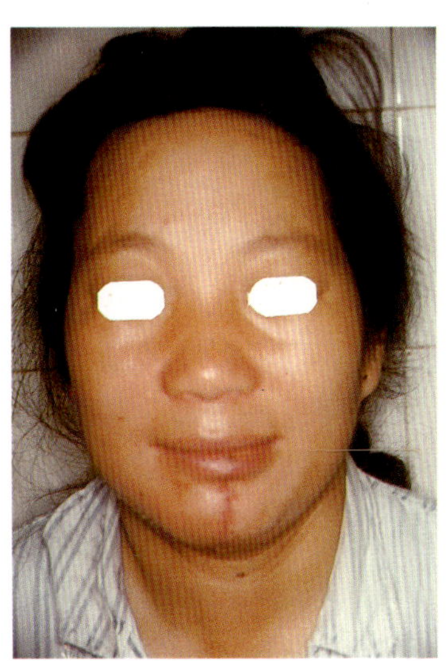

图 634

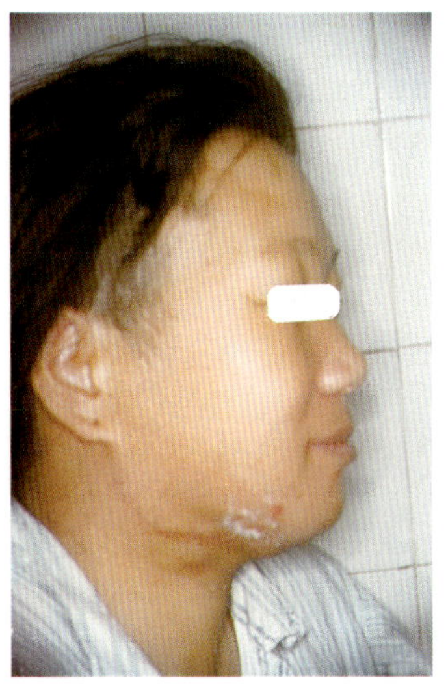

图 635

图 634, 635 术后 10 天患者正面及侧面观示创口愈合良好。

Fig. 634, 635 Frontal and lateral views of the patient 10 days after operation show that the wound healing is fine.

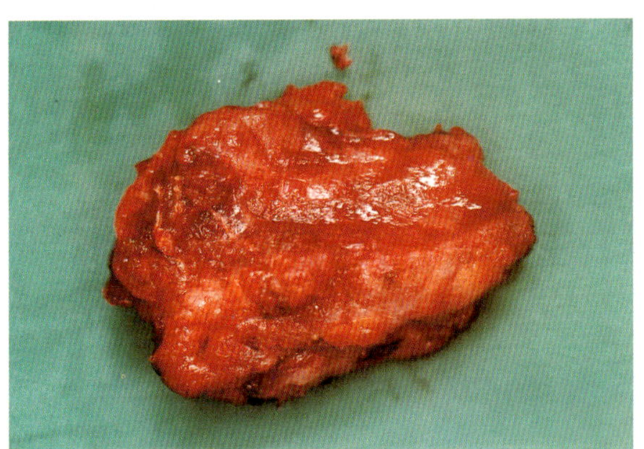

图 636

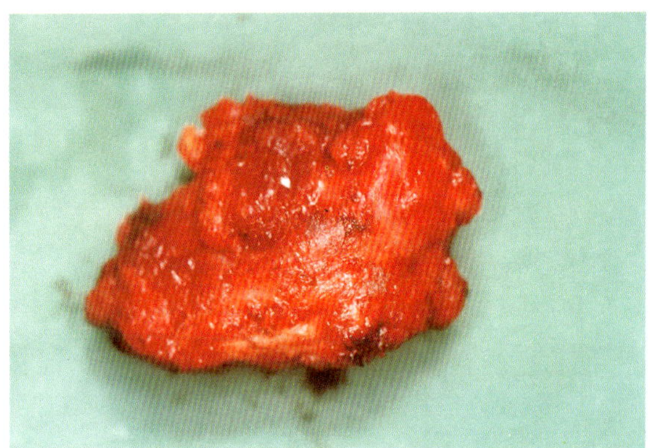

图 637

图 636, 637 术后肿瘤的外、内侧面观。

Fig. 636, 637 External and internal surface views of postoperative specimen.

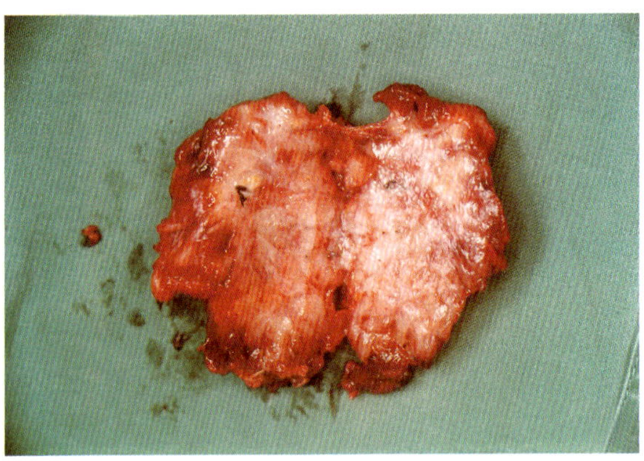

图 638

图 638 肿瘤剖面观。

Fig. 638 View of the cut surface of the tumor shows firm and greyishwhite.

# 40. 颌下腺腺样囊性癌颌颈联合根治术

# 40. Combined operation of radical neck dissection with resection of mandible for the adenoid cystic carcinoma in the submandibular gland

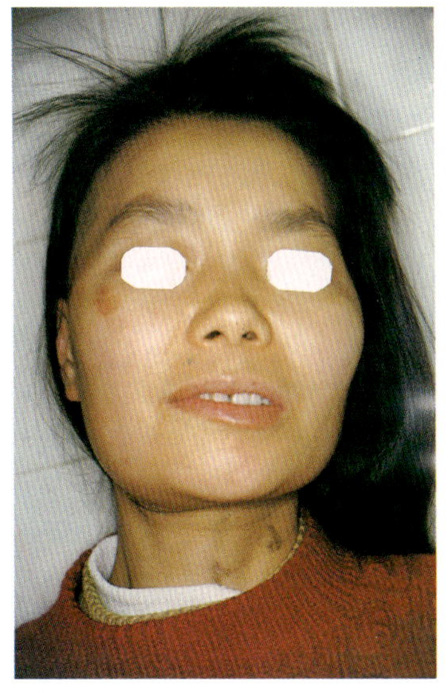

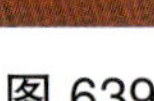

图 639

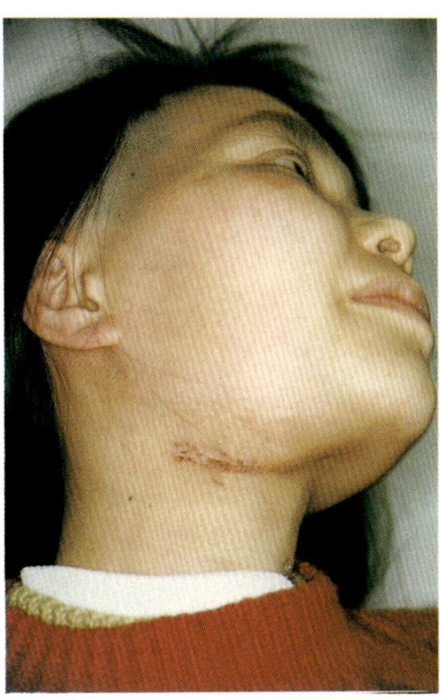

图 640

**图 639，640** 患右颌下腺囊性腺样癌的 36 岁女性患者的正、侧面观。

正面观显示右颌下区明显膨隆，表面皮肤上有长条形瘢痕，肿块与下颌内侧骨膜粘连；侧面观显示右颌下膨隆，皮肤手术瘢痕明显。

**Fig. 639, 640** Frontal and lateral views of a 36-year-old female patient with adenoid cystic carcinoma in the right submandibular gland.

Frontal view shows obvious expansion of the right submandibular region. There is a long scar on the submandibular skin. The tumor is attached to internal periosteum of the mandible. Lateral view shows the right submandibular expansion and the operative scar on the skin is obvious.

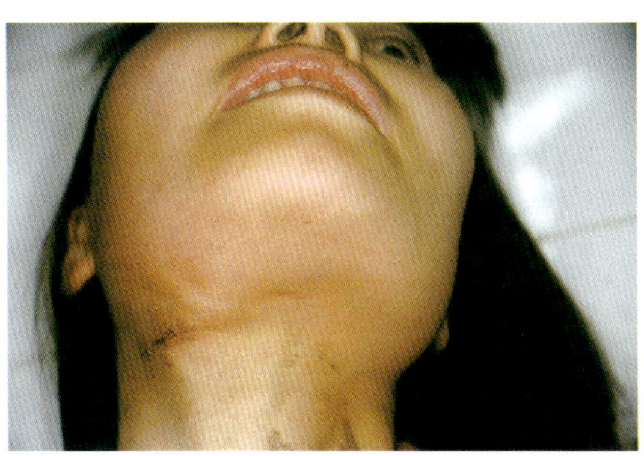

图 641

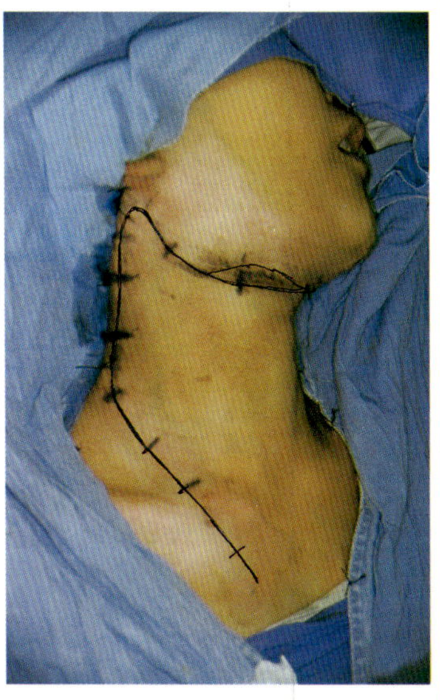

图 642

**图 641** 仰面观显示双侧颌下区不对称，右侧明显膨隆，皮肤上有一横形长约 4cm 的瘢痕。

**图 642** 颈淋巴清扫术的切口设计，用亚甲蓝标出切口线。

**Fig. 641** Submental view shows bilateral submandibular region are asymmetry, the right submandibular region is obvious expansion. There is a horizontal 4 cm scar on the submandibular region.

**Fig. 642** Incision design of neck radical dissection is marked out with methylene blue.

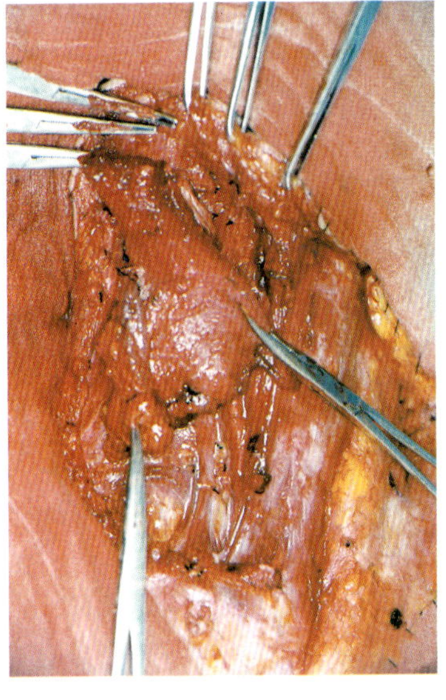
图 643

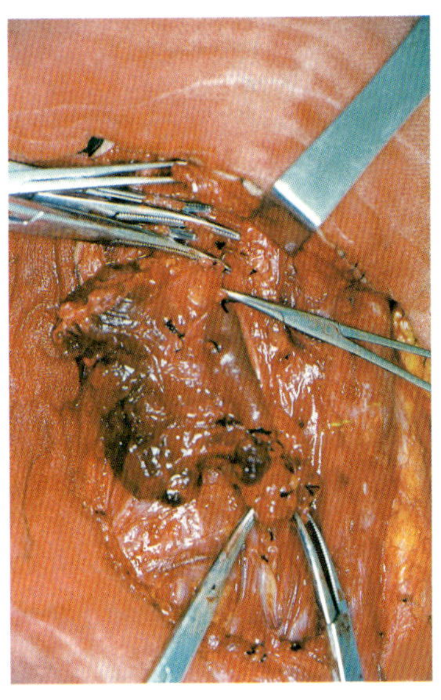
图 644

**图 643** 按颈淋巴清扫术的常规操作方法行颈淋巴清扫术。

**图 644** 显示颈淋巴清扫术进行至胸锁乳突肌上端时，用血管钳分别夹住胸锁乳突肌上端后将其剪断，用 4 号丝线缝扎；图 644 显示颈淋巴清扫术进行至颌后区时，用血管钳夹住颈内静脉上端，将其用 7 号、4 号丝线结扎，然后用 1 号丝线缝扎。

**Fig. 643** A radical neck dissection is performed in the usual manner.

**Fig. 644** Shows when the neck dissection is reached to upper end of the sternocleidomastoid muscle, the sternocleidomastoid muscle is severed at the mastoid process. Fig644 shows when the radical neck dissection is performed to the upper end of the internal jugular vein, the vein is exposed by elevating or reflecting the posterior belly of the digastric muscle and carefully dividing the loose fascial envelope surrounding the vein beneath the muscle, the vein is divided and ligated opposite the palpable prominence of the transverse process of the atlas.

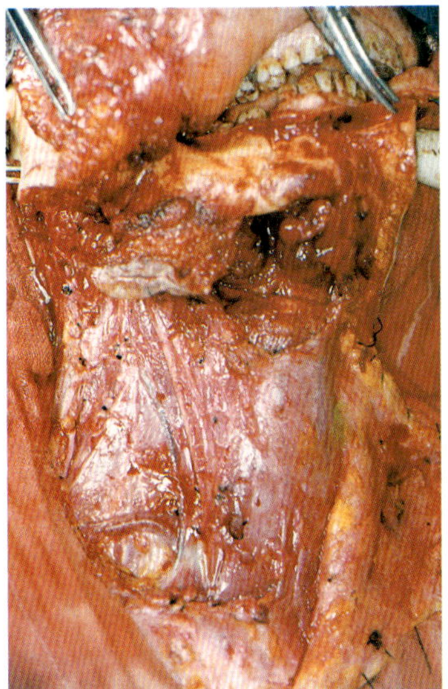
图 645

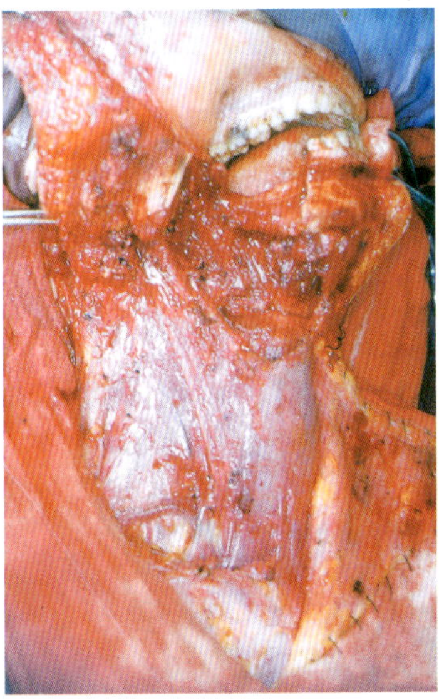
图 646

**图 645** 按常规完成颈淋巴清扫术后，在下唇正中将下唇切开，然后沿口内龈颊沟靠颊侧切开龈颊沟粘膜并沿下颌体部锐性解剖，掀起颊瓣，暴露下颌骨体部。

**图 646** 拔除4|，用线锯将右侧下颌骨体部锯开，此时下颌骨后段已被游离。在下颌角部锯断下颌后部。一旦下颌骨骨段已经被游离，绕肿瘤周围的切口便可以被确定，一般在肿瘤周围正常粘膜 1cm 内切除。切口通过口底的深层肌肉，此时，口内的肿瘤和下颌骨已经与周围附着组织完全分离，将其去除。用细线结扎出血的血管后，创面用生理盐水冲洗。

**Fig. 645** After radical neck dissection has been completed, the lower lip is split in the midline and a cheek flap is elevated by an incision in the gingivobuccal gutter and dissection along the body of the mandible.

**Fig. 646** The mandible is divided well anterior to the lesion with a Gigli saw. The first premolar tooth is extracted before the mandible is divided. Once the segment of mandible has been freed posteriorly, an incision is outlined around the tumor, leaving at least 1.0 cm of normal mucosa on all its edges. The incision is carried through the deep musculatures of the floor of the mouth. Posteriorly, the mandible is sectioned at the angle. The tumor and mandible have now been freed from all attachments above. The tumor, the attached segment of mandible, and the neck contents are removed en masse. Hemostasis is obtained by ligating all bleeding vessels with ties of fine chromic catgut. The wound is thoroughly irrigated with saline solution.

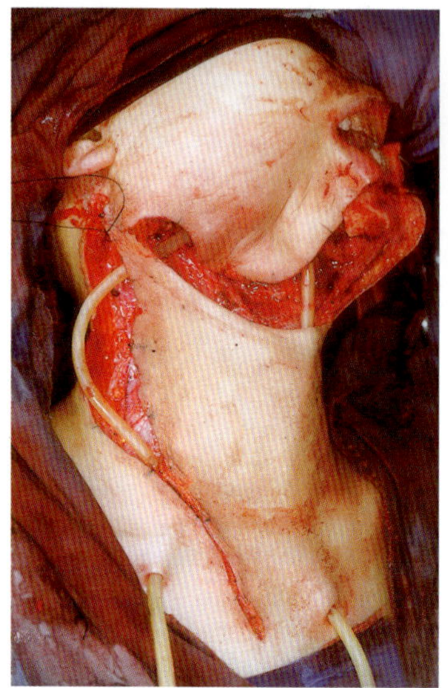

图 647

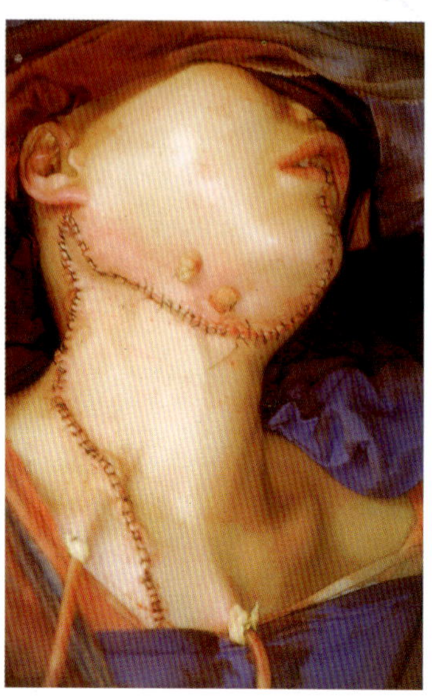

图 648

**图647** 将颊粘膜与口底粘膜及剩余下颌骨断端牙龈粘膜相缝合。为了防止唾液渗漏于口底创口内，在缝合的粘膜深层再将颊部肌层与口底肌层缝合。分层缝合切开的下唇及颏部组织，此时应特别注意红唇皮肤交界缘的对合。

**图 648** 按常规方法在颈部创区放置橡皮引流管 2 根后分层缝合颈阔肌、皮下组织及皮肤，颈部轻压包扎。

**Fig. 647** The mucosal edges are jointed with interrupted sutures of 4 – 0 silk, the knots being tied within the mouth. To prevent a leak, this suture line must be reinforced by deep sutures wherever possible. This is accomplished by suturing the muscle of the floor of the mouth to the deep surface of the cheek flap with interrupted sutures of 3 – 0 chromic catgut. The lip is reconstructed with buried chromic sutures in the orbicularis muscle and fine silk sutures in the skin and mucosa. Care is taken to align accurately the vermilion – skin junction.

**Fig. 648** The neck wound is drained and closed in the usual manner. A bulky pressure dressing is applied.

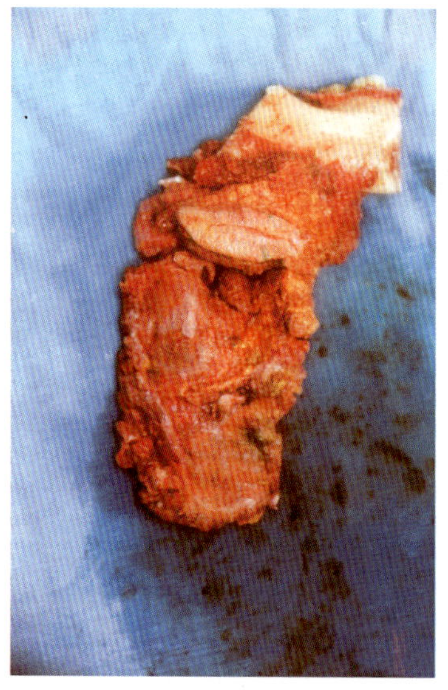

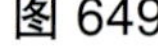

图 649

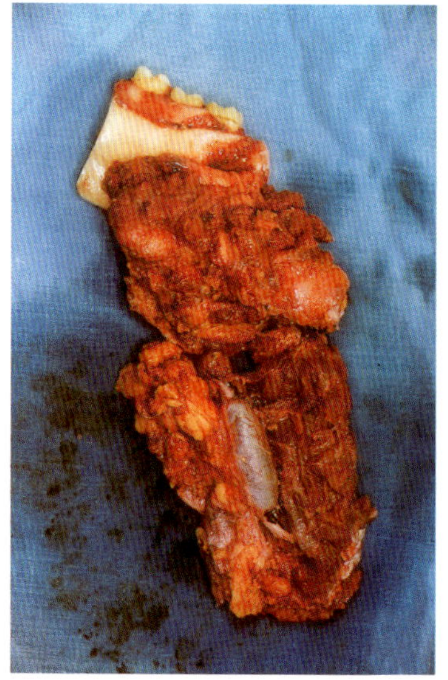

图 650

**图 649, 650** 术后标本的外、内侧面观。

**Fig. 649, 650** External and internal surficial views of the postoperative specimen.

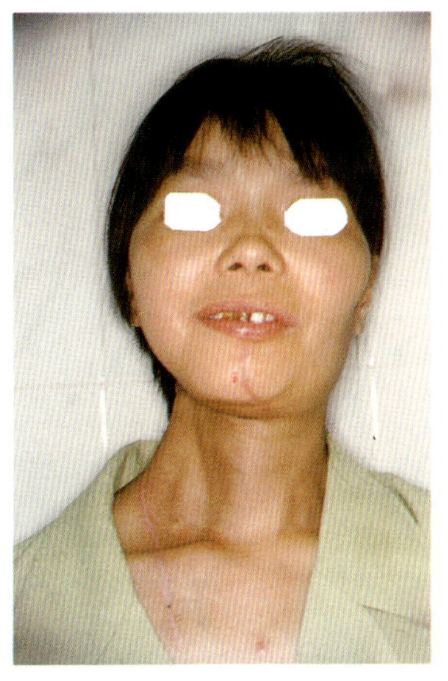

图 651

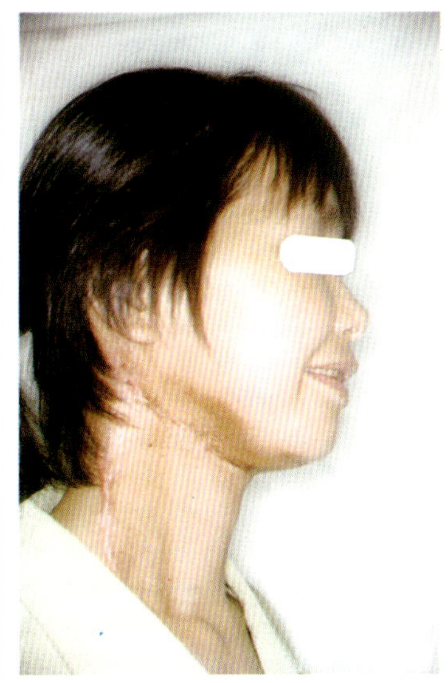

图 652

图 651, 652 患者术后 6 个月的正、侧面观。

Fig. 651, 652 Frontal and lateral views of the patient's postoperative 6 months.

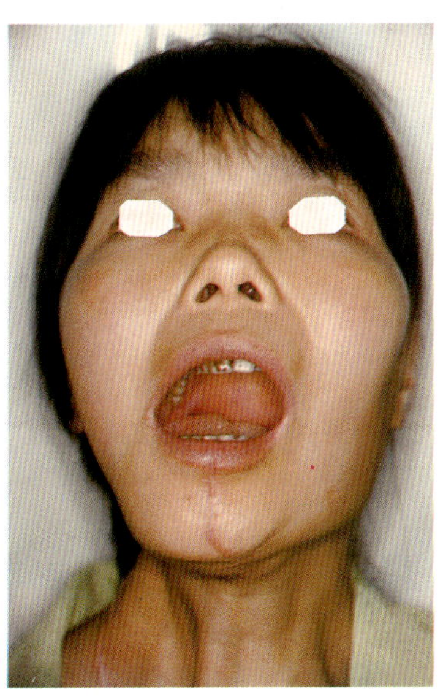

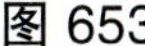

图 653

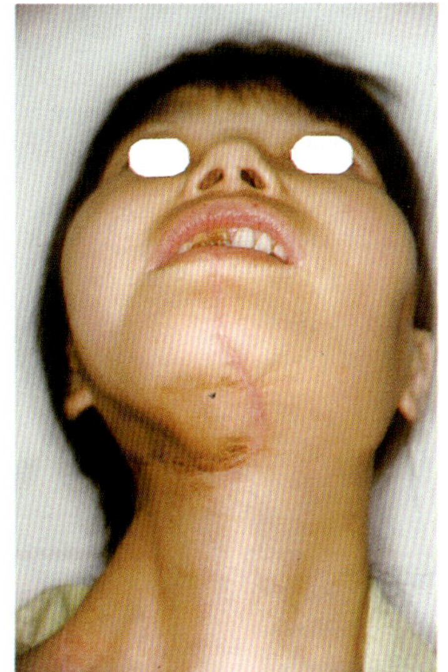

图 654

图 653 患者术后 6 个月的张口情况 .
图 654 患者仰面观情景。

Fig. 653 The condition of opening mouth after the patient's postoperative 6 months.
Fig. 654 The condition of the patient's submental view.

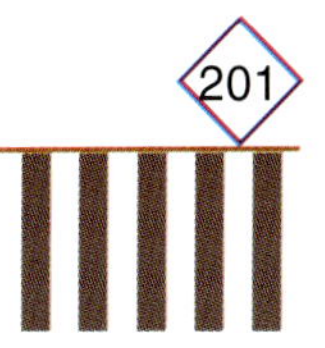

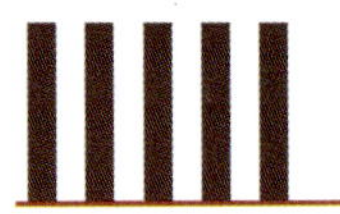



# X．颏及颈部肿瘤

41．颏颈血管瘤摘除术
42．甲状舌管囊肿摘除术
43．鳃裂囊肿摘除术
44．面颈部巨大淋巴管瘤摘除术

# X．Chin and neck region tumors

41．Excision of haemangioma in the chin and the neck
42．Excision of thyroglossal cyst
43．Excision of branchial cleft cyst
44．Excision of giant lymphangioma in the facial and neck regions

# 41. 颏颈血管瘤摘除术

# 41. Excision of haemangioma in the chin and the neck

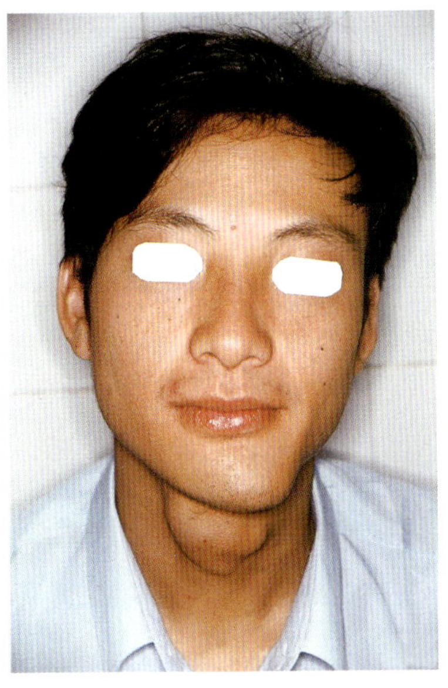

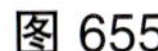

图 655

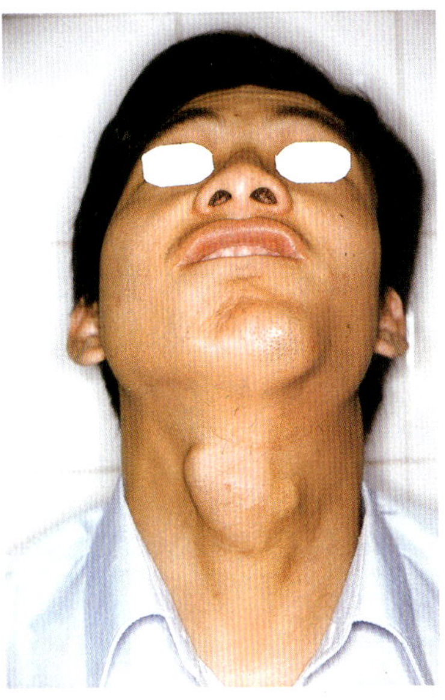

图 656

**图 655，656** 患颏颈部血管瘤的 27 岁男性患者的正、仰面观。

正面观显示颏及颈正中上部明显膨隆，扪及有压缩性，穿刺有鲜血。仰面观显示颈正中部血管瘤。

**Fig. 655, 656** Frontal and submental views of a 27-year-old male patient with haemangioma in the chin and the neck.

Frontal view shows obvious expansion of the chin and the upper midline of the neck. There is compresion by palpation and blood by aspiration. Submental view shows haemangioma in upper midline of the neck.

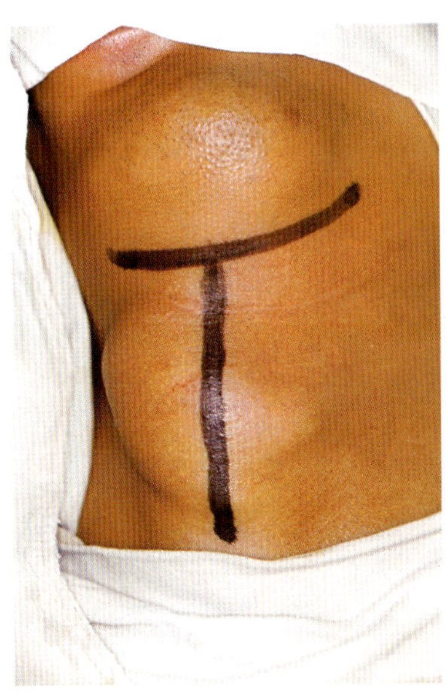

图 657

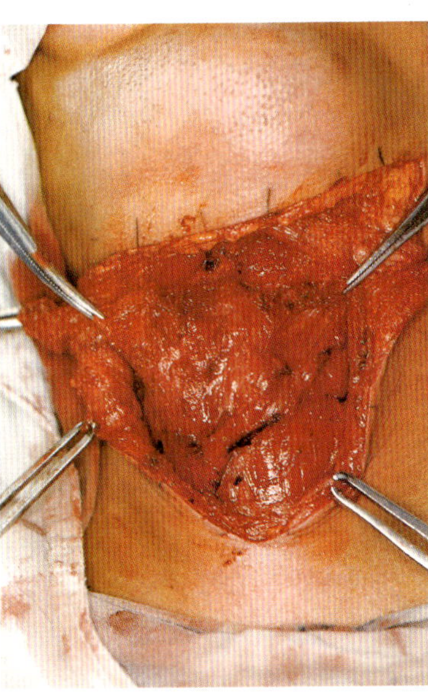

图 658

**图 657** 用美蓝在颏下及颈部画切口线。

**图 658** 按切口线切开皮肤、皮下及颈阔肌，翻开颈部肌皮瓣，暴露血管瘤的浅面，然后分离血管瘤的左、右侧界及上极，在深面由上向下分离，摘除血管瘤。

**Fig. 657** Incision lines are marked out by methylene blue.

**Fig. 658** According to incision line marked out, the skin and the platysma are incised. The skin flap is elevated from the muscles of the neck, exposing surficial portion of haemangioma, then blunt dissection is made around the tumor. The tumor is excised completely.

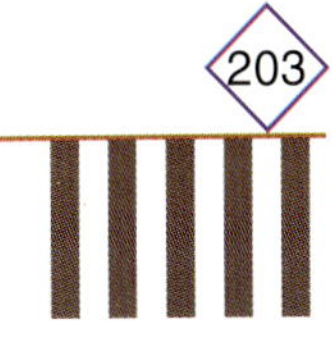

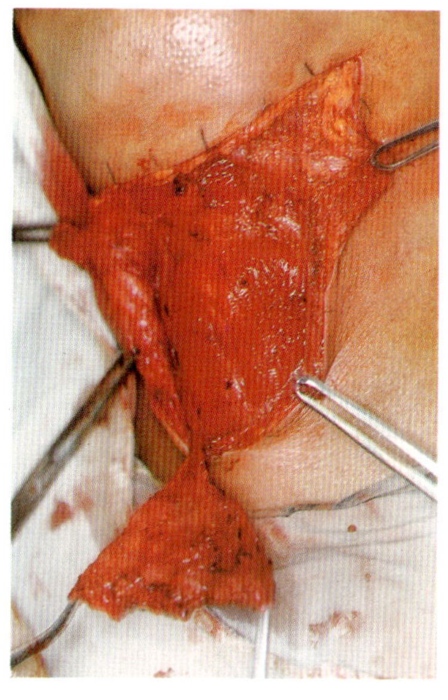

图 659

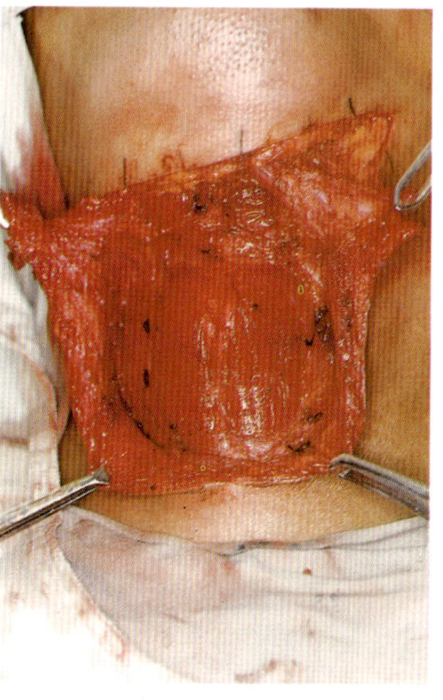

图 660

**图 659** 颈部的血管瘤被切除后，用结扎和电凝彻底止血。

**图 660** 显示颈部血管瘤被切除后的情景。

**Fig. 659** After haemangioma in the neck has been excised, the bleeding vessels are ligated or electrocoagulation .

**Fig. 660** Shows the condition after haemangioma in the neck is excised.

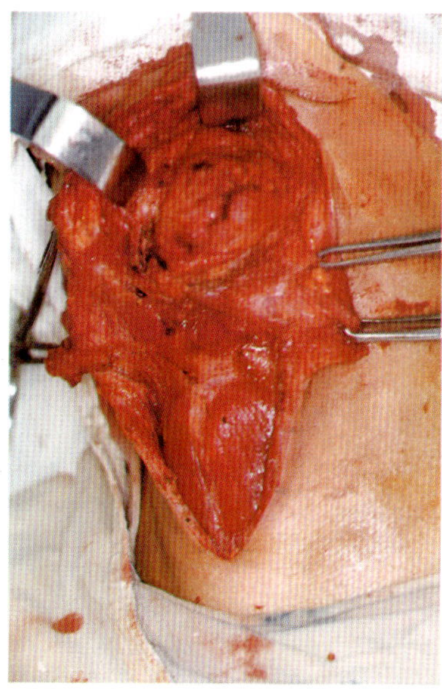

图 661

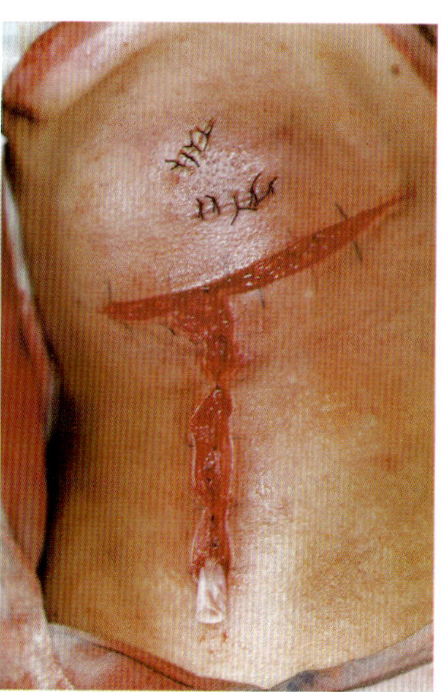

图 662

**图 661** 钝性分离颏部皮瓣，暴露颏部的血管瘤表面。在血管瘤的边缘，由下向上分离血管瘤深层组织，完整切除颏部血管瘤后彻底止血。生理盐水冲洗创面。

**图 662** 将组织瓣还回，分层缝合颈阔肌、皮下组织及皮肤。留置橡皮引流条 48 小时。

**Fig. 661** The skin flap on the chin is elevated with blunt dissection, exposing surficial portion of haemangioma in the chin. At the border of the haemangioma, the deep tissues are separated from the tumor from inferiorly to superiorly, the haemangioma in the chin is removed completely. The wound is irrigated with saline solution.

**Fig. 662** The skin flaps are returned in place and the sutures are performed in layers. The skin is sutured with interrupted silk sutures and a drain is maintained for 48 hours.

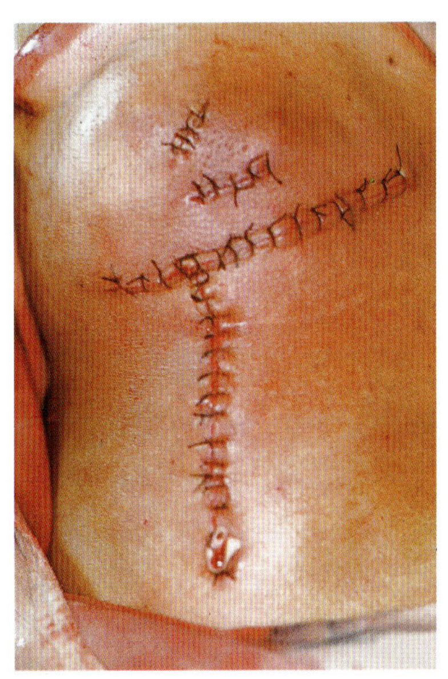

图 663

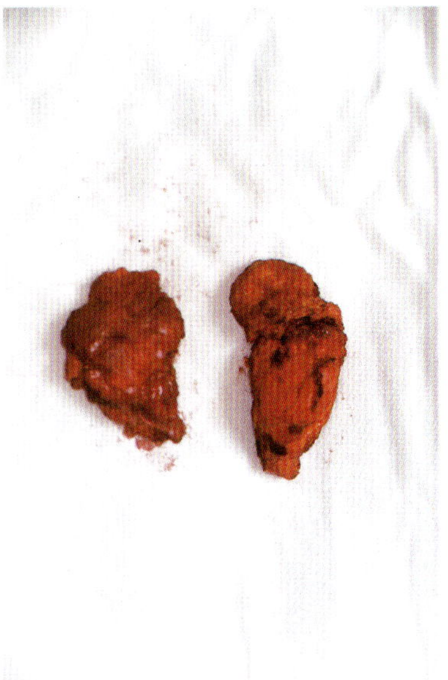

图 664

图 663 皮肤缝合后情景。
图 664 手术后血管瘤标本。

Fig. 663 Condition after the skin has been sutured with interrupted silk sutures.
Fig. 664 Postoperative haemangiomatic specimen.

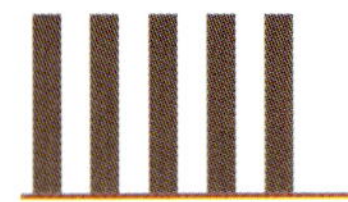



# 42. 甲状舌管囊肿摘除术

# 42. Excision of Thyroglossal Cyst

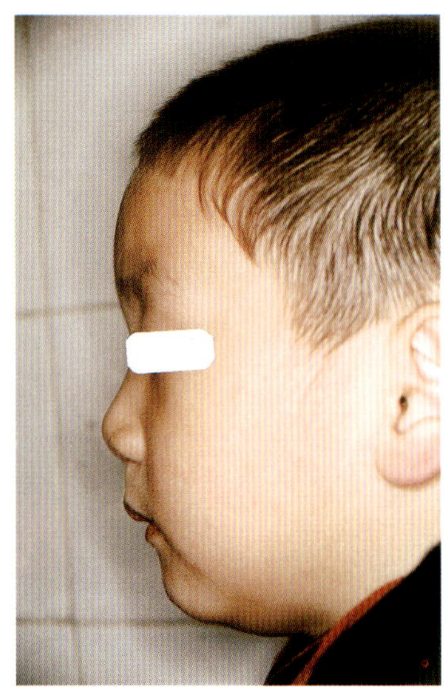

图 665

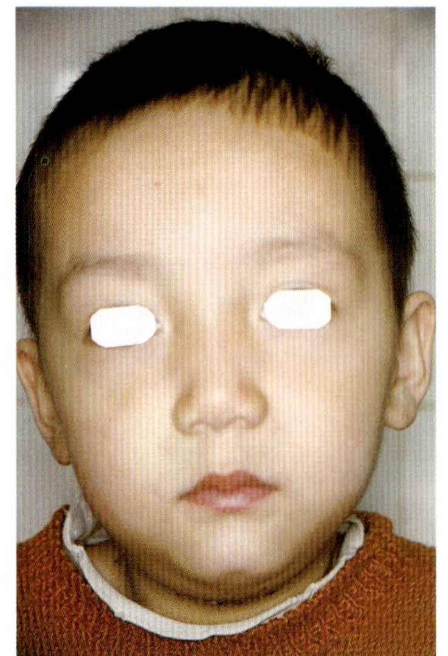

图 666

**图 665，666** 患有颏下区甲状舌管囊肿的患者手术前侧面观及手术后正面观。

**Fig. 665，666** Preoperative lateral view and postoperative frontal view of patient with thyroglossal cyst in the submental region.

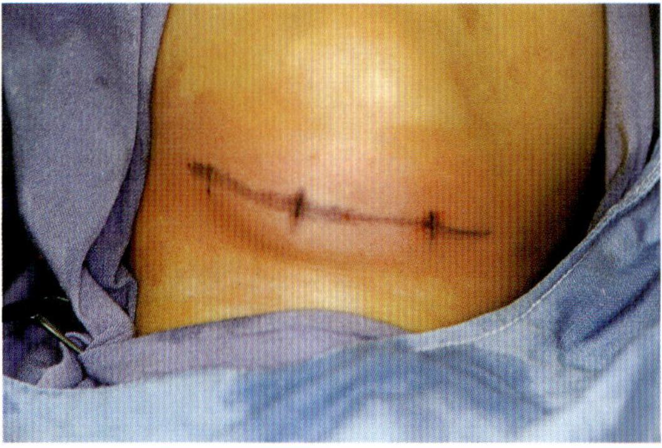

图 667

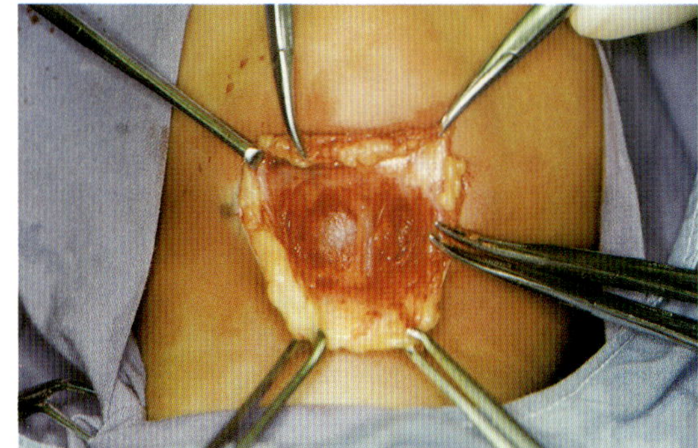

图 668

**图 667, 668** 沿颈部皮肤于囊肿表面最隆起部用美蓝画出切口线。切口经过囊肿表面，其两端超过囊肿边缘，如为瘘管，则绕瘘口做一横梭形切口，将瘘口周围粘连的皮肤一并切除。切口长度一般为 5～8cm。沿切口设计线，切开皮肤、皮下组织和颈阔肌，显露囊肿或瘘管。

**Fig. 667，668** The incision，5～8 cm in length，extends transversely over the cyst parallel to the hyoid bone. Flaps of skin and platysma are elevated to expose the cyst. It may lie above or below the superficial layer of the deep cervical fascia. Occasionally it lies beneath the pretracheal fascia.

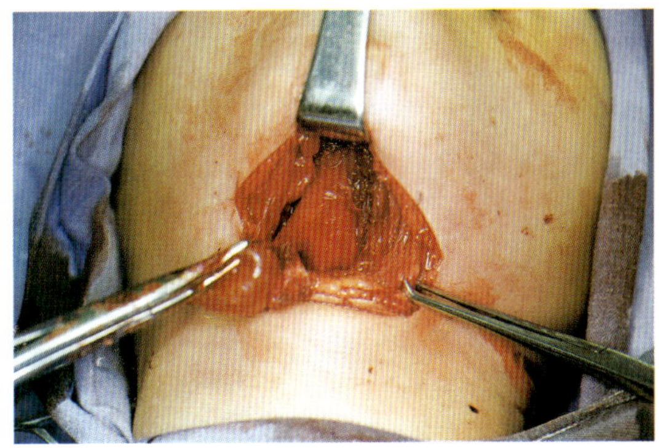

图 669

**图 669** 沿囊肿表面向舌骨方向剥离囊肿至舌骨体。分离囊肿底部及后上极时，应仔细寻找可能存在的管状物，而避免损伤其深面的甲状舌骨膜及其外侧走行的喉上神经。分离囊肿至舌骨体下缘时，在囊肿与舌骨体粘连的两侧，切开舌骨膜及其肌肉附着，用骨剪剪断舌骨，此时，囊肿与舌骨体中段即可一并游离。截除的舌骨体长约 1cm。

**Fig. 669** The inferior and lateral aspects of the cyst are freed. Superiorly, dissection proceeds cautiously so that the tract leading upward from the cyst may be identified. Dissection is now carried to the broad central portion of the hyoid bone. The bone is drawn forward into the wound and its central portion freed of muscle insertions, using a scalpel or sharp periosteal elevator. The hyoid bone is divided with a bone-cutting forceps on each side of its central part to which the cyst or its tract is attached.

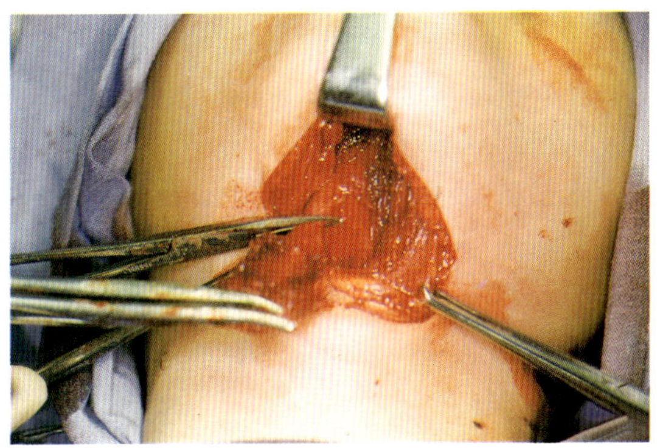

图 670

**图 670** 在舌骨体上方，沿中线切断下颌舌骨肌部分肌纤维，分离颏舌骨肌，由助手将食指伸入患者舌根部，将舌盲孔推向前方，缩短盲孔至舌骨的距离，便于手术操作。轻提已切断之中部舌骨，由舌骨至舌盲孔处，连同囊肿周围 2～3mm 的肌肉组织作一柱状整块切除。

**Fig. 670** The assistant's finger is placed in the patient's mouth and the midline of the base of the tongue is pushed forward toward the operative field. A core of muscle tissue of the tongue is excised exactly in the midline, extending from the hyoid bone to the base of the tongue, a surprisingly short distance of about 2.5 cm. The specimen consisting of the cyst and the central part of the hyoid bone attached to a core of midline tongue muscle is removed.

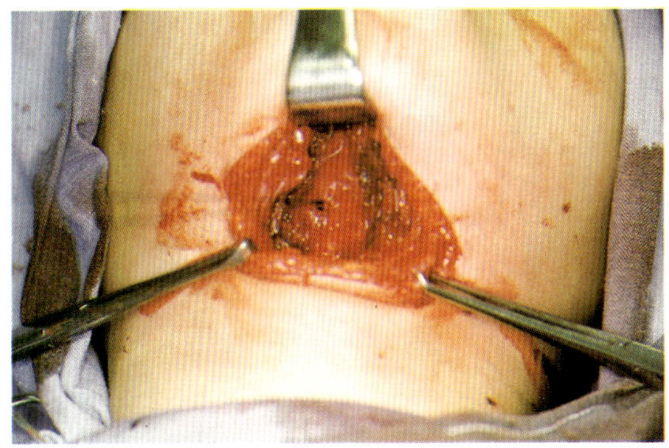

图 671

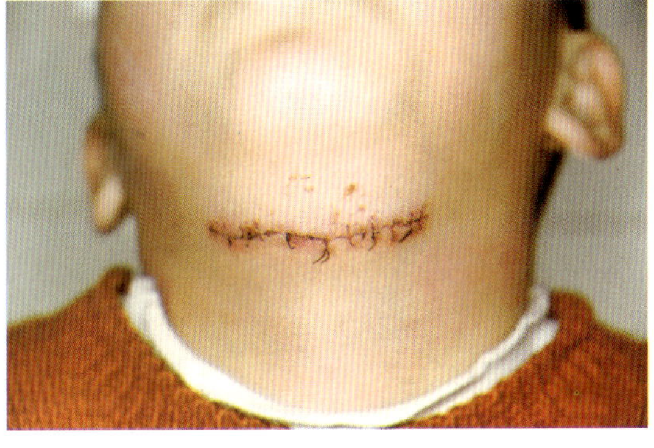

图 672

**图 671, 672** 在手术分离至囊肿末端时，先用弯血管钳将末端夹住，再行切断并予以贯穿缝扎，继用细肠线在粘膜下行荷包缝合，消除死腔。缝合切断的舌骨。创腔内放橡皮引流条，分层缝合颈阔肌及皮下组织及皮肤，轻压包扎。

**Fig. 671, 672** The pharynx is opened below the base of the tongue and is closed with a few fine chromic sutures. The incision is closed by approximating the platysma and the skin around a small rubber drain placed at one angle of the wound. It is unnecessary to suture the divided hyoid bone or tongue muscle.

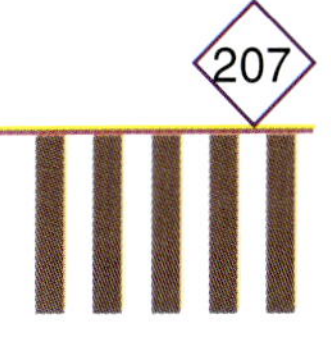

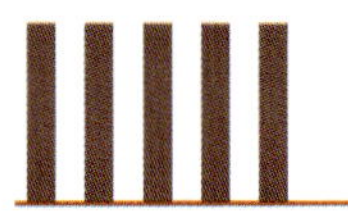



# 43. 鳃裂囊肿摘除术

# 43. Excision of branchial cleft cyst

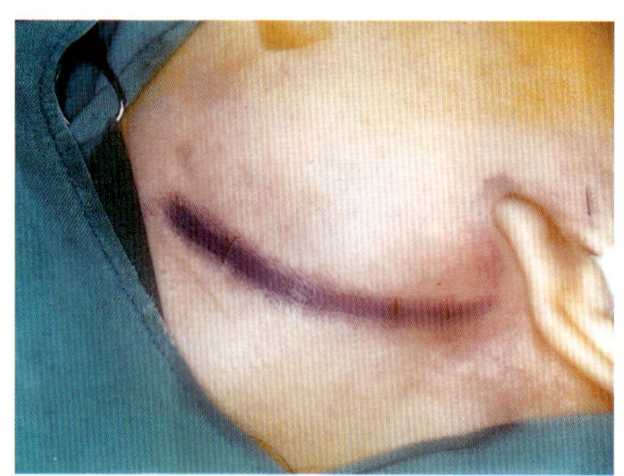

图 673

图 673　一般可在局部浸润麻醉下施行手术，囊肿位置较深时，可考虑采用全麻。手术体位以仰卧、头偏向健侧为宜，肩部还需垫高。

Fig. 673　Branchial cleft cysts should be treated by total excision.　Incision and drainage of the cyst is justified only occasionally as a temporary measure in suppuration.　Removal of the cyst from its usual location beneath the upper end of the sterno-cleidomastoid muscle should be a carefully planned procedure, using general endotracheal anesthesia.　The spinal accessory nerve is needlessly damaged far too often during surgery for branchial cleft cysts.　This nerve and other important structures around the cyst must be identified and protected.

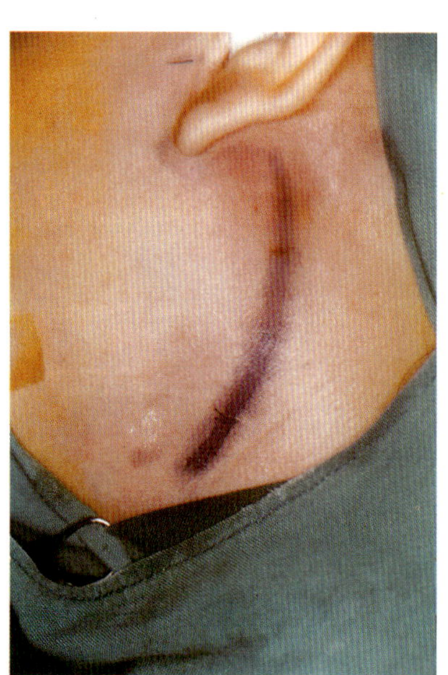

图 674

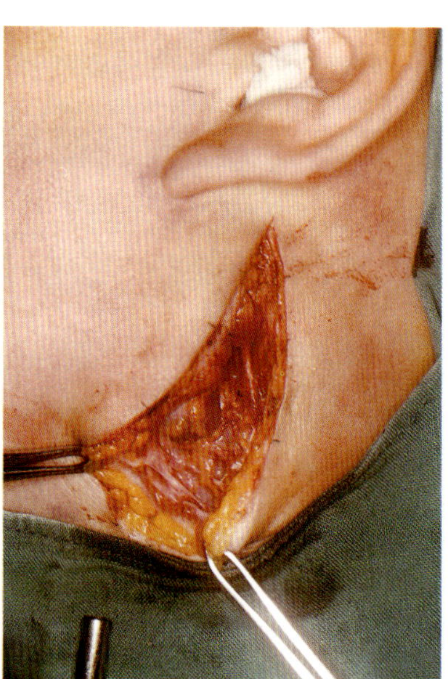

图 675

图 674, 675　沿胸锁乳突肌前缘做纵行切口，切口长度与囊肿大小相当或稍长，也可在下颌角下方、囊肿表面做横形的弧形切口。逐层切开皮肤、皮下组织及颈阔肌。

Fig. 674,　675　The incision is made along the anterior border of the sternocleidomastoid muscle and extends from the tip of the mastoid process downward over the cyst to the middle third of the neck.　The incision is deepened through the platysma and skin flaps including platysma are retracted.　The cyst lies beneath the upper half of the sternocleidomastoid muscle and the fibers of this muscle are stretched over its surface.　The external jugular vein lies superficial to the cyst and the greater auricular nerve may cross the upper third of the cyst wall.

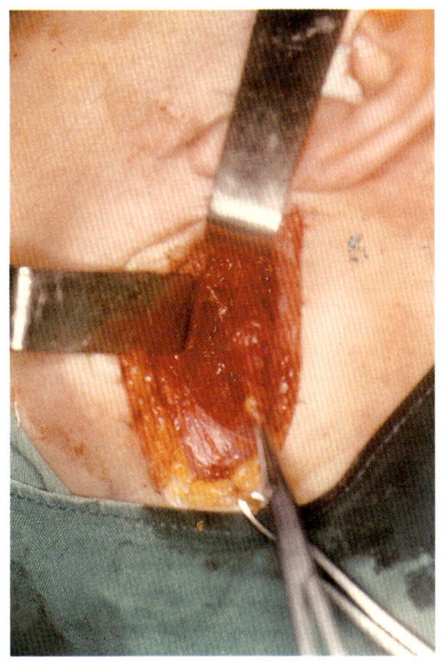
图 676

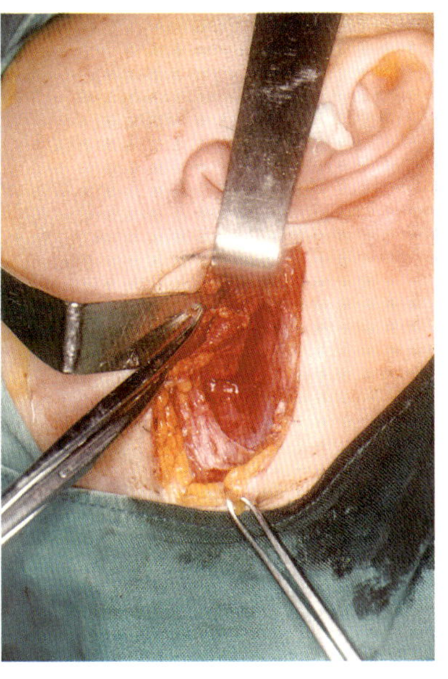
图 677

**图 676, 677** 向两侧牵开皮肤及颈阔肌，结扎、切断经过其中的颈外静脉，继由胸锁乳突肌前缘分离覆盖囊肿之胸锁乳突肌，并向后牵引，使居其深面的囊肿显露。

**Fig. 676, 677** The sternocleidomastoid muscle is dissected from the superficial surfaces of the cyst and retracted posteriorly. The dissection is now carried close to the cyst wall and is the best commenced at its lower angle. In this region, the internal jugular vein and the common carotid artery are identified and found to lie on the undersurface of the cyst. The common facial vein is closely adherent to the anterior cyst wall. All these structures are dissected free and protected. The posterior belly of the digastric muscle is now identified.

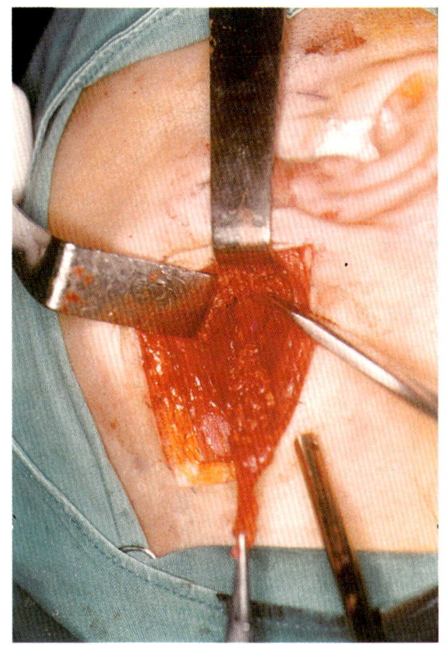
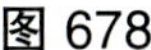
图 678

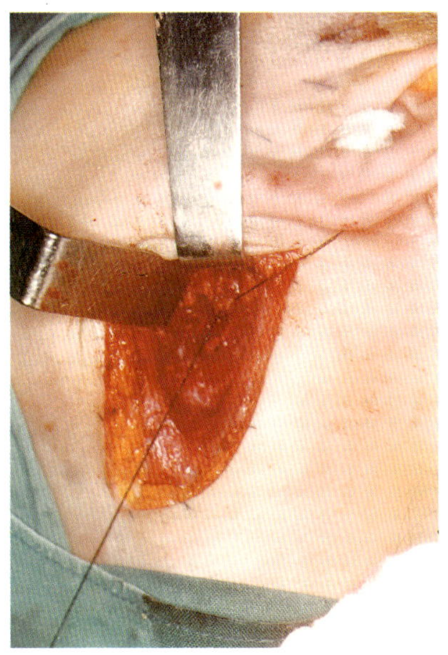
图 679

**图 678, 679** 先从囊肿下方开始，逐步分离显露囊肿深面的颈内静脉和颈动脉，然后沿囊壁逐渐向上分离。因囊壁常与颈内静脉粘连，故宜施行钝性分离，且应小心仔细，避免损伤颈内静脉、颈总动脉、颈内外动脉及迷走神经。在分离囊肿与胸锁乳突肌上部后方深面时，还需避免损伤副神经。囊肿前壁与面总静脉有时有粘连，故分离前壁时也应小心谨慎，必要时也可结扎切断面总静脉。分离至二腹肌深面时，需将囊肿与二腹肌分开，并注意避免损伤舌下神经。如此继续分离，即可完整摘除囊肿。

**Fig. 678, 679** The digastric muscle is freed from the deep anterior border of the cyst and the spinal accessory nerve is identified lying on the undersurface of the upper third of the sternocleidomastoid muscle. In all cysts in this location, emphasis must be laid on the identifying, isolating, and protecting the spinal accessory nerve.

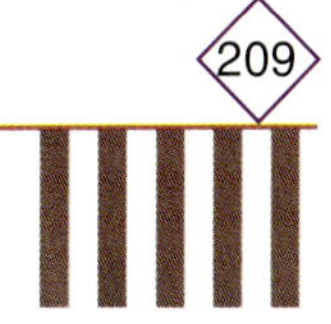

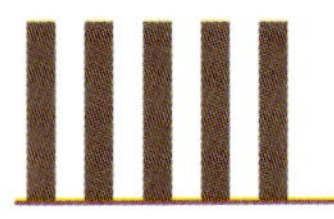



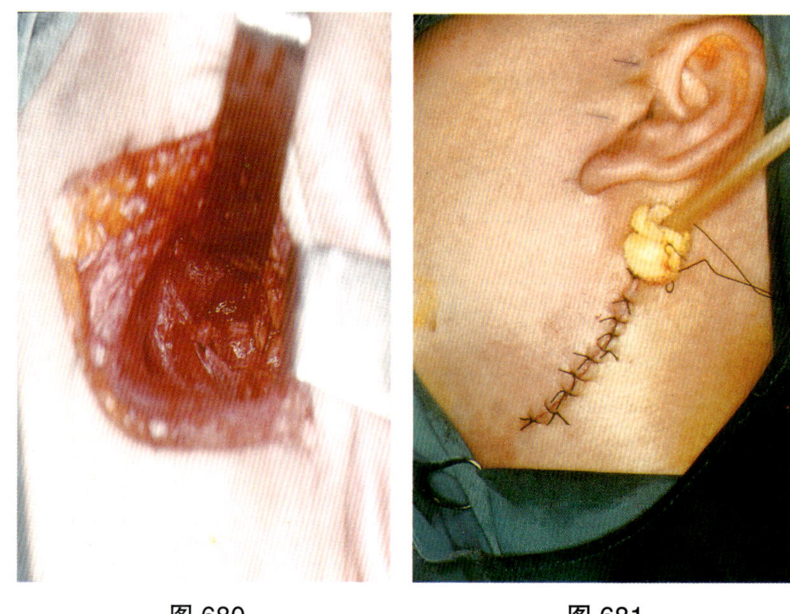

图 680　　图 681

**图 680, 681** 冲洗创腔，彻底止血后，创腔内置放橡皮引流条，分层缝合创口。

**Fig. 680, 681** Following removal of the cyst, the incision is closed by approximating the platysma with fine chromic sutures. A small Penrose drain is placed in the lower angle of the wound and the skin closed.

# 44. 面颈部巨大淋巴管瘤摘除术

# 44. Excision of giant lymphangioma in the facial and neck region

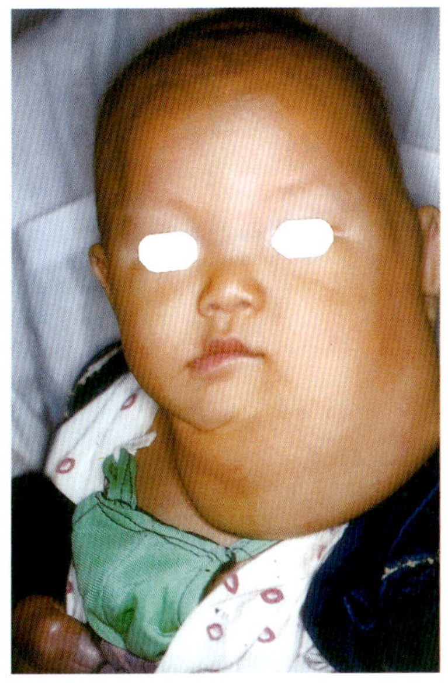

图 682

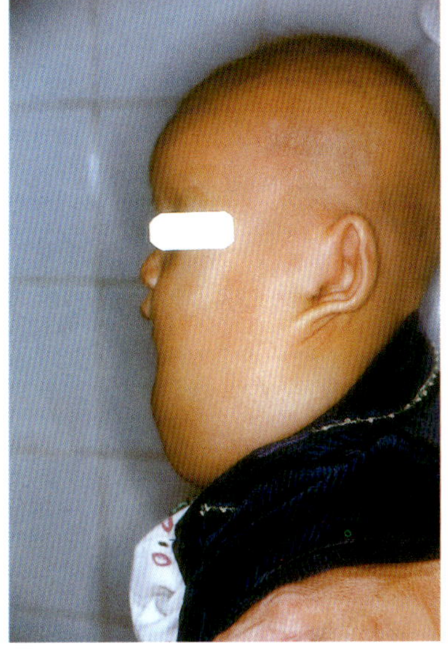

图 683

图 682, 683 患左面颈部巨大淋巴管瘤的 3 个月男性婴儿的正、侧面观。

正面观示左侧面颈部明显膨隆，表面皮肤正常，肿瘤巨大；侧面观淋巴管瘤侵犯整个左半侧面颈部。

Fig. 682, 683 Frontal and lateral views of a 3-month-old male infant with giant lymphangioma in the left facial and neck region.

Frontal view shows obvious expansion in the left facial and neck region. The tumor is giant and superficial skin normal. Lateral view shows that lymphangioma involved whole left facial and neck region.

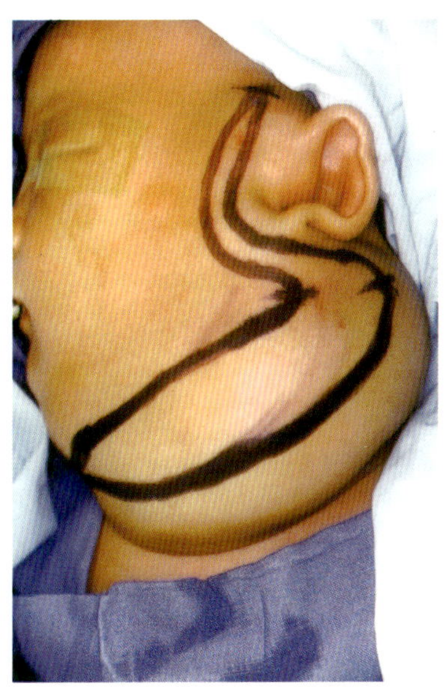

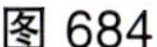

图 684

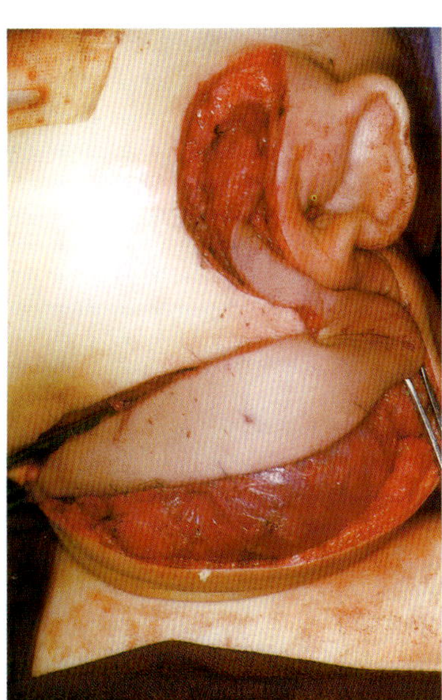

图 685

图 684 用美蓝画出手术切口线，两切口线之间皮肤为切除之皮肤。

图 685 按设计之切口线切开皮肤、皮下组织及颈阔肌，此时，部分肿瘤的浅面已暴露在手术野中。

Fig. 684 The incision line is marked out with methylene blue, the skin between two incision lines is removed.

Fig. 685 According to marked incision line, skin and platysma are incised, The superficial portion of the tumor has been exposed in the operative field at the same time.

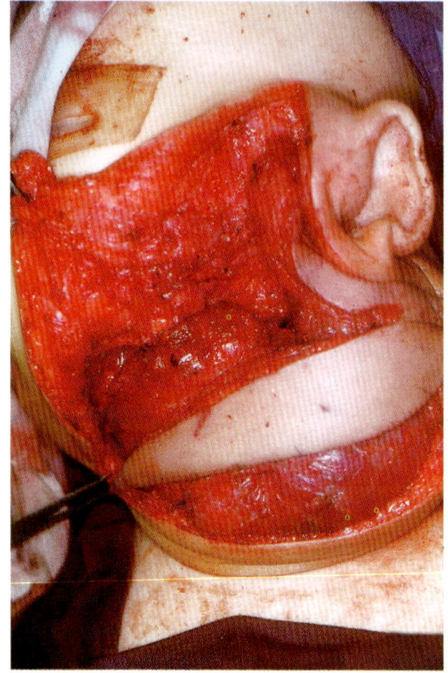

图 686

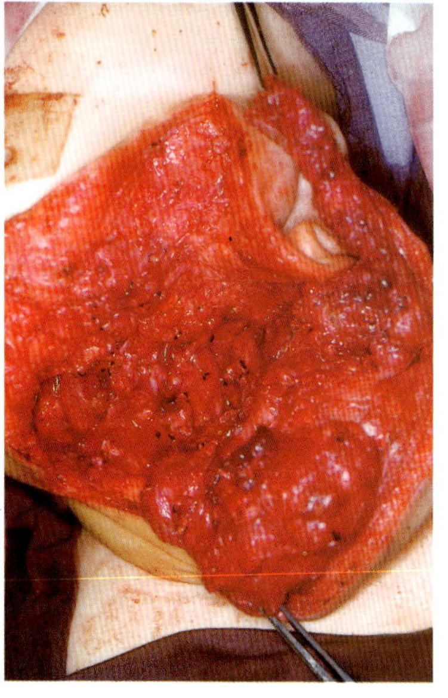

图 687

图 686, 687 在腮腺下极的浅面，肿瘤上极的边缘，由上向下分离淋巴管瘤的深面至下颌下缘。分离肿瘤前份深面，然后在胸锁乳突肌浅面，由上向下分离淋巴管瘤后界深面。

Fig. 686, 687 The superficial portion of the lower pole of the parotid gland and the upper border of the tumor are dissected. The deep portion of lymphangioma is separated to the lower rim of the mandible from upperiorly to inferiorly.

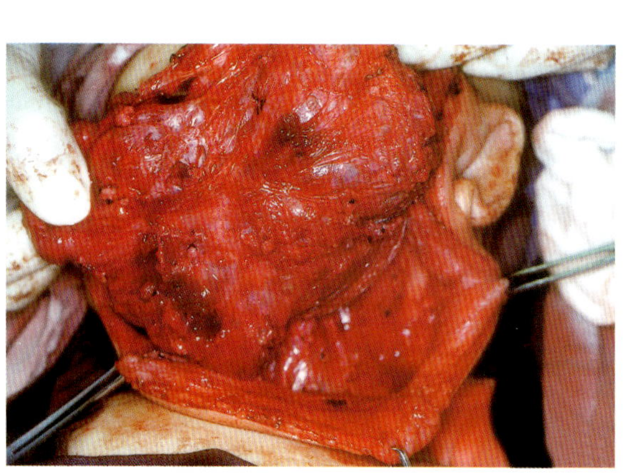

图 688

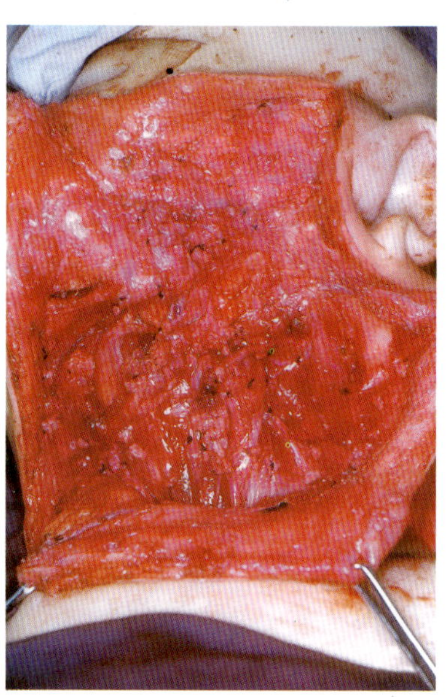

图 689

图 688 将颈部皮肤牵开，用电刀将肿瘤与皮肤分离，逐渐由浅入深，此时可见到颈外静脉后分支，将其分离结扎。继续由后向前解剖肿瘤组织，使整个淋巴管瘤组织与颈部正常组织分离，去除淋巴管瘤。

图 689 面颈部淋巴管瘤被完整摘除后的情景。

Fig. 688 The skin of the neck is retracted posteriorly and the lymphangioma is pulled forward. The lymphangioma is separated from the skin with electric knife. At the same time, the posterior branch of the external carotid vein may be seen and divided and ligated. The total lymphangioma is dissected from normal tissues in the neck from posteriorly to anteriorly and is removed.

Fig. 689 The condition after the lymphangioma has been excised.

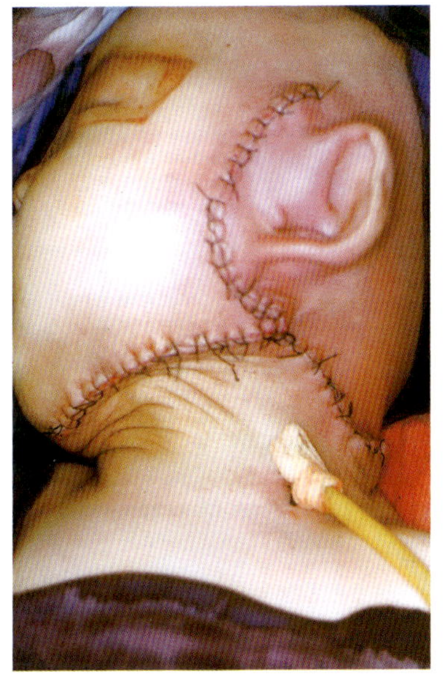

图 690

**图 690** 用生理盐水冲洗整个创口，分层缝合颈阔肌、皮下组织和皮肤。在切口的下端颈部将引流管穿出接上负压引流。

**Fig. 690** Total wound is irrigated with saline solusion. Platysma and skin are sutured with interrupted sutures in layers. A rubber tube is placed in the parotid bed and brought out through the inferior angle of the wound.

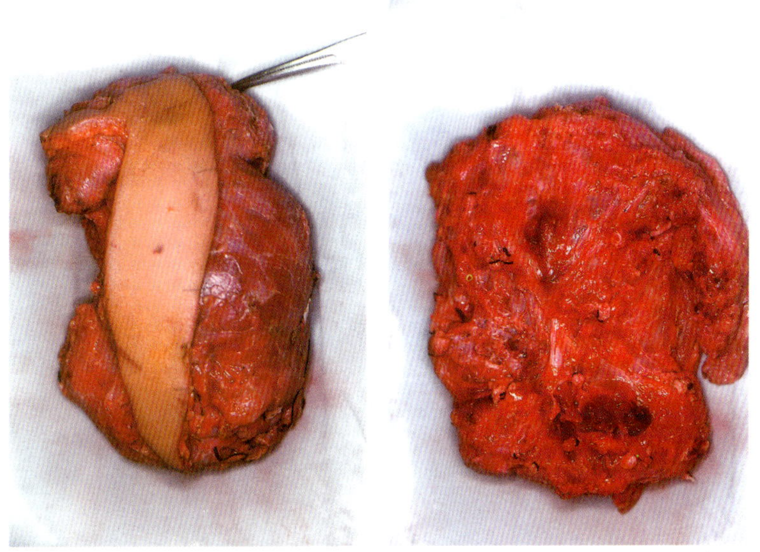

图 691　　图 692

**图 691, 692** 术后标本的正面及侧面观。

**Fig. 691, 692** Frontal and lateral views of postoperative specimen.

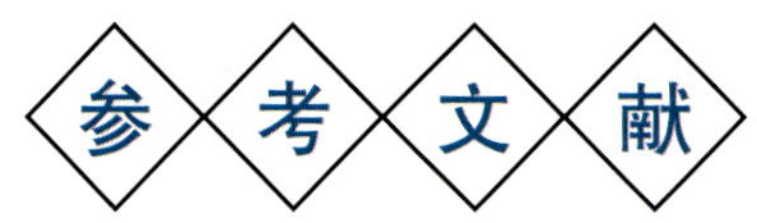

# 参考文献

## References


1. Pieper DR, Al-Mefty O.: Management of intracranial meningimas secondarily involving the infratemporal fossa: Radiographic characteristic, pattern of tumor invasion and surgical implications. *Neurosurgery*. 45(2): 231–238, 1999.
2. Jian XC, Chen XQ, and Wang CX.: A surgical approach to extensive tumors in the pterygopalatine fossa extending into the maxillary sinus. *J. Oral Maxillofac Surg*. 56: 578–584, 1998.
3. Cocke EW, Robertson JH, Robertson JR, et al.: The extended maxillotomy and subtotal maxillectomy for excision of skull base tumors, *Arch Otolaryngol Head Neck Surg*. 116: 92–104, 1990.
4. Biller HF, Shugar JMA, Krespi YP.: A new technique for wide-field exposure of the base of the skull, *Arch Otolaryngol*. 107: 698–702, 1981.
5. Janecka IP, Sen CN, Sekhar LN, et al. Facial translocation: A new approach to the cranial base. *Otolaryngol Head Neck Surg*. 103: 413–419, 1990.
6. Janecka IP. Classification of facial translocation approach to the base. *Otolaryngol Head Neck Surg*. 112: 579–585, 1995.
7. Catalano PJ, Biller HF.: Extended osteoplastic maxillotomy: A versatile new procedure for wide access to the central skull base and infratemporal fossa, *Arch Otolaryngol Head Neck Surg*. 119: 394–400, 1993.
8. Sekhar LN, Schrann VL, Jones NF. Subtemporal-preauricular infratemporal fossa approach to large lateral and posterior cranial base neoplasms. *J. Neurosurg* 67: 488–499, 1987.
9. Guinto G, Abello J, Molina A, et al: Zygomatic-transmandibular approach for giant tumors of the infratemporal fossa and parapharynged space. *Neurosurg*. 45: 1385–1397, 1999.
10. Jian XC.: Surgical excision of lymphangiomatous macroglossia: A case report. *J. Oral Maxillofac Surg*. 55: 306–309, 1997.
11. Zhan FH, Jian XC, and Shen ZH.: Giant hemangioma of the sternocleidomastoid muscle: Report of a case. *J. Oral Maxillofac Surg*. 55: 190–193, 1997.
12. Dufresne C, Cutting C, and Valauri F, et al.: Reconstruction of mandibular and floor of mouth defects using the trapezius osteomyocutaneous flap. *Plast Reconstr Surg*. 79(5): 686–696, 1987.
13. Donohue WB.: Immediate mandibular reconstruction following resection. *J. Canad Dent Asso*. 39(10): 720–727, 1973.
14. Hoopes JE, Edgenton MT.: Immediate forehead flap repair in resection for oropharyngeal cancer. *Am J Surg*. 112: 527–533, 1966.
15. Leonard AG.: The forehead flap: minmising the secondary defect by preservation of the frontalis muscle. *Brit. J. Plast Surg*. 36: 322–326, 1983.
16. Persky MS, and Daly JF.: The forehead flap for mucosal resurfacing. *Laryngoscope*. 89: 493–495, 1979.
17. Bertotti JA.: Trapezius-musculocutaneous island flap in the repair of major head and neck cancer. *Plast*

*Reconstr Surg*. 65(1): 16 – 21, 1980.

18. Chicarilli ZN.: Sliding posterior tongue flap. *Plast Reconstr Surg*. 79(5): 697 – 700, 1987.
19. Wagner JD.: Preoperative assessment and preparation for mandible reconstruction. Operative Technique. *Plast Reconstr Surg*. 3(4): 217 – 225, 1996.
20. Eppley BL.: Nonvascularized methods of mandible reconstruction. Operative Technique. *Plast Reconstr Surg*. 3(4): 226 – 232, 1996.
21. Anthony JP, and Foster RD.: Mandibular reconstruction with the fibula osteocutaneous free flap. Operative Technique. *Plast Reconstr Surg*. 3(4): 233 – 240, 1996.
22. Hidalgo D.: Refinements in mandible reconstruction. Operative Technique. *Plast Reconstr Surg*. 3(4): 257 – 263, 1996.
23. Samman N, Cheung KL, and Tideman H.: The buccal fat pad in oral reconstruction. *Int. J. Oral Maxillofac Surg*. 22(1): 2 – 6, 1993.
24. Stuzin JM, Wagstrom L, and Kawawoto HK, et al.: The anatomy and clinical applications of the buccal fat pad. *Plast Reconstr Surg*. 85: 29 – 37, 1990.
25. Tideman H, Bosanquet A, and Scott J.: Use of the buccal fat pad as a pedicled graft. *J. Oral Maxillofac Surg*. 44: 435 – 400, 1986.
26. Vuillemim T, Ravth J, and Ramon Y.: Reconstruction of the maxilla with bone grafts supported by the buccal fat pad. *J. Oral Maxillofac Surg*. 46: 100 – 105, 1988.
27. Vogel JE, Mulliken JB, Kaban LB,: Macroglossia: A review of the condition and a new classification. *Plast. Reconstr. Surg*. 78: 715 – 721, 1986.
28. 翦新春,编著:口腔颌面部畸形缺损外科学,湖南科学技术出版社. 2000, P: 28 – 104.
29. 翦新春、黄晓元、王承兴, 等: 游离下腹直肌肌皮瓣全舌再造术, 临床口腔医学杂志. 17(2): 99 – 101, 2001.
30. 翦新春、郭峰、蒋灿华等: 舌前滑行组织瓣修复半侧舌中份缺损, 上海口腔医学杂志. 11(1): 81 – 83, 2002.
31. 陈新群、翦新春、粟红兵等: 婴幼儿腮腺区血管瘤的手术治疗, 中国现代医学杂志. 11(8): 60 – 62, 2001
32. 翦新春、粟红兵、陈新群: 巨舌症 2 例手术治疗报告, 中华整形烧伤外科杂志. 5(3): 229, 1989.
33. 翦新春、李正本、郭峰等: Attenborough 与改良 Barbosa 手术进路对翼腭窝肿瘤暴露与术后功能影响的研究, 口腔医学研究, 18: 316 – 318, 2002.
34. 翦新春、刘志敏、郭峰等: 淋巴管瘤或淋巴血管瘤性巨舌症的外科手术治疗, 临床口腔医学杂志, 18: 367 – 368, 2002.
35. 翦新春、胡延佳、刘景平等: 切除翼上颌及颅中窝底肿瘤的一个新手术进路(5 例报告), 口腔颌面外科杂志, 12: 300 – 302, 2002.
36. 刘志敏、翦新春、粟红兵等: 巨大型面侧深区肿块摘除手术进路探讨, 医学临床研究, 19: 343 – 345, 2002.

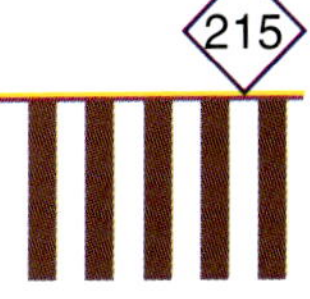